CANCER
OF THE
COLON AND RECTUM

Its Diagnosis and Treatment

CANCER
OF THE
COLON AND RECTUM

Its Diagnosis and Treatment

SECOND EDITION

BY

FRED W. RANKIN
B.A., M.A., M.D., LL.D., Sc.D., F.A.C.S.

Surgeon, St. Joseph's and Good Samaritan Hospitals, Lexington, Kentucky
Clinical Professor of Surgery, University of Louisville, Louisville, Kentucky

AND

A. STEPHENS GRAHAM
M.D., M.S. (in Surgery), F.A.C.S.

Surgeon, Stuart Circle Hospital, Richmond, Virginia
Associate Professor of Surgery, Medical College of Virginia

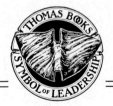

CHARLES C THOMAS · PUBLISHER
Springfield · Illinois · U. S. A.

CHARLES C THOMAS · PUBLISHER
BANNERSTONE HOUSE
301–327 EAST LAWRENCE AVENUE, SPRINGFIELD, ILLINOIS, U.S.A.

Published simultaneously in The British Commonwealth of Nations by
BLACKWELL SCIENTIFIC PUBLICATIONS, LTD., OXFORD, ENGLAND

Published simultaneously in Canada by
THE RYERSON PRESS, TORONTO

Printed in the United States of America

PREFACE TO THE SECOND EDITION

Progress in treatment of cancer of the lower gastrointestinal tract by surgical methods has continued apace over the last quarter century with an accentuation upon certain features during the last decade which have added materially to it. Considering operation as a single step in a planned program, surgery for malignancy of the colon and rectum has approached a state of ideal standardization insofar as the preoperative and postoperative measures are concerned. However, it should be emphasized that individualization of cases still determines in a large measure mortality and morbidity statistics because judgment based upon long experience, which means the performance of surgical procedures in a large group of cases, unquestionably remains the deciding factor in success or failure in the vast majority of instances.

Now-a-days, because of better preparatory measures and the judicious utilization of chemotherapeutic agents and antibiotics, patients come to the operating room in a state more nearly approaching physiological equilibrium than hitherto. A longer preparatory period permits adequate decompression and cleansing and sterilization of the bowel. The use of whole blood, high caloric diet, attention to protein and electrolyte balance and the co-operative assistance of internists and cardiologists, particularly in this period, have immeasurably forwarded surgery in this field. It is because of these factors, as well as the fact that a larger number of well-trained surgeons are operating upon these cases, that mortality figures have been reduced in expert and trained hands to well below 5 per cent—one might almost say to below 3 per cent as an average among mature surgeons.

Moreover, the same processes operate to permit the utilization of one-stage procedures with satisfaction in a very high percentage of cases. It is our belief that practically all of the cancers of the right and transverse colon can be removed in one stage with immediate restoration of the gastrointestinal continuity either by open or aseptic anastomosis, as the surgeon is inclined. In the left colon we believe that obstructive resection is the operation of choice in the vast majority of cases, although the ideal operation of resection and immediate end to end anastomosis may be carried out in 25 to 30 per cent of the cases.

It is emphasized that when an anastomosis in this portion of the colon is undertaken, two criteria must be adhered to: (1) visualization of adequate blood supply to the cut ends of the bowel, and

(2) adequate decompression must have been accomplished prior to resection. Any anastomosis in the face of even moderate obstruction is very likely to result fatally. Whether one does an aseptic maneuver or not is a matter of little importance apparently, and the tendency to do more and more open operations is very properly wide spread. We have used an aseptic type of anastomosis over a three-bladed clamp for many years, but recently find ourselves employing the open type of procedure more and more.

The trend towards one-stage operations in the rectum is fully developed and we heartily concur in the utilization of the Miles procedure or some modification of it in the vast majority of rectal cancers. Gabriel has developed a satisfactory perineo-abdominal operation which many surgeons utilize advantageously. It must be recognized that there are rectal cancers in certain patients who have coexisting debilitating diseases and who are unable to withstand formidable procedures. This is a very small group, one must admit, but no one operation is sufficient to apply to all cases of malignancy anywhere in the body, and it is our belief that occasionally a Lockhart-Mummery operation is advisable or even a local operation such as that of Harrison-Cripps or of Quénu-Tuttle.

Within recent years there has been developed a not inconsiderable advocacy of the preservation of the rectal sphincter in rectal and rectal-sigmoidal cancers which are not closer to the sphincter muscle than three to four centimeters. For this type of operation or any of the recently rediscovered "pull through" procedures, we have small enthusiasm. Certainly this latter view is shared by a large group of widely experienced surgeons both here and abroad, and it will remain for time and especially end-results to prove the validity of the contention that as high a percentage of five years' freedom from recurrence will result from such operations. We emphasize that measurements by proctoscope are inaccurate and not satisfactory in locating a tumor's relationship to the pelvic peritoneum. There are great differences in the types of pelves in the human race, and certainly the peritoneal reflection differs widely in patients and for many reasons. It is our feeling that no cancer of the rectum which is below the peritoneal reflection should be submitted to a sphincter-saving operation. Here the abdominoperineal operation is the procedure of choice.

When a growth is somewhat above the peritoneal fold, anastomosis, if it may be done readily, certainly is a feasible procedure. It is no great feat to sew together two pieces of bowel low down in the pelvis. Usually, although one can not be sure of the blood supply collateral, circulation takes care of the rectal end and the anastomosis heals quickly. The crux of the situation, however, is not the degree of technical skill involved in such a gymnastic feat but whether or not one may, by employing such a procedure, carry out the cardinal requisite of all cancer operations, namely removal of gland-bearing tissues in juxtaposition to the growth and sufficiently far away to insure the highest percentage of cure. That is the goal we believe may be accomplished more satisfactorily by the acceptance of a colostomy than otherwise, save only when the growth is definitely inside the peritoneum.

In the diagnosis of lesions of the lower gastrointestinal tract, progress has kept pace with the strides which have developed in preoperative and postoperative care as well as technical maneuvers of great magnitude. The diagnosis of all cancers of the rectum, it must be repeated time and again, can be made by: (1) digital examinations, (2) proctoscope examination, and (3) biopsy. The diagnosis of practically all lesions of the colon and their accurate localization is readily made by our roentgenological colleagues, provided only that they are permitted to examine the patient with a clean bowel and to introduce the medium per rectum. Despite long continued repetition of this necessary step, all surgeons are from time to time confronted with a case of acute intestinal obstruction produced by oral administration of the opaque medium thus superimposing an acute lethal condition, unless relieved, upon a malignancy and gravely compromising the individual's opportunity for cure. These lessons must be continually impressed upon the profession by the unfortunate surgeons who are compelled to deal with them.

We are indebted to the editors and publishers of *Surgery, Annals of Surgery, Surgery, Gynecology and Obstetrics, The New England Medical Journal*, and to W. B. Saunders Company for permission to reproduce charts and illustrations. Moreover, we wish to record our sincere thanks to the many surgeons who gave so generously of their time in answering our questionnaire and in preparing for us detailed statistical data. Particularly do we wish to thank Dr. R. W. Postlethwaite, Dr. Fred A. Coller, Dr. Alton Ochsner, Dr. William H. Daniel, Drs. R. K. Gilchrist and Vernon C. David, Dr. Thomas E. Jones, Dr. Robert S. Grinnell, Dr. I. S. Ravdin, Dr. Claude F. Dixon and his associates at The Mayo Clinic, and Dr. Richard B. Cattell, for their valuable contributions of unpublished material.

To Mr. Charles C Thomas, our publisher, and his son, Payne E. L. Thomas, we wish to express appreciation for their hearty co-operation.

FRED W. RANKIN

PREFACE TO THE FIRST EDITION

Cancer is the major lesion of the large bowel and rectum for which surgery is done. Because of this fact it has seemed desirable to incorporate in the volume our own experiences with cancer of the lower gastrointestinal tract, and to correlate and record the work of other surgeons interested in this field, both in this country and abroad.

Progress in diagnosis and treatment of cancer of the large bowel has been one of the outstanding accomplishments in surgery of the past quarter century. More efficient methods of diagnosis, more meticulous co-operative preparatory efforts, and a broadening experience in the application of special surgical maneuvers to these cases have resulted in a comfortable reduction of mortality and more satisfactory statistical data as to prognosis.

In 1932, with two of my former associates, I published a volume on diseases of the colon, rectum and anus. Because of the large amount of space required for discussion of other lesions, abbreviation of the discussion of cancer was necessarily practiced to some extent. Since that time there have been few fundamental changes made in the treatment of malignant disease in this location, yet an increasing experience has reluctantly forced an abandonment of some steps hitherto deemed most essential and has accentuated the value of other maneuvers. It is now commonly accepted that the co-operative management under the care of internists and surgeons has enormously forwarded the treatment of surgical diseases in many parts of the body. Certainly in dealing with cancer of the large bowel and rectum, one makes no exception but is convinced that one of the most potent factors of success is adequate preliminary decompression and rehabilitation. To these are added other safety factors which are discussed in detail in this volume.

One practice which we feel was in former years given undue prominence in the discussion of surgical attack on cancer of the colon and rectum, we have reluctantly abandoned, namely, the routine use of intraperitoneal vaccine. This has been done hesitatingly and we acknowledge with gratitude efforts of many earnest and scientific workers in an attempt to forward methods of increasing peritoneal resistance against contamination, for peritonitis is the greatest single lethal factor in the casualty list of operations for any intra-abdominal cancer. Suffice it to say that in our experience and with the methods which were being used in our service, we were forced to the conclusion that intraperitoneal vaccination was not the huge factor in reduction of mortality that we once felt it to be.

Along with this deletion in routine management of colonic and rectal lesions, there have been many additions to the preoperative care which have seemed to influence noticeably not only the prognosis, but likewise the immediate satisfaction of both patient and surgeon. These we have attempted to describe and illustrate as clearly as possible.

Accompanying the progress in diagnosis and offensive maneuvers against cancer of the lower gastrointestinal tract, great strides forward have necessarily been made in the technic of the roentgen-ray. Roentgenoscopic examinations of the large bowel are now considered to be as accurate and efficient as those done for lesions in other parts of the body, and assisted by palpatory manipulation, permit accurate localization and recognition of the pathologic type in more than 95 per cent of the lesions of this segment. The great efficiency of the radiologist in the accurate localization and recognition of disease of the colon has been uniformly progressive and has made us rely more and more upon his interpretations. These advances have been of inestimable value and it is a pleasure to acknowledge the surgeon's debt to his radiologic confrere.

It is a great pleasure to thank Dr. Fred M. Hodges for the contribution of a chapter on radiotherapy. Dr. Hodges, whose observations during years of experience and research have rendered him especially capable of expressing definite conclusions, takes a very conservative view of radiotherapy and discusses its advantages and disadvantages from the standpoint of palliation and cure in an authoritative manner.

Dr. A. C. Broders, so eminently known for his work in pathology, has graciously contributed photomicrographs illustrating the four grades of his classification. We can affirm in this connection that one of the factors which influences us most in the selection of the type of operation for individual cases is the knowledge of the grade of growth. In this problem Broders' index of malignancy is a constant source of help.

To Mr. W. B. Gabriel, of London, we most gratefully acknowledge indebtedness for materials furnished from a volume of his on this same subject which is now in publication. The sound, constructive thought which runs through the writings of British surgeons on cancer therapy is forcefully evident in the lucid descriptions and timely suggestions gleaned from the experiences of Mr. Gabriel.

In discussing the anatomy and physiology of the large bowel

and rectum, some of the most important considerations involve the blood supply. Some years ago a former associate of mine, Dr. J. A. Steward, did a most excellent piece of original work on the blood supply of the lower gastrointestinal tract, and from his very conclusive experiences and observations many practical and useful applications have resulted. This work has been drawn on in no small measure in this book, feeling as we do that our knowledge of the vascular patterns of the large bowel and rectum has been materially increased by his efforts.

We also take cognizance of the heightened value which the clear and graphic illustrations of the artist, Miss Dorothy Booth, have lent the manuscript. Likewise, it is a pleasure to acknowledge the valuable work of Miss Kate Lee McLeod whose untiring efforts and ardent interest in the preparation of the manuscript have aided materially in its publication.

During the past five years relatively few changes in technic of resection of segments of the large bowel or the rectum itself have been introduced, but two very definite variations have been used and found to be exceedingly desirable. The first one relates to the accomplishment of the obstructive resection for cancer of the middle and left colon. We are still firmly convinced that one does a more radical procedure and removes wider areas of mesentery and gland-bearing tissues if there is no attempt at a primary reestablishment of the gastrointestinal continuity. Likewise, we have felt that the obstructive resection continues to accomplish a radical maneuver without losing too much time in convalescence. Recently it has been my plan to routinely accompany this type of extirpative procedure by a complementary cecostomy. The desirability of this will immediately evidence itself to anyone adding this further step to his operative maneuver, and the ease and simplicity of making a cecostomy adds little to the surgical risk.

In dealing with cancer of the rectum we have more and more abandoned for the sturdy or average risks, all operative maneuvers in favor of the one-stage combined abdominoperineal resection, and in about one-third of the cases, especially the bad risks, the continued use with satisfaction of the graded procedure of Lockhart-Mummery, colostomy and posterior excision. These changes are described and illustrated in full and we feel that the arguments supporting them warrant their acceptance in the surgery of this field.

A careful study of statistical data representing the ultimate end-results by the different maneuvers and in the hands of both American and British surgeons is incorporated in this volume, and we think it demonstrates beyond peradventure a progress in dealing with cancer of the lower gastrointestinal tract, which is encouraging. Again, we acknowledge the great debt which our foreign colleagues, interested in surgery of the colon, have placed upon us in permitting the publication of the outcome of their efforts.

We wish also to make grateful acknowledgment for the use of materials and pictures to the editors and publishers of *Surgery, Gynecology and Obstetrics, Annals of Surgery,* the *Journal of the Southern Medical Association,* the *British Journal Surgery,* and to W. B. Saunders Company, and H. K. Lewis & Company, Ltd. Finally, we wish to record our sincere thanks to Mr. Charles C Thomas, our publisher, for his hearty co-operation and constructive suggestions.

Emboldened to record our own work and the work of others in a special field of surgical endeavor, it will be sufficient gratification and reward if this volume succeeds in creating constructive thought and criticism which will further forward efforts toward both cure and palliation of a lamentable malady.

FRED W. RANKIN

CONTENTS

Part I

GENERAL CONSIDERATIONS

Part II

TREATMENT

Part III

OPERATIVE PROCEDURES

CANCER
OF THE
COLON AND RECTUM

Its Diagnosis and Treatment

PART I

GENERAL CONSIDERATIONS

CHAPTER I

ANATOMY AND PHYSIOLOGY

COLON

The colon, which derives its name from the Greek word meaning to impede, extends from the terminal ileum to the rectum. Developmentally and functionally, the right and left divisions of the large bowel differ. From that portion of the primitive intestinal tube known as the mid-gut, the right half of the colon approximately to the middle of the transverse segment is developed, whereas the distal arm, including the rectum, evolves from the primitive hind-gut. Functionally, as Keith has pointed out, the cecum resembles a second stomach, and the right half of the large bowel simulates from this standpoint that portion of the small in-

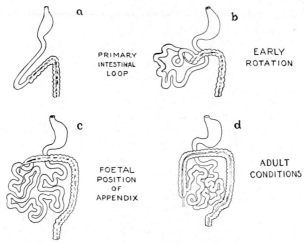

FIG. 1. Changes in enteric canal from period of primary intestinal loop to establishment of adult condition; note rotation of intestinal tract about the superior mesenteric vessels (from Livingston).

testine which develops with it, and the true function of the large intestine begins in the transverse colon, near the splenic flexure. This developmental and functional difference not only influences, markedly, the pathologic type of neoplasm encountered, but alters materially the symptomatology in the two segments, the type of operation selected, the prognosis, and end-results.

In its beginning the colon lies low in the abdominal cavity and its progress is from below upwards, toward the left (Fig. 1). By the fourth month of intra-uterine life the cecum has rotated toward the right, crossing the median line and lying directly under the liver, using the superior mesenteric vessels as an axis about which rotation takes place. From this position normally, the head of the colon descends into the right iliac fossa to its semi-fixed position of adult life, to become attached along the lateral abdominal parietes by

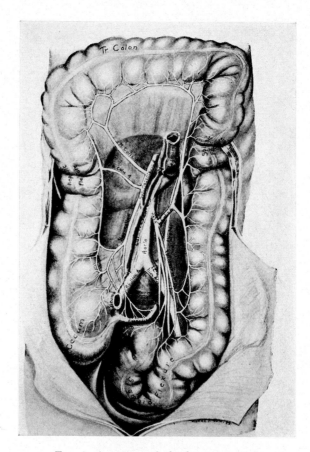

Fig. 2. Anatomy of the large intestines
(from Cunningham).

fusion of the peritoneum of its outer layer with the lateral parietal peritoneum. From this circumstance, the blood vessels are entirely mesial along the whole course of the large bowel and the outer half of the mesentery may be divided freely with no fear of hemorrhage.

The adult colon may be traced from the pouch-like structure in the right iliac fossa, ascending vertically and being fixed under the liver by ligamentous attachments. Thence, the colon crosses the abdomen from the right to left costal arch. Between these two points of fixation the transverse colon is festooned across the abdomen, usually around the level of the umbilicus. From the splenic flexure the descending colon normally falls away more or less in a straight line and at the brim of the pelvis assumes the shape of a letter S (the sigmoid), which becomes continuous with the rectum (Fig. 2). In 52 per cent of adult bodies there is neither an ascending nor a descending mesocolon (Treves).

The colon measures about 130 cm., or approximately one-fourth of the whole extent of the intestinal canal. Its diameter gradually diminishes from the cecum to the sigmoid, that of the former being about 7.5 cm., and of the latter 3 cm. The narrowest point of this segment of bowel is at the junction of the sigmoid with the rectum and, as has been pointed out by Treves, it is significant that this is the point at which stricture is the most common. Moreover, the tendency to stricture increases as one proceeds from the cecum to the anus. The colon differs from the small intestine in its greater size, its more fixed position, and its sacculated or pouch-like form. The latter is due to the peculiar arrangement of the longitudinal muscular coat, which, instead of being evenly distributed over the surface of the bowel, as is the case with the small intestine, is arranged in three narrow bands, the taenia coli, which are equidistant from one another. These muscular bands are shorter than the other coats of the intestine, consequently the intervening bowel pouches out to give a characteristic appearance to the colon. Attached to the colon, chiefly to the transverse and sigmoid portions, are numerous pedunculated peritoneal sacs, the appendices epiploicae.

RECTOSIGMOID, RECTUM, AND ANUS

Anatomists generally have adopted the third sacral vertebra as a convenient landmark for defining the upper end of the rectum. Gray states that it commences opposite the left sacro-iliac symphysis, passes obliquely downward from left to right to the middle of the sacrum, forming a gentle curve to the right side; then regaining the middle line, it descends in front of the lower part of the sacrum and coccyx, and, near the extremity of the latter bone, inclines backwards to terminate in the anus, being curved both in the lateral and anteroposterior direction. The rectum is cylindrical, not sacculated like the rest of the large intestine; it is narrower at its upper part (rectosigmoid) than the sigmoid flexure, gradually increases in size as it descends, and immediately above the anus presents a considerable dilatation (ampullary portion) capable of acquiring an enormous size (Fig. 3).

In textbooks on surgery of the rectum writers are in the habit of quoting different figures as to the length of the rectum. Yeomans, and also Edwards, stated that the rectum is from 12 to 15 cm. in length; Pennington gives the length of from 13 to 16 cm.; Cripps from 15 to 20 cm., and Tuttle from 9 to 15 cm. The length is greater in males than females, greater in the aged than in the young, and it may be increased at any time by distention.

The serous coat, derived from peritoneum, partially invests the anterior surfaces of the upper portion of the rectum to form in the

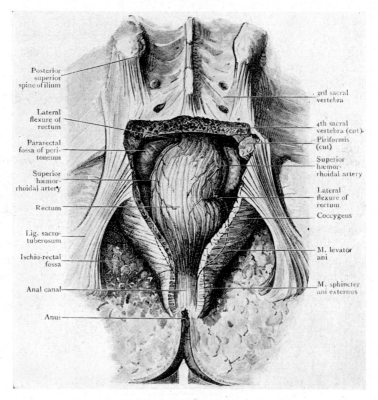

FIG. 3. Anatomy of the rectum (from Cunningham).

male the recto-vesical pouch, which reaches within about 7.5 cm. of the anus, and in the female the recto-uterine pouch, which reaches a somewhat lower level. On the posterior surface there is no peritoneum below a point about 12.5 cm. from the anus.

From a functional as well as a morphological point of view, according to Treves, the rectum is divided into two parts—an upper, in relationship with the peritoneum and the recto-vesical pouch, dilatable, and before defecation, laden with feces; and a lower which is beyond the peritoneum and serves merely for the passage, not the storage, of feces. The lower part, generally considered the ampulla of the rectum, is encased in a dense layer of extraperitoneal tissue, lies in a rectal channel, bound by a layer of pelvic fascia which encloses, above and in front, the prostate gland and seminal vesicles, or the vagina. Behind and below, the pelvic fascia covers the coccyx and anococcygeal body, and on each side, the levator ani muscles.

Above the base of the prostate the anterior wall of the rectum, at the junction of the upper and lower parts, is folded within the lumen of the bowel to form the inferior valves of Houston, or plica transversalis recti.

Rectosigmoid.—The portion of the large intestine at the juncture of the sigmoid and rectum has long been of particular anatomic and surgical interest, both as regards the bowel and its blood supply. In this region the longitudinal bands of muscle spread to form a complete coat; the mesosigmoid is at first markedly shortened, and a few centimeters farther it disappears entirely, leaving the bowel with peritoneum on the anterior surface only. In the last few decades this region has been referred to as the rectosigmoid, and although the term is anatomically descriptive, it is necessarily loosely used because of the variation in position and length of the two parts involved. The point at which the sigmoid ends and the rectum begins has been widely discussed. Treves, in 1885, located the beginning of the rectum opposite the third sacral vertebra and assigned the upper portion to the pelvic colon. Jonnesco, in 1889, confirmed Treves' observations, and since then anatomists for the sake of exactness have adopted the third sacral vertebra as a convenient landmark for defining the upper end of the rectum. Gant uses the third, or O'Beirne's sphincter, to define the juncture of the rectum and sigmoid, but Symington doubted the existence of such a structure, and Hyrtl, although believing in the sphincter physiologically, was often unable to demonstrate it in carefully executed dissections. Again, attempts have been made to determine the upper limit of the rectum by means of Houston's valve. Jones, as well as Paterson, advocated the use of the third valve of Houston, or the superior rectal fold, as the upper limit of the rectum. These folds are admittedly variable in form and position and are no landmarks except when seen through a proctoscope.

It has not been definitely proved despite frequent assertions that there is a sphincteric mechanism in the rectosigmoid. Reeves, in 1917, dissected out the rectum and rectosigmoid from 46 cadavers and found that a terminal constriction was present in 80 per cent. More recently, Martin and Burden in a study of 31 specimens concluded that "as a rule, the sigmoid has a well-developed musculature exhibiting no local increment of circular fibers to suggest an anatomical sphincter, nor is there a constant perceptible narrowing in the rectosigmoid juncture" (Fig. 4).

Anus.—The anal canal originates from the proctoderm, or skin infold. The final stages in its development consists of union of the postallantoic gut with the proctodeum, and invagination of the epiblast at a point in the anal membrane where later the anus is formed. Absorption of this septum makes the rectum and anus continuous. The anal canal is lined with pavement epithelium, has no mucous membrane, and is in no way a part of the rectum. The anal canal begins at the level of the levator ani muscles and, at rest, is directed downward and backward; it measures about 3.5 cm. Di-

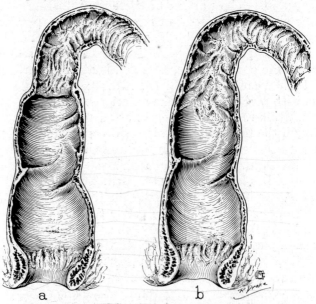

FIG. 4. Rectum and variations in the form of the recto-sigmoid: *a*, sharply defined juncture; *b*, gradual transition from sigmoid to rectum (after Martin and Burden).

rectly in front of the canal is the apex of the prostate gland and behind and a little above is the tip of the coccyx.

The anal canal is surrounded by the external and internal sphincter muscles and at its upper limits also by the levator ani muscles. The external sphincter ani, which encases the lower segment of the canal and spreads out in a spindle shape from the tip of the coccyx to the central point of the perineum, is a thick, potent voluntary muscle, on which fecal continence chiefly depends. It extends outward from the mucocutaneous juncture. The anterior surface of the anal canal in the female is in relation to a mass of adipose and muscular tissue known as the perineal body; in the male, to the bulb of the urethra and the base of the urogenital diaphragm. Posteriorly, between the coccyx and the anal canal, is situated a fibromuscular mass known as the anococcygeal body. And on either side is situated the ischiorectal fossa, which because of its content of loose adipose tissue, permits distention of the anal canal during defecation.

BLOOD SUPPLY

The basis for this description of the blood supply of the large intestine is a report made in 1933 by Steward and Rankin, follow-

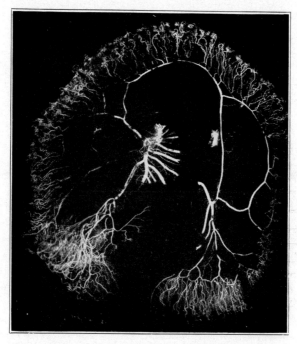

FIG. 5. Specimen injection with opaque material showing: (1) the anterior cecal artery as the first branch of the ileocolic artery; (2) anastomosis between the branches of the ileocolic artery; (3) the origin of the right colic artery from the ileocolic artery, and (4) slight anastomosis between the ileocolic and right colic arteries (Steward and Rankin).

ing the study of tissue at necropsy. Forty specimens in which the blood supply of the entire part could be determined exactly, and casts or roentgenograms preserved, were used in their report, which follows:

COLON

The arteries of the colon are derived from the superior and the inferior mesenteric. The former supplies the cecum, the ascending and the transverse colon, and a varying amount of the descending colon. The supply of the latter is completed by the inferior mesenteric which is also distributed to the sigmoid flexure. The general plan includes a series of anastomoses between neighboring branches by which long arterial arches run near the border of the gut, to which they give off irregular twigs (Piersol). Following this general description, the blood supply of the colon may be divided into three parts, the main arteries, the anastomosing loops or marginal artery, and the terminal arteries.

Main arteries.—The arteries to the colon derived from the superior mesenteric artery are: ileocolic, right colic, and middle colic, and from the inferior mesenteric, the left colic. Each of these arteries will be described separately (Figs. 5 to 8).

The *ileocolic artery* is generally described as the last artery given off on the right side of the superior mesenteric artery and as one of its two terminal branches. The terminal branches of the ileocolic artery are designated: (1) a colic branch which ascends along the wall of the colon; (2) an ileac branch which continues downward and then to the left along the terminal portion of the ileum to anastomose with the last intestinal artery and enclose the avascular area of Treves; (3) an anterior cecal artery which courses downward to the anterior surface of the cecum; (4) a posterior cecal artery which passes to the posterior surface of the cecum, and (5) the artery to the appendix. The artery to the appendix, although usually originating from the posterior cecal branch of the ileocolic artery, may be given off by one of the other branches, or may have an independent origin directly from the ileocolic artery. In regard to the ileocolic artery, it may be concluded: (1) the existence of the artery is constant; (2) its course is toward the ileocolic valve and varies slightly with the position of the valve, and (3) the terminal branches of the artery vary in their origin.

The *right colic artery* is described as the second artery from the right side of the superior mesenteric artery. Its course is to the right, below the mesocolon to the region of the hepatic flexure of the colon. The right colic artery is the most inconstant of the colic arteries. Early anatomists, such as von Haller, failed to describe it. A consideration of its existence becomes academic when a particular origin is insisted on before naming the artery. In the specimens studied its variations were marked. The artery originated from the superior mesenteric in 40 per cent of the cases, from the middle colic in 30 per cent, from the ileocolic in 12 per cent, whereas in 18 per cent there was no artery that corresponded in course or distribution to the right colic artery. It may be concluded that the right colic artery is extremely variable in presence, origin, and size.

The *middle colic artery* is described as the first artery coming from the right side of the superior mesenteric artery. It runs to the right between the layers of the mesocolon, then divides, its branches supplying the transverse colon and anastomosing with the right and left colic arteries. Some remarkable variations of the middle colic artery have been reported. It may be concluded that the middle colic artery does not occur constantly, that it varies in the number of branches, and through large branches, or by accessory middle colic arteries it supplies the left side of the transverse colon and splenic flexure in 37 per cent of the cases.

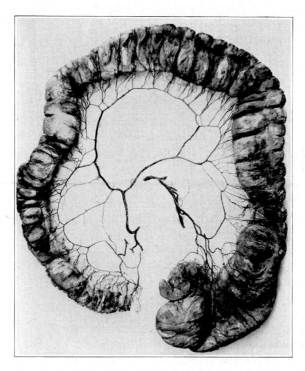

Fig. 6. Posterior view of celluloid cast of a specimen showing: (1) the anterior cecal branch (broken) as the first branch of the ileocolic artery, and (2) the absence of the middle and right colic arteries, replaced by the left colic artery (Steward and Rankin).

The *left colic artery* is described as the first branch of the inferior mesenteric artery. It passes transversely to the left and divides into an ascending branch and a descending branch which supply the descending colon and anastomose respectively with the left branch of the middle colic artery and the first sigmoid artery. It may be concluded that there is marked variation in the size, course, and distribution of the branches of the left colic artery, and that in most cases the ascending branch extends above the splenic flexure to the transverse colon. This artery is almost invariably present.

Marginal arteries.—The first comprehensive description of the blood supply of the colon by von Haller drew attention to the anastomosis of the adjacent colic arteries near the wall of the bowel. Since von Haller's description, anatomists have acclaimed the significance of the anastomosis along the wall of the colon as the only connection between the superior and inferior mesenteric

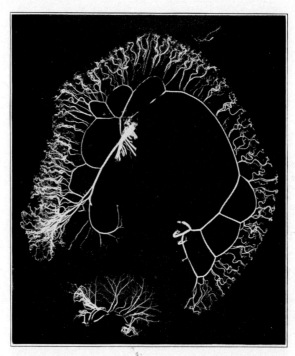

FIG. 7. Specimen injected with opaque mixture showing: (1) the anterior cecal artery as the first branch of the ileocolic artery; (2) multiple ascending colic branches from the anterior cecal branch, and (3) the origin of the right colic from the ileocolic artery (Steward and Rankin).

arteries. If the anastomosing loops are considered as an entity, the main colic branches may be considered simply as the source of supply for the artery. Although the existence of the arterial arcade along the colon has long been recognized, descriptions by anatomists have been meager. This neglect may be due to the variations of the arcade.

With the growth of surgery, the significance of the anastomosis of the colic arteries has become more apparent. At present, in spite of the reported failures of anastomosis between the colic arteries and the protests of Desmarest, and Jamieson and Dobson, surgeons successfully ligate individual colic arteries as the occasion demands and rely on vascularization through the marginal artery. Study of the marginal artery in the injected specimens emphasized its value as a source of blood supply to the colon. The marginal artery was continuous from the ascending colon to the sigmoid in all but 5 per cent, and in these there was failure of anastomosis between the ileocolic and the right colic arteries.

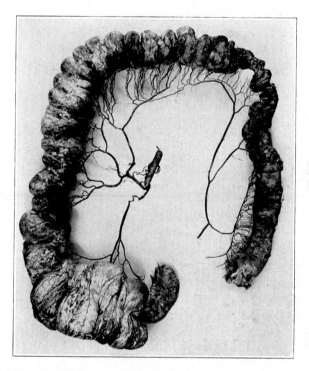

Fig. 8. Celluloid cast of a specimen showing: (1) tri-furcation of the middle colic artery and (2) anastomosis between the left and middle colic arteries effected by a slender branch (Steward and Rankin).

In more than 100 specimens in which this particular area was examined there was no failure of anastomosis of the left colic and middle colic arteries. This fact deserves particular emphasis because of the prevalent, hazy statement to the contrary. The distance of the marginal artery from the wall of the colon is inconstant. A general estimate should not be made, as the distance varies in each specimen, and in the different parts of the same specimen, from a fraction of 1 to 8 cm. As a rule, the artery is farthest from the wall at the points of bifurcation of the main artery; the larger the marginal artery at a particular point, the more distant it is likely to be from the bowel. Usually the marginal artery is nearer the left half of the transverse and the descending portion of the colon than the right half of the colon.

The secondary arcades are also inconstant. They are most common at the points of bifurcation of the main arteries or their subdivisions, but there is no regularity in their presence. Tertiary loops are occasionally found. Secondary loops give a more flexible blood supply to a colon, but their existence is not constant enough so that the surgeon may safely place any degree of reliance on them.

It may be concluded that a marginal artery occurs quite constantly, failing only in rare cases along the ascending colon in the presence of a profuse supply from the direct branches; that it runs

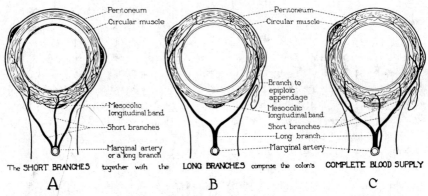

FIG. 9. Diagram of the terminal arteries of the colon: *A*, short branches; *B*, long branches, and *C*, complete supply by both long and short branches (Steward and Rankin).

at varying distances from the wall of the colon; and that it may have secondary loops in different positions in its course.

Terminal arteries.—The branches of the terminal arteries usually originate independently from the marginal artery and proceed directly to the colon, but occasionally two branches may have a common origin. Anastomosis between terminal branches before they reach the colon is rare. Terminal arteries are most numerous in the cecum and ascending colon. The size of the terminal arteries in the transverse and descending colon is slightly smaller, and the number of vessels per centimeter is less than in the ascending portion. The branches vary slightly with the size of the subject, but there is no difference in the size of the arteries in the dilated and the contracted portions of the colon in the same specimen.

The terminal arteries to the colon are of two types: long and short branches, a combination of the two types affecting the complete supply to the wall (Fig. 9). The long branches divide near the mesocolic taenia, one branch courses in the haustra of the anterior aspect, and the other on the posterior aspect of the wall of the colon. In this part of their course the arteries lie in the serosa and give off short branches to the mesocolic portion of the colon, small twigs to the serosa and peritoneum and arteries to the epiploic appendages.

Near the amesocolic or distal longitudinal bands the long branches divide and pass deeply beneath the longitudinal muscle and through the circular muscle to the submucosa. In this position they continue their course sending small branches upward to the muscle and peritoneal covering. In the submucosa anastomosis is established with the short branches and a relatively scanty anastomosis with the long branch from the opposite side of the colon.

Regarding the terminal arteries of the colon, it may be concluded that: (1) they are of two types, long branches which supply the amesocolic or distal third of the colon and short branches which supply the mesocolic or proximal two thirds of the colon; (2) the mesocolic taenia portion of the colon has most of the blood supply; (3) the course of the terminal arteries is in general perpendicular to the axis of the bowel, and (4) there is little anastomosis between the terminal vessels except in the submucosa.

Anastomosis of arteries between the omentum and colon.—Cruveilhier, Gray, Cunningham and Piersol stated that the transverse colon receives its blood supply from the omental arteries. Surgeons have not verified the anastomosis between the arteries of the omentum and those of the colon. Lardennois and Okinezye stated that twigs do not exist which merit a ligature when the omentum is separated from the colon, and one finds that only one artery near the splenic flexure need be tied in separating the two structures. Lardennois pointed out that all important vessels of the omentum run on the anterior layer. It may be concluded that the anastomosis between the arteries of the omentum and the transverse colon is normally through a few branches from the terminal arteries of the colon and that the anastomosing branches are about equal to large peritoneal twigs.

Veins.—It may be stated in general that the veins of the colon follow directly the course of the corresponding arteries. The left colic vein is a distinct exception to this orderly return of the colic veins along the arterial courses.

Sigmoid.—The arteries to the sigmoid usually arise from the lateral aspect of the inferior mesenteric artery and spread fanlike to the mesosigmoid toward the bowel (Fig. 10) supplying not only the sigmoid, but in cases to which the left colic artery is small or has a high course, the lower part of the descending colon as well. The number of sigmoid arteries varies. The arterial branches anas-

tomose with those in their vicinity to form a network in the mesosigmoid, ramifying the marginal artery. The marginal artery,
which is continuous with that of the descending colon, may lie from
a fraction of a centimeter to several centimeters from the sigmoid
wall. The distance of the marginal artery from the wall, as in the
case of the colon, has no relation to the length of the mesosigmoid.

From the marginal artery to the sigmoid the terminal arteries
are sent to the wall of the bowel. These are similar in kind (long
and short) and course to those of the colon. Frequently in the lower

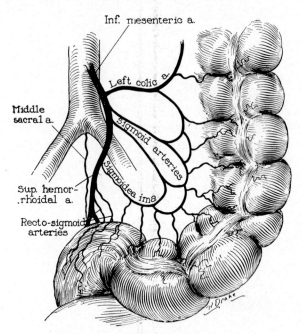

FIG. 10. Arteries to the sigmoid and rectosigmoid
(Steward and Rankin).

portion of the sigmoid and sometimes in the middle portion the
longitudinal fibers spread outward from the longitudinal bands and
form a complete investment of the bowel. In such cases the long
arteries pass beneath the longitudinal fibers near the mesosigmoid
portion of the bowel. The veins follow the general course of arteries
in all the smaller ramifications until the large veins are formed.
These take an upward course, uniting near the base of the mesosigmoid, and finally joining with the left colic from the inferior mesenteric vein.

RECTOSIGMOID, RECTUM, AND ANUS

Below the level of the left common iliac artery, the inferior
mesenteric artery, lying in the base of the mesosigmoid, becomes

the superior hemorrhoidal artery. The artery proceeds toward the median line and downward to its point of bifurcation. The point of bifurcation is generally said to be at the third sacral vertebra and is one of the criteria used to determine the upper end of the rectum. However, the point of bifurcation is in some dispute. Cripps found that the artery divides from 10 to 11 cm. above the anus, whereas Rubesch gives the point of division at from 17 to 20 cm. from the anus. Lockhart-Mummery's observation seems most logical: that the point of division of the superior hemorrhoidal artery varies considerably, as a rule at the upper end of the rectum, but that it is not rare to find a low bifurcation.

The branches of the superior hemorrhoidal artery in its short course from its beginning at the level of the left common iliac artery to its bifurcation have been extensively studied. In the ordinary case the branches generally consist of a vessel which sends a branch upward along the pelvic sigmoid to anastomose with the last sigmoid artery and several (from two to four) branches which run downward more or less parallel with the bowel.

Because of the mechanical difficulties encountered in this region and the occasional occurrence of gangrene following surgical procedures, the anastomosing artery from the superior hemorrhoidal to the sigmoid has commanded considerable attention. Numerous studies of the vessel have been made by injection. Sudeck, in 1907, was the first to emphasize the anastomostic value of the vessel. He found that the vessels of the rectum become filled with injected material from the inferior mesenteric artery by traversing the marginal artery when a ligature was placed on the superior hemorrhoidal artery above the origin of the last branch to the sigmoid. If the ligature were placed below the origin of the artery, few if any of the rectal vessels were injected. Sudeck therefore established the origin of the last sigmoid artery as the critical point for maintaining the blood supply to the rectum in cases in which it was necessary to ligate the superior hemorrhoidal artery to obtain mobility. This experiment was substantiated by Hartmann two years later. However, Rubesch, in 1910, studying this region by the same method, called attention to the fact that the last sigmoid artery, which he calls the sigmoidea ima, may be given off below the bifurcation of the superior hemorrhoidal artery, and that the so-called critical point is not exactly situated but may be encountered within a range of from 13 to 20 cm. from the anus. Manasse emphasized the feebleness of the border vessels in the lower portion of the sigmoid and stated that the last sigmoid artery does not participate in it to a great extent. Drummond, in 1914, studied by injection and roentgenograms the inferior mesenteric artery of twenty specimens. The results of this work are convincing. In eight of the cases the last sigmoid artery and its proximal anastomosis was very small, and in two cases the artery was not even present. The examples of carefully injected specimens in the articles of Pope and Buie, and Pope and Judd confirm the variation in position and number of vessels in this region.

Notwithstanding these findings, there is a growing tendency to question the significance of the so-called critical point of Sudeck. In the past decade anterior resection of the rectosigmoid with immediate anastomosis has been carried out in hundreds of instances without circulatory disturbances resulting from ligation of the superior hemorrhoidal and marginal arteries. In 1944, Dixon said that it could be "definitely stated that the superior hemorrhoidal artery can be ligated and removed and even some of the marginal artery can be resected, as of necessity must be done in removing some of the lower left portion of the colon and the first portion of the sigmoid, without significantly damaging the blood supply to the remaining portion of the descending colon, rectosigmoid or rectum. It is, in brief, safe to assume that all the colon which lies below the brim of the true pelvis will remain viable without the marginal or superior hemorrhoidal arteries. The blood supply to this distal portion of the bowel is adequately cared for in my experience by means of the middle and inferior hemorrhoidal arteries. I base this statement on experience in more than 100 anterior resections in which both the superior hemorrhoidal artery and a portion of the marginal artery were removed without any difficulty arising from inadequate blood supply to the distal segment of bowel."

Rectum.—The rectum is supplied by a variable number of small arteries from the superior hemorrhoidal artery before its division, by the right and left branches of the superior hemorrhoidal artery, by the middle and the inferior hemorrhoidal arteries and by a variable amount from the middle sacral artery.

For many years anatomists have described the arterial supply of the upper part of the rectum as coming only from the right and left branches of the superior hemorrhoidal artery. These small vessels supply the bowel in the gap between the termination of the marginal artery in the lower portion of the sigmoid and the division of the superior hemorrhoidal artery (Fig. 10). Their course is at once encircling toward the anterior aspect of the bowel and downward, coursing more or less parallel with the longitudinal axis of the rectum on its lateral and anterior aspect. The vessels vary in number from one to five and both number and size are proportional to the anatomic variations encountered in this region, that is, a high, small, or absent last sigmoid artery, or a low-dividing superior hemorrhoidal artery. They are to be regarded as supplemental and irregular vessels.

The superior hemorrhoidal artery divides near the upper end

of the rectum into two branches, a right and a left superior artery (Fig. 11). The point of bifurcation is not constant, but usually is opposite the second and third sacral vertebra and, in many instances, is marked by absence of the mesosigmoid. Pope and Judd found that the point of bifurcation is 18 cm. from the origin of the inferior mesenteric artery. The branches course downward along the rectum, gradually encircling it from the posterior aspect. The two branches are seldom equal in size. Quénu, in a meticulous study

of the arteries in thirteen specimens, found that the right branch is usually the larger, and frequently furnishes a large branch to the posterior surface of the rectum. Branches of the arteries are given off irregularly to pierce the thick musculature of the rectum at an acute angle and ramify in the submucosa. Among the lowest branches are some which anastomose with middle hemorrhoidal and prostatic or vaginal arteries.

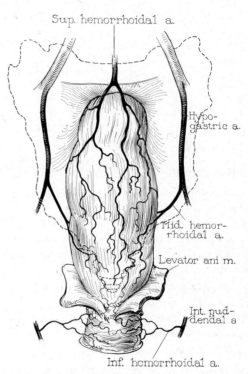

FIG. 11. Arteries to the rectum; posterior view (Steward and Rankin).

The middle hemorrhoidal arteries are the first vessels to the large bowel to be derived from outside the splanchic circulation. Their origin is variable, coming either directly from the anterior division of the internal iliac artery, or from a common trunk with the middle vesical, vaginal, prostatic or internal pudic artery. The arteries course forward to the lateral aspect of the rectum along which they descend, sending into it small irregular branches, some of which anastomose with the branches of the superior hemorrhoidal and some with the vaginal, vesicle, or prostatic arteries. The middle hemorroidal vessels are inconstant in size, distribution, and anastomosis. Particular interest has been centered on the anastomosis of the middle with the superior hemorrhoidal artery. Drummond encountered a case in which there were no middle hemorrhoidal arteries, and Quénu in his more detailed study found the anastomosis extremely irregular. In the thirteen cases examined by Quénu there was complete failure of anastomosis between the middle and superior hemorrhoidal arteries in one case, the anastomosis was through one side only (most frequently the left) in eleven cases, and was bilateral only once.

Formerly, owing to these studies, it was believed that no great reliance could be placed on the anastomosis between the superior and middle hemorrhoidal arteries. Practical experience, however, with anterior resection of the rectosigmoid in hundreds of cases in recent years has demonstrated the adequacy of such anastomosis.

The last artery to the large bowel is the inferior hemorrhoidal. These arteries, usually one on each side, arise from the internal pudic artery during its course through Alcock's canal in the perineum. The vessels subdivide irregularly into three or four smaller branches which circle the anus anteriorly and posteriorly. The vessels supply the musculature of the anus and by fine twigs anastomose with the middle hemorrhoidal artery.

In specimens of the rectum in which the arteries are carefully injected, an anastomosis with the middle sacral artery is seen. This small vessel originates at the bifurcation of the aorta and descends along the anterior surface of the sacrum. Quénu particularly has noted this vessel, and found that it furnishes two or three small branches directly to the posterior wall of the rectum. Pope and Buie included it in the retrorectal plexus. The artery is small, its branches are inconstant, and its value as a supply to the rectum is negligible.

The *veins* of the rectum have received considerable attention from anatomists because of the anastomosis between the portal and caval systems. The rectal veins correspond in name, number, and general course of the arteries. The inferior hemorrhoidal veins drain the region of the anus and sphincter and communicate not only with the middle hemorrhoidal veins above, but also with the veins of the perineum and scrotum. The blood is gathered into several large branches from a perineal plexus, and these branches usually unite before emptying into the internal pudic vein in Alcock's canal.

The middle hemorrhoidal veins are the most important in anastomosing the caval and portal venous systems. Through their connections they communicate both submucosally and perimuscularly with the inferior hemorrhoidal vein, drain the region of the rectum immediately above the internal sphincter, and have free submucosal anastomosis with the superior hemorrhoidal vein. Their branches also anastomose freely with the prostatic or vaginal plexus and in some cases the middle hemorrhoidal vein becomes one of the principal veins to return blood from the urinary vesicle. From many ramifications the veins gather into larger branches on each side of the rectum, and, following the course of the middle hemorrhoidal artery upward, the final single trunks join the internal iliac veins.

The largest of the rectal veins are the superior hemorrhoidal. From as low in the rectum as the columns of Morgagni, the blood is collected by a large mucosal and submucosal plexus and returned upward in the submucosa. In this course the vessels unite to form larger twigs which eventually penetrate the thick muscularis of the rectum at an angle and then continue upward parallel to it. As higher branches from the mucosa penetrate the muscle they join the original veins which also receive branches from the perirectal tissues. Near the upper end of the rectum, large right and left veins are formed which accompany the corresponding branches of the superior hemorrhoidal artery. The veins receive small vessels from the region of the rectosigmoid and pelvic colon. The vessel continues upward to the left of the median line, becoming the inferior mesenteric vein at the level of the left common iliac artery.

Surgical considerations.—The primary purpose of the study of the blood supply of the large intestine was to apply it practically to surgery. Operations on this part of the intestinal tract are fraught with the danger of sepsis, even when most carefully performed, because of the type of bowel and nature of its contents; and the added peril of gangrene in the wall of the bowel from ischemia has undoubtedly been a contributing factor to the hospital death rate. With this thought in mind, an attempt has been made to apply the anatomic facts relating to the blood vessels to the operations usually performed on the large bowel. A description of the technic of the operation, aside from its application to the blood supply, has been purposely avoided, for this is considered in the chapter on operative procedures.

The colon and its blood vessels are roughly similar to a rubber-tired wheel with a few irregularly placed spokes. The spokes represent the named colic arteries, and the rim represents the marginal artery from which the colon is supplied by the terminal branches. It is important in handling the blood supply of the colon to keep in mind that the arterial pattern of each colon is original. The present study has established a few facts, such as the continuity of the marginal vessel and the percentage of occurrence of the various named arteries; but the outstanding fact emphasized is the variability of the arterial pattern, making it essential to deal with each case as a variant. The fact that single colic arteries may be ligated experimentally or by mishap during an operation and the supply to the bowel maintained by the marginal artery should not be an excuse for carelessness. These arteries should be ligated purposefully and only when occasion demands. The arteries of the colon are variable in size and position, and the two adjacent vessels should be investigated before one artery is occluded. The importance of this cannot be more emphatically proved than by reference to the celloidin cast shown in figure 6. Here ligation of the inferior mesenteric artery would inevitably result in ischemia and gangrene of more than half of the colon. The vessels to the portion of the bowel involved should be identified in all surgical procedures. Identification may be difficult in the presence of excessive fat or adhesions; however, a knowledge of the approximate situation of the vessels and palpation for their pulsations will usually establish their situation.

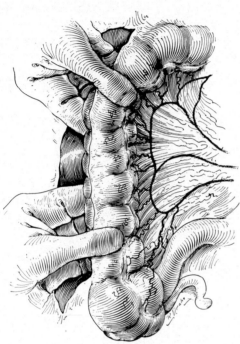

FIG. 12. Colon elevated after incision of the peritoneum along line of its lateral reflection (Steward and Rankin).

Mobility.—Mobility of the colon is a decided advantage in dealing with the blood supply. If the part of the bowel involved can be lifted so that the mesocolon is vertical to the posterior wall, the blood vessels are easily identified even in the presence of moderate obesity. There is nearly always mobility in the transverse portion of the colon, and although we have found a mesocolon to be present in the ascending and descending portions of the colon more frequently than Treves' classic figures indicate, it is usually too short to allow any appreciable upward manipulation. To obtain mobility, the peritoneum should be incised along the lateral side of the colon. There is usually slight thickening of the peritoneum at the line where the upward reflection from the posterior wall takes place, and the resulting white streak may be incised throughout its entire length without danger of encountering vessels. The bowel may be lifted mesially and upward and the centrally situated blood supply brought into prominent relief (Fig. 12).

Insufficient mobilization of the colon, in the course of a procedure in which the bowel is to be fixed, may have several detrimental effects on the blood vessels. Undue pull on the colon will tend to stretch the vessels to that part longitudinally and thereby decrease the diameter of their lumen. This is particularly true of the marginal and the terminal vessels. Another danger is that acute angulation of more distantly attached vessels may occur, especially at the points where the colon is permanently fixed by ligaments. The blood vessels of the colon lie beneath a loose peritoneal covering which allows considerable movement, and their attachments are only through their inosculations and terminal branches. For this reason, angulation of a vessel several centimeters distant may be caused by tension on the colon, thereby reducing the anastomotic supply at a point where it is most necessary. This trouble is particularly likely to be encountered in operations in which the bowel is fixed to the wall of the abdomen, such as colostomy, and will be referred to again when these procedures are considered.

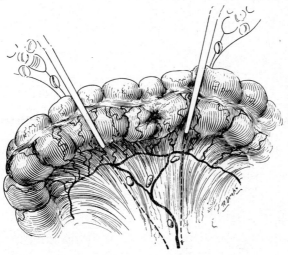

FIG. 13. Colon cut across at angle to preserve the meso-colic, vascular portion (Steward and Rankin).

The wall of the colon.—In the study of the terminal vessels to the colon, we have stressed several important facts: (1) the comparatively scanty anastomosis between the small terminal arteries; (2) the greater vascular supply to the mesocolic two-thirds of the bowel, and (3) the subserosal position of the long arteries before they pass beneath the two amesocolic taenia to supply the relatively avascular third portion of the colon. These anatomic peculiarities give us several guides in surgical procedures on the wall of the bowel. The slight anastomosis of the arteries demands greater care in handling the large intestine than the small. When the bowel is to be cut across, as for end-to-end anastomosis, a greater part of the vascular mesocolic portion of the colon should be retained than the amesocolic third. This is accomplished by cutting the bowel at an angle (Fig. 13). If the colon is cut perpendicular to its axis, the incision may just include one of the long terminal branches to the amesocolic portion, thus destroying for perhaps 2.5 cm. the only supply to a naturally impoverished portion of the bowel. Pauchet, without considering the course of the vessels, advocated cutting the colon at an angle of 45 degrees. So great an angle might make it difficult to obtain sufficient mobilization to avoid pull on the amesocolic part of the anastomosis in cases in which the colon was large and would result in a sharp angle in the lumen. A more rational rule would be to cut a bowel at less acute angles, so that the two ends will most closely coincide in diameter. Cutting the colon at an angle has the added advantage of producing a larger opening at the anastomosis.

When a longitudinal incision in the colon is necessary, it should be placed in the center of the amesocolic third of the bowel (Fig.

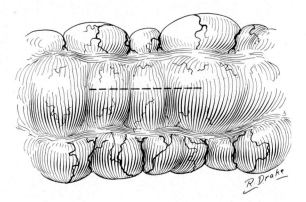

Fig. 14. The dotted line indicates the proper site for a longitudinal incision in the colon (Steward and Rankin).

14). The closer a longitudinal incision is made to the mesocolic taenia, the greater will be the area of colon between the incision and the outer point on the circumference of the bowel to be furnished by the feeble anastomosis of the encircling arteries of the opposite side and the adjacent terminal vessels. The direct supply to the area will have been sacrificed, and the danger of gangrene will be commensurate with the length of the incision. Fortunately for patients and surgeons, the amesocolic section of the colon is usually the most accessible and the least encumbered with fat, and therefore is the place usually selected for ileocolostomy and insertion of enterostomy tubes. If the anatomy of the terminal vessels to the colon is kept in mind, the surgeon will make only longitudinal incisions in the colon parallel with, and exactly between, the amesocolic longitudinal bands.

The subserosal course of the long terminal arteries exposes them to considerable danger when an effort is made to clear fat away from the colon. These arteries furnish branches to the epiploic appendages before passing beneath the longitudinal muscles to the amesocolic section of the wall. In elevating and clamping fat tabs, it is easy to include the long artery, especially if the colon is contracted, and there is increased redundancy of the arteries. Since these arteries are the sole supply to the outer third of the colon, their value cannot be overestimated. As an experiment, the long arteries have been intentionally included when cutting off the epiploic appendages of colostomy loops which are later to be trimmed off and remain as permanent colonic stomas. In one case in which the long arteries were ligated on opposite sides of the colon at the same point, necrosis of the wall between the longitudinal bands occurred for about 2.5 cm., the opening, which appeared on the fifth day, being circular. Although there may have been slight impairment of the circulation to the colostomy loop, the resulting necrosis can be regarded only as evidence of the avascularity of this part of the colon and emphasizes the advantage of leaving the long terminal vessels intact. To avoid injury to the blood supply, the epiploic appendages should not be pulled outward too vigorously, and the clamp

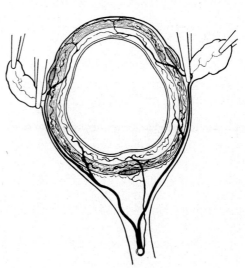

FIG. 15. The correct (left) and incorrect (right) method of clamping epiploic appendages (Steward and Rankin).

should be placed on the neck of the tab, parallel to a tangent at the longitudinal muscle band (Fig. 15). The mesocolic fat should be removed by blunt dissection.

The marginal artery.—This artery has been found to be a continuous vessel present in all colons. In a small number of ascending colons (5 per cent), it is replaced by profuse single branches. The distance of the artery from the wall of the bowel varies from a half to several centimeters, and the presence of secondary loops is uncertain. In position and function, the marginal artery is comparable to the water main in a city street. Whenever possible, the artery should be left intact. However, its presence assures the colon of a distal as well as proximal blood supply, and whenever the occasion demands, the surgeon should have no hesitancy in resecting the marginal artery of the part of the intestine being removed. In fact, it may be desirable in cases of malignant conditions when it is recalled that the second set of lymph nodes, the paracolic nodes, follows its arcades down to the main arteries. When the marginal artery is resected, care should be taken that the remaining artery extends beyond the cut edges of the colon which it supplies (Fig. 13). The principle of the wedge or fan-shaped resection applies to resection of the mesocolon with its blood vessels quite as much as to that of the mesentery of the small bowel. Should the wedge of mesocolon include one of the main colic arteries, the artery itself should be made the apex of the resected wedge and ligated as close to its source as is compatible with proper peritonealization of the posterior wall. In this way the resection would include the third set of lymph nodes, the intermediate nodes, which follows the course of the colic arteries.

Colostomy.—The oldest operation on the colon is colostomy. Regardless of the type or position of the colostomy, there are a few fundamental rules which should be remembered with regard to the blood vessels. The colon must be sufficiently mobilized to allow the bowel to extend above the skin of the abdomen without undue pull upward on the peritoneal attachments. This may be accomplished by incising along the lateral peritoneal reflection as described. With the colon freed to allow exteriorization of a small loop without undue pull on the underlying arteries, the immediate vessels must be considered. The marginal artery will be found running more or less parallel with the wall of the colon at a distance varying from a half to several centimeters. This vessel should always be left intact when colostomy is performed as it is the immediate source of supply to the colon and the important anastomosis between the arteries of the colon. In the types of colostomy in which it is desirable to make an opening in the mesocolon, either to draw components of the abdominal wall together below the loop or simply to fix the loop in position on a tube or rod, the opening should be made between the colon and the marginal artery (Fig. 16). In order to obtain an opening of sufficient size, it may be necessary to ligate several of the terminal vessels, but this is preferable to ligating the marginal artery or making the opening beneath it. Ligation of the vessel may rob the colon proximal to the colostomy of a valuable anastomotic blood supply, whereas an opening below the artery adds to the first danger a second from the embarrassing amount of bleeding produced by the relatively simple process of cutting across the colostomy opening.

Some surgeons customarily sew the peritoneum to the elevated colon after performing colostomy. Although we believe that sewing into the colon should be avoided whenever possible, we wish to emphasize here only a point regarding the blood supply. In the mesocolic portions of the colon, the vessels lie loosely beneath the serosa and are often covered with fat. In sewing the peritoneum to the wall of the colon, it is easy to injure or ligate several of the long terminal branches.

Resection.—Resections of parts or all of the colon must be adjusted to the nature of the lesion. There is no advantage in removing the marginal vessel and the main arteries in cases of benign lesions such as polyposis or ulcerative colitis. The handling of the wall of the colon and the marginal artery n resection has been considered and we wish here merely to advocate primary ligation of the main arteries to the part to be removed. In any case in which an appreciable portion of the colon is to be removed, the operation can be greatly simplified and shortened by ligating the vessels to the part in their central position before an attempt to remove the bowel is made. This necessitates careful identification of vessels and may not be feasible if the patient is obese. For example, in the removal of the right portion of the colon after ileo-

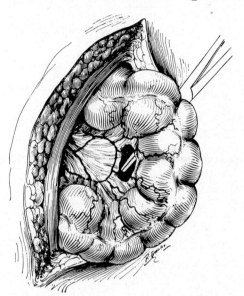

FIG. 16. Opening between the colon and marginal artery in performing colostomy (Steward and Rankin).

colostomy has been performed, if the ilecolic, the right colic, and the marginal arteries just distal to the anastomosis are ligated first, resection can be made without further clamping and only a negligible amount of blood will be encountered in the distal vessels (Fig. 17).

Resection of the splenic flexure frequently offers great difficulty from the technical standpoint. It has been shown that the marginal artery is present in this region, at least before operation, and that there is no lack of blood to the part. However, the splenic flexure lies high, and is deeply placed within the abdomen in the form of a long, inverted U. The blood vessels to the region, through the marginal artery, are almost parallel and close together. If resection of this part is attempted from the median aspect, the marginal arteries are in grave danger of being injured at points proximal to the site of resection. The attack must be lateral to the colon, freeing the splenic flexure along the white line of the peritoneal reflection, severing any connection between the omentum and the spleen and any peritoneal attachments of the colon to the posterior wall. The entire splenic flexure may then be brought mesially and upward with the arteries uninjured, and the resection may proceed as conditions indicate.

The sigmoid offers the most favorable site for operation on the large bowel from the standpoint of dealing with blood vessels. The mesosigmoid allows easy exposure of the affected part; the arterial supply is adequate and flexible, due to the secondary loops usually present below the marginal artery, and in addition the sigmoid is low in the abdomen where infection is less dangerous than near the diaphragm. The rules that apply to handling the blood supply of the colon are applicable in operations on the sigmoid.

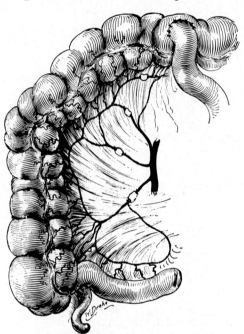

FIG. 17. Primary ligation of the vessels in removal of the right portion of the colon (Steward and Rankin).

LYMPHATICS

Knowledge of the lymphatic structures of the large intestine is due chiefly to: (1) the exceptionally thorough researches of Jamieson and Dodson on the lymphatic vessels of the colon; (2) the careful clinical observations of the lymphatic vessels of the rectum by Miles; and (3) the extensive treatise on the subject by Poirier, Cuneo, and Delamere. For a detailed consideration of the lymphatic apparatus of the large intestine the reader is referred to these works.

Colon.—The distribution of the lymphatic vessels of the colon is not uniform, the cecum, for example, being more freely supplied with these structures than is the splenic flexure or descending colon. The intimate relationship of the lymphatic glands to the blood vessels is important because the lymphatic vessels entering them uniformly follow the course of the blood vessels supplying the different segments, and in order to remove widely the lymphatic structures, in cases of carcinoma of the colon, frequently it is necessary to ligate the blood supply close to its origin (Fig. 18).

Jamieson and Dobson describe each chain of lymphatics, accompanying its blood vessels of like name, as being composed of

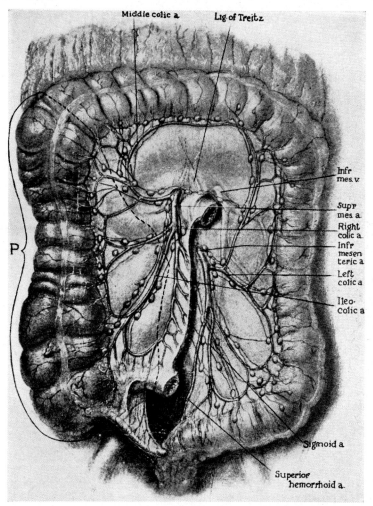

FIG. 18. The mesenteric lymph nodes (from Printy).

epicolic, paracolic, intermediate, and main groups of glands. The lymphatic vessels arise from plexuses in the submucous and subperitoneal coats, which have the same disposition as in other parts of the alimentary canal. The deeper vessels escape chiefly along the entering blood vessels, and those from the outerside of the gut curve behind the gut to join those from the front. Many are interrupted almost immediately in the epicolic glands in the appendices epiploicae or on the sacculi. The efferents of these glands, with other uninterrupted vessels, pass inwards and meet the paracolic glands which intercept the great majority, but some vessels slip between the paracolic glands and reach the intermediate glands

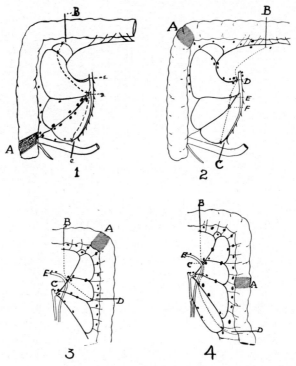

FIG. 19. Excision of growths situated in different parts of the colon and their "lymphatic areas" (after Jamieson and Dobson). A, growth; B and D, line of section of colon and mesocolon; C line of section of ileum. The points of ligation of the ileocolic, middle, right and left colic arteries are indicated.

(lying on the vessels in the mesocolon) in company with the epicolic and paracolic efferents; in some cases these vessels run directly to the main group of glands, situated at the base of the blood vessels supplying the different segments of colon.

Rectum.—The observations of Handley, Miles, and others have tended to show that the intramural lymphatic vessels of the rectum and colon are of little practical significance. Miles has never observed carcinoma to spread within the wall of the intestine, while Handley observed such spread in the lymphatic vessels of the submucous plexus on two occasions. However, he emphasized the rarity of such occurrences.

Poirier, Cuneo, and Delamere described three main collecting trunks of lymphatic vessels for the anus and rectum: (1) inferior group, which drain the skin of the margin of the anus, the efferent vessels terminating in the superficial inguinal glands; (2) middle group, which drain the anocutaneous area; some of efferent vessels perforate the rectal wall slightly above the levator ani, ascend on the lateral wall of the rectum, traverse the para-rectal glands, and join the efferents from the upper part of the rectum which terminate in nodes of the mesorectum, others ascend in the columns of Morgagni and terminate in the rectal mucosa, whereas occasionally these efferent vessels ascend the middle hemorrhoidal vessels or pass beneath the levator ani vessels onto the inferior hemorrhoidal vessels; and (3) superior group, which pass through the muscular coat of the rectum at different levels, usually as satellites of the vessels, and coursing obliquely upwards and backwards, terminate in nodes of the mesorectum. The superior group corresponds to the superior hemorrhoidal artery, the middle group to the middle and inferior hemorrhoidal homologue in the arterial system (Fig. 19).

Carcinoma cells reaching the extramural lymphatic vessels may according to Miles, spread downward, laterally, or upward: "The general scheme of the extramural lymphatic channels is represented in figure 49. The various tissues traversed by these vessels are vulnerable to metastatic deposits. Corresponding to the three lymphatic areas there are three zones of spread: (1) the zone of downward spread, which includes the peri-anal skin, the ischiorectal fat, and the external sphincter muscle; (2) the zone of lateral spread, which embraces the levatores ani muscles, the retrorectal lymph glands, the internal iliac glands, the base of the bladder, and the vesiculae seminales, and, in the female, the posterior wall of the vagina, the cervix uteri, and the base of the broad ligament with Poirier's gland; and (3) the zone of upward spread, which includes the pelvic peritoneum, the pelvic mesocolon in its entirety, the paracolic lymph glands, and the group of lymph glands at the bifurcation of the left common iliac artery. The most vulnerable of these are the ischiorectal glands and the pelvic mesocolon. Therefore, these tissues must be freely removed in an operation for cancer of the rectum."

NERVES

The large intestine receives its innervation from both sympathetic and cerebrospinal nerves (Fig. 20). Filaments of the latter anastomose with the sympathetic ganglia to form nerve plexuses, and the spinal nerves pass to the colon indirectly through the ganglia. Accurate knowledge of the sympathetic nerve supply to the distal part of the colon and rectum is significant from the standpoint of surgical procedures for the relief of pain in the event of pelvic recurrences and vesical atony following resection of the rectum (see Palliative and Miscellaneous Procedures); also for the relief of megacolon. Rankin and Learmonth have described this innervation in the following manner:

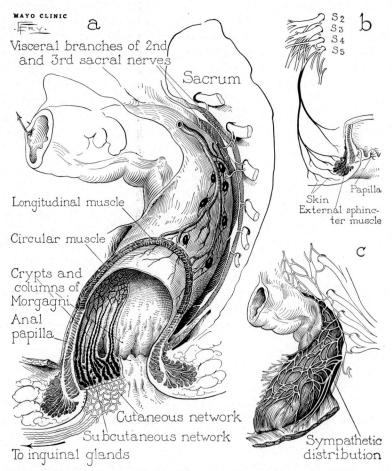

FIG. 20. Diagrammatic sketch showing in detail the character of the lymphatic network above and below the pectinate line and also the nerve supply to the rectum and anus (from Buie's "Proctologic Examination," courtesy of W. B. Saunders Co.).

The sympathetic nerves which pass to the distal part of the colon have for their immediate origin the intermesenteric plexuses. These networks of nerves descend on the anterolateral aspects of the abdominal aorta, from the level of the origin of the superior mesenteric artery downward. On each side there are two or three large trunks which are made up of nonmyelinated fibres, arising from: (1) the semilunar ganglion and celiac plexus; (2) an anastomotic loop which crosses the aorta transversely, below the origin of the superior mesenteric artery; and (3) the aorticorenal ganglion, or the renal periarterial plexus.

The intermesenteric plexus is joined on each side by branches from the first and second lumbar ganglia. These branches contain myelinated fibres; those on the right side pass between the vena cava and the aorta to reach the front of the latter vessel. The fibres which form the intermesenteric plexuses are thus derived from two sources; their original fibres spring from that part of the abdominal sympathetic system connected with the thoracic splanchnic nerves, while the branches which the plexus receives as it descends along the aorta spring from the lumbar ganglia or trunks. There is a difference of opinion among anatomists concerning the extent to which the lumbar fibres mingle with those of the intermesenteric plexus proper. According to Delmas, Laux, and others, the mesially-directed lumbar communicating branches, constituting the pelvic splanchnic nerves, remain distinct in the outer part of the plexus, and ultimately form the lateral roots of the presacral nerve of Latarjet (superior hypogastric plexus of Hovelacque). On the other hand, Hovelacque holds that those lumbar communicating branches actually contribute to the intermesenteric plexus (Fig. 21). The point is one of great significance. If the former view were correct, lumbar ramisectomy and ganglionectomy would affect only that portion of the bowel innervated through the presacral nerve; namely, the lower part of the rectum and the internal sphincter of the anus; if the latter arrangement were the true one, it would affect, but only partly, the descending and sigmoid portions of the colon, as well as the rectum and the internal sphincter of the anus. The beneficial results of lumbar ramisectomy in cases of megacolon strongly favor the view that the branches which join the intermesenteric plexus from the first and second lumbar ganglia do have a share in the innervation of the colon.

Immediately below the level of the origin of the inferior mesenteric artery, a large branch leaves the intermesenteric plexus of each side, and passes inward, on the aorta, to reach the inferior mesenteric artery about 1.5 cm. from its origin (Fig. 21). Finally these two trunks unite, and give rise to three or four large branches which course along the lateral borders of the vessel, communicating at intervals with each other. Fortunately for the surgeon, the nerves associated with the inferior mesenteric artery retain their individuality, and neither form so close a network, nor possess such an intimate relationship with the wall of the vessel, as do the nerves supplying other viscera. From these nerves subsidiary trunks arise at the levels of the main divisions of the artery.

Soon, however, they abandon the vessels, and anastomose with one another in avascular parts of the mesosigmoid. From this network the final nerves of distribution are derived; these slender filaments cross the juxtacolic vascular arcades and enter the wall of

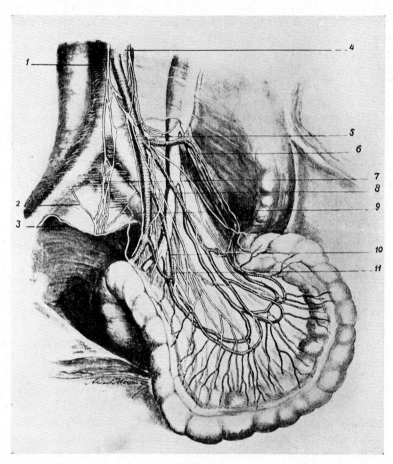

Fig. 21. The inferior mesenteric nerves: 1, intermesenteric nerves of the right side; 2, branch from right fourth lumbar ganglion to presacral nerve; 3, cut edge of peritoneum; 4, intermesenteric nerves of the left side; 5, inferior mesenteric nerves; 6, inferior mesenteric vein; 7, presacral nerve; 8, sigmoid artery; 9, branch from left fourth lumbar ganglion to presacral nerve; 10, sigmoid artery, and 11, sigmoid artery (from Hovelacque).

the bowel between the terminal branches of the vessels. Two or three large branches accompany the superior hemorrhoidal artery, and invest the lateral and posterior walls of the rectum in a plexiform manner. Their terminal twigs join the hypogastric ganglia. The distribution of the inferior mesenteric nerves corresponds to that of the inferior mesenteric artery, and toward the end of the transverse colon, where the left colic artery anostomoses with the middle colic, branches of the inferior mesenteric plexus communicate with filaments derived from the superior mesenteric plexus.

It has been seen that the inferior mesenteric nerves are formed in greater part of post-ganglionic fibres. If the lumbar communicating branches contribute to the plexus there should be a ganglion about the root of the artery, in which their myelinated fibres effect synapses. There is no doubt that there are ganglionic masses in this area, but they are most inconstant, both in position and in size. In some cases of megacolon the dilatation of the large bowel extends to the internal sphincter of the anus, so that it has been suggested that this structure may offer undue resistance to the expulsion of the contents of the bowel. In vertebrates the internal sphincter of the anus is innervated through the thoracicolumbar sympathetic outflow. In man, there are two possible paths by which thoracicolumbar fibres might reach the sphincter: (1) by way of the inferior mesenteric nerves, their hemorrhoidal branches, and the branches of distribution of the hypogastric ganglia; and (2) by way of the presacral nerve (superior hypogastric plexus), and the branches of distribution of the hypogastric ganglia. The first route has been described. The presacral nerve is a complex nerve, lying in the angle between the common iliac arteries. It has three roots: On each side, succeeding branches arising from the first to the fourth lumbar ganglia join to form its lateral roots, which converge toward the anterior aspect of the fifth lumbar vertebra. Into the angle between the two lateral roots descends the third or middle root. Weinstein in a recent (1942) report, based on 150 personal dissections of the superior hypogastric plexus, demonstrated a wide variation in the configuration of this plexus and the relative rarity of a single presacral nerve (4 per cent). The nerve descends into the pelvis, and at the level of the first sacral vertebra divides into the two hypogastric nerves, which join the corresponding hypogastric ganglia. From these, post-ganglionic fibres of distribution pass to the pelvic viscera, including the lower part of the rectum and the internal sphincter of the anus.

The external sphincter of the anus, the mucutaneous lining of the anal canal, and the perianal skin are abundantly supplied with sensory nerve endings, derived from the cerebrospinal system, through the third and fourth sacral nerves, and the pudic nerve by its hemorrhoid branch. Motor, sensory, and sympathetic filaments are contained in (Fig. 19) branches of these structures. Above the pectinate line, however, the rectum is relatively free of sensory endings, consequently the rectal mucosa is relatively insensitive to tactile and thermal stimuli, whereas the smallest break in the continuity of the anal mucosa will elicit pain, and in instances of neoplasms situated here the pain may become excruciating.

PHYSIOLOGY

Nature, it has been asserted, is interested in function rather than appearance, in physiology rather than anatomy. The value and effectiveness of surgical measures depend very largely upon the functional end-results obtained. It is insufficient, therefore, that the surgeon think in terms of anatomy alone, and particularly is this true in regard to surgery of the colon (Livingston).

In man, the most important function of the colon is probably that of a storehouse to accommodate feces until they can be conveniently eliminated. The next most important function appears to be that of returning to the blood the water which has been poured into the small intestine during the progress of digestion. Impairment of this function, as in the presence of diarrhea, leads to dehydration and the inability of the colon to serve as a storehouse for fecal residue. That the colon is not an indispensable organ has been shown many times by surgeons who have removed it in its entirety. Usually after a short interval the terminal portion of the ileum becomes adapted to a retention of fecal matter; in fact, one of our patients even became constipated and required an occasional laxative in less than three months following the establishment of an ileostomy preliminary to resection of the colon.

A study of the physiology of the large intestine leads one to conclude that it is a bifunctional organ and, indeed, when one considers its embryologic development such a conclusion is obvious. The right half of the colon is the absorbing half, and is comparable in function to the small bowel with which it has a common embryologic beginning. From the papilla of Vater approximately to the middle of the transverse colon the large intestine develops with the small intestine from the mid-gut, and the function of this whole division is digestion and absorption. Beyond the middle of the transverse colon the large bowel is developed from the hind-gut, and its duty is one of storage. The two halves not only differ structurally, they derive their blood supply from different sources, the superior mesenteric artery supplying the digestive or absorptive part of the gastrointestinal tract, the inferior mesenteric the distal half. These differences are significant in that they decidedly influence the symptoms produced by lesions situated in the two segments. Notwithstanding the tendency to become large fungating growths, the liquid nature of the fecal current and the greater diameter of the lumen in this segment prevents obstruction by carcinomas in the right half of the large bowel. The symptoms are chiefly due to some perverted or inhibited physiologic function of the mucous membrane which permits the absorption of toxin from the extensive infected surface of the growth and neighboring segment of bowel, giving rise to a characteristic profound secondary anemia. On the other hand, in the distal segment of the large bowel carcinomas usually are scirrhous and annular and the fecal matter of a solid nature; and there, obstruction—chronic, subacute, or acute—almost invariably develops.

It is well known that the feces in the cecum and ascending colon are liquid, in the transverse and descending portions, more solid, and by the time they reach the rectum are often in the form of inspissated balls. The feces of constipated persons float, whereas, if the stools are loose much of the matter settles to the bottom of the toilet bowl. In other words, the specific gravity of the feces is so near that of water that the colon can be said to float in the abdomen, and the mesentery serves more as a guy-rope than a support. It is a mistake, therefore, to speak of the colon as being weighted down with feces.

It is very probable that some mild, long-continued, and unexplained diarrheas are due to failure of the mechanism which normally removes water from the feces; conversely one may explain some cases of constipation on the basis that the mechanism is too efficient. Many experiments and considerable clinical observations have shown that, besides water, only dextrose and salt can be absorbed in appreciable quantities from the greater part of colonic mucosa. For this reason the so-called nutrient enema of eggs, beef-juice, cream, etc., has fallen into disrepute. As is well known, when drugs are given by rectum the amounts are generally twice those that are effective by mouth. The fate of glucose solution, even, administered by rectum is quite problematic. McNealy and Willems list these possibilities: It may stay in situ indefinitely; it may be expelled; its character may be changed by bacterial or other action; absorption in the colon may take place; or it may pass into the small bowel. The latter is generally conceded to be the more likely alternative if the glucose is utilized, absorption occurring in the lower ileum.

The ease and rapidity with which solutions placed in the rectum reach the cecum and even the ileum, as can readily be demonstrated in instances of cecostomy, would appear to contraindicate such a practice following operations on the colon or ileum. There is an abundance of experimental and clinical data (Drummond, Friedenwald and Feldman, Alvarez, Rolleston and Jex-Blake, Bline and Schmoll, and others), which clearly demonstrates that nutrient enemas, and even simple glucose solution, frequently hinder emptying of the stomach, inhibit normal peristalsis, or, occasionally, initiate reverse peristalsis and, eventually, vomiting of a fecal

nature. Such data and our own observation have thoroughly convinced us that the rectal instillation of fluids following operations
on the intestine is unphysiologic, even dangerous. It is rare indeed
that an adequate fluid intake cannot be maintained orally, subcutaneously, or by the intravenous route.

Alvarez has shown that the mucous membrane of the colon
functions as an efficient barrier in preventing the passage of toxins
into the circulation. One of the factors that tends to protect the
body from intestinal auto-intoxication is the dryness of the feces
in the left half of the colon. Most of the toxic end products of protein digestion which are supposed to cause symptoms are either
blocked by the mucosa of the colon, or changed as they pass
through it; those that do get through are possibly changed in the
liver or during their passage through the capillaries of the lung. It
is obvious that any material that succeeds in running the gauntlet
must trickle into the general circulation in quantities too minute
to have an effect. In many sensitive persons the distention of the
rectum with cotton or a balloon gives rise at times to nausea, sleepi-
ness, mental haziness, and depression. When the distending body
is fecal material the impression of the patient is that he is suffering
from auto-intoxication but it would seem obvious that the symptoms cannot be due to absorption of toxins, as they disappear almost immediately on removal of the distending body, whereas
relief from circulating toxins would not come until they had been
eliminated by the slow process of excretion. No doubt intestinal
auto-intoxication does occasionally occur, but most students of the
subject agree that it is far more likely to be present with diarrhea
than with constipation. Indeed, it has been the exception, in our
experience, to observe symptoms of toxic absorption in cases of
chronic obstruction produced by carcinoma of the colon, even when
obstruction had reached the stage in which flatus alone was expelled. In these cases it has been almost the rule to find the blood
chemistry normal.

A function of the colon about which little is known is the excretion of heavy metals and other substances which have been absorbed higher in the bowel. Quite possibly some of the hypersensi-
tiveness of the colon, so frequently observed, is due to irritation
caused by the excretion of a toxic substance, the nature of which
is not known. Many investigators have found various products of
excretion in the intestinal secretions, such as aluminum iron, magnesium, bismuth, calcium, and phosphates. Ulceration of the large
bowel so commonly associated with mercury poisoning indicates
that the metal probably is excreted by this route. Peola's studies
have led him to believe that sugar might be eliminated by the colon

in cases of diabetes, thus giving rise to the diarrhea occasionally noticed in these cases.

The principal secretion of the colon is mucus, and it serves as a lubricant to the feces and as a protective agent to the lining of the colon. Although it possesses no anti-bactericidal power it probably acts as a mechanical barrier to infection. It is noteworthy that of the salivary glands the parotid is the only one frequently subject to inflammation and few mucus-producing cells are found in this structure. In the submaxilliary and sublingual glands mucus is secreted in considerable quantities.

The term mucous colitis has originated because of the presence of an excess of mucus in and about the stool. Bargen states that no one has ever demonstrated pathologic data sufficient to allow this condition properly to be called colitis. The literature on this subject is vast and there is much difference of opinion as to its character and etiology. The preponderance of evidence favors the view that the condition is purely neurogenic and the mucus produced is a hypersecretion. The idea prevails—especially among laymen, but also among some physicians—that the colon is a constant source of danger because of the presence of bacteria or of toxins produced by decomposition of foods, and that these must be responsible for many ills of man; and it is often difficult to convince a patient that certain intestinal disturbances could be the result of a disordered nervous state. All of the 200 consecutive cases studied by Bargen had definite symptoms of neurosis. Often there was a history of much nervous strain, anxiety, worry, intolerance of the presence of crowds, excessive physical and mental effort, introspection, insomnia, unhappiness with their lot, family difficulties, excessive use of tobacco or liquor, and dissipation in one form or another. Nervous phenomena tended to precipitate attacks of the abdominal symptoms. Our observations are in full accord with those of Hurst who has pointed out that "not the slightest sign of inflammation is observed in the mucous membrane of patients with so-called mucous colitis unless they have been treated with irritating enemas."

The various types of peristaltic movements in the colon are of considerable interest to the gastro-enterological investigator, but the scope of this work will not permit their consideration in detail. Of more practical significance is the reflex mechanism generally termed appetite reflex or gastrocolic reflex, in which the placing of food into the empty stomach is followed by activity in the colon. The so-called mass movements which ordinarily precede defecation are most likely to take place immediately after breakfast when the bowel is most sensitive after the night's rest. It is well known that one of the causes of constipation and probably the chief one is the tendency of many persons to disregard this call. After weeks and months of such neglect the lower colon and rectum become less sensitive to the presence of feces, and less able to respond with a defecatory reflex.

Many investigators have shown that distention of the colon retards emptying of the stomach and gives rise to loss of appetite, nausea, and even vomiting. Inflammatory lesions in the ileocecal region, appendicitis for example, may produce all grades of back pressure even to vomiting of large amounts of fluids. Moreover, Cannon has shown that intestinal injury, such as incising or handling the bowel, will retard the emptying time of the stomach. It is conceivable that a protective mechanism exists for the purpose of holding back food until the bowel becomes healed. The presence of formed fecal material in the rectum will, after abdominal incision, often inhibit peristalsis until evacuated. This has been strikingly revealed to us on a number of occasions.

No attempt has been made in this brief consideration of the subject to discuss all the facts pertaining to the physiology of the colon and rectum. For a more comprehensive consideration the reader is referred to the investigations of Alvarez, Cannon, Bargen, and more recently (1933) the illuminating treatise of Larson, which has been freely drawn on in the preparation of this chapter.

REFERENCES

1. ALVAREZ, W. C.: The mechanics of the digestive tract. Ed. 2. New York, Paul B. Hoeber, Inc., 447 pp.
2. BARGEN, J. A.: Conditions commonly called colitis. *Am. Jour. Roentgenol. and Radium Therap.*, **25**: 308–313 (March), 1931.
3. BARGEN, J. A.: Modern concept of intestinal function. *Jour. Am. Med. Assoc.*, **132**: 313–316 (Oct.), 1946.
4. BARGEN, J. A.: Modern management of colitis. Springfield, Charles C Thomas, 1943.
5. BLINE and SCHMOLL: Quoted by Larson and Bargen.
6. CANNON: Quoted by Larson and Bargen.
7. CUNNINGHAM, D. J.: Text-book of anatomy. Ed. 5, New York, William Wood and Company, 1921.
8. DIXON, CLAUDE F.: Anterior resection for carcinoma low in the rectosigmoid. *Surgery*, **15**: 367–377 (March), 1944.
9. DRUMMOND, HAMILTON: Some points relating to the surgical anatomy of the arterial supply of the large intestine. *Proc. Roy. Soc. Med.* (Sect. Proct.), **7**: 185, 1914.
10. DRUMMOND, HAMILTON: The arterial supply of the rectum and pelvic colon. *Brit. J. Surg.*, **1**: 677, 1914.
11. FRIEDENWALD and FELDMAN: Quoted by Larson and Bargen.
12. GRAY, HENRY: Anatomy of the human body. Philadelphia, Lea & Febiger, 1924.

13. HANDLEY, W. S.: The dissemination of rectal cancer. *Brit. Med. Jour.*, **1**: 584 (March 15), 1913.
14. JAMIESON, J. K., and DOBSON, J. F.: The lymphatics of the colon. *Ann. Surg.*, **50**: 1077 (Dec.), 1909.
15. KEITH, A. Diverticula of the alimentary tract of congenital or of obscure origin. *Brit. Med. Jour.*, **1**: 376–380 (Feb. 12), 1910.
16. LARSON, LAWRENCE M., and BARGEN, J. A.: Physiology of the colon. *Arch. Surg.*, **27**: 1–50 (July), 1933.
17. LIVINGSTON, E. M.: A clinical study of the abdominal cavity and peritoneum. New York, Paul B. Hoeber, Inc., 1932.
18. MARTIN, EDWARD, and BURDEN, V. G.: The surgical significance of the rectosigmoid sphincter. *Ann. Surg.*, **86**: 86–91 (July), 1927.
19. MILES, W. E.: Cancer of the rectum. London, Harrison and Sons, Ltd., 1926, pp. 4–18.
20. McNEALY, R. W., and WILLEMS, J. S.: The absorption of glucose from the colon: a preliminary study of the glucose enema. *Surg., Gynec., and Obst.*, **49**: 794–798 (Dec.), 1929.
21. PENNINGTON, J. R.: A treatise on diseases of the anus, rectum and pelvic colon. Philadelphia, P. Blakiston's Son & Co., 1923.
22. PEOLA: Quoted by Larson and Bargen.
23. POIRIER, P., CUNÉO, B., DELAMERE, G.: The lymphatics. London, Constable and Co., Ltd., 1913, 301 pp.
24. POPE, C. E., and BUIE, L. A.: A description of the arterial blood supply of the pelvic colon. *Tr. Am. Proct. Soc.*, 1929, p. 78.
25. POPE, C. E., and JUDD, E. S.: The arterial blood supply of sigmoid, rectosigmoid, and rectum. *S. Clin. North America*, **9**: 957 (Aug.), 1929.
26. RANKIN, F. W., and LEARMONTH, J. R.: Section of the sympathetic nerves of the distal part of the colon and the rectum in the treatment of Hirschsprung's disease and certain types of constipation. *Ann. Surg.*, **92**: 710–720 (Oct.), 1930.
27. ROLLESTON and JEX-BLAKE: Quoted by Larson and Bargen.
28. STEWARD, J. A., and RANKIN, F. W.: Blood supply of the large intestine: Its surgical considerations. *Arch. Surg.*, **26**: 843–891 (May), 1933.
29. TUTTLE, J. P.: A treatise on diseases of the anus, rectum, and pelvic colon. New York, D. Appleton and Company, 1906.
30. WEINSTEIN, B. BERNARD: The surgical anatomy of the superior hypogastric plexus. *Surg., Gynec., and Obstet.*, **74**: 245–255 (Feb.), 1942.
31. YEOMANS, F. C.: Proctology. New York, D. Appleton and Company, 1929.

CHAPTER II

INCIDENCE, OCCURRENCE AND ETIOLOGY

INCIDENCE

According to mortality statistics compiled by the U. S. Bureau of the Census, carcinoma of the large intestine represents about 15 per cent of all cancers of the body. In 1944 there were 171,171 deaths from cancer. Of this number, 58,888 were from cancer of the gastro-intestinal tract, and 29,909 (or 17.4 per cent) were from cancer of the bowel, including the small intestine. Cancer in general has become second only to heart disease as a cause of death: in 1900 it was seventh place, being preceded in the order named by tuberculosis, heart disease, influenza and pneumonia, chronic nephritis, enteritis, and cerebral hemorrhage. The rise of cancer to second place was due more to decline in the death rate of other diseases than to an increase in the cancer death rate. Nevertheless, during this period the rate for cancer has increased slowly but continuously from 64.0 to 129.1 per 100,000 of population in 1944. There has been also a corresponding increase in the incidence of deaths from cancer of the large intestine. In the period between 1920 and 1929, of all deaths from carcinoma, deaths from carcinoma of the intestinal tract showed the most pronounced increase. Carcinoma of the intestine (excluding the rectum) increased from 7.1 to 9.4 in each 100,000 inhabitants and carcinoma of the rectum increased from 3.2 to 4.2. Similarly, in England and Wales, during the same period, carcinoma of the intestines increased from 6.8 to 13.6 and carcinoma of the rectum from 6.8 to 8.3 in each 100,000 inhabitants. In judging this increase it is not easy to distinguish the actual from the apparent increase. Cancer being largely an old-age disease, no accurate measures of rates can be determined without making allowances for the age constitution of the population. Because of a prolongation of the span of life from an expectancy of forty years in 1850 to forty-eight in 1900 and sixty-four in 1945 larger numbers now reach the "cancer age" who formerly would have died of diseases now preventable or controllable. In this connection, Pennington's analysis of 7,313 cases of cancer of the large intestine is significant. Of this number, 4,886 occurred in persons aged more than fifty years.

There are other factors equally important in their effect on the rates. Improvement in diagnosis undoubtedly accounts for some of the apparent increase. In the case of cancer of the colon, its more frequent recognition may be attributed to the increased accuracy of roentgenologic diagnosis and the more general employment of roentgenograms in the diagnosis of suspected lesions of the intestinal tract. The present difference in the death rates from cancers for cities and those for rural districts tend to confirm this view. In 1932 rates for cities were higher than those for the rural districts by 47.8 per cent. The obvious explanation lies in the fact that hospital and other facilities for diagnosis of the disease are greater in the cities than in the rural districts. Greater accuracy in death certificates must also explain in part this increased incidence of cancer. According to Lubarsch, the diagnostic error of internal cancer, as determined by 8,301 necropsies in Germany (1920 and 1921), was 32.44 per cent. And records from other countries show similar results.

Statistics on the incidence of cancer from various sources show considerable variations. On the whole, however, they reveal that death rates from directly visible cancers—skin, buccal cavity, and breasts—decreased, while those of cancers of the intestinal organs increased. The inference to be drawn is that the increasing death rates of internal cancer may reflect the advances in diagnostic methods rather than a real increase in cancer incidence and mortality. Visible cancers were almost as readily diagnosed twenty years ago as today, and being free of handicaps of diagnostic difficulties, medical progress has been reflected in declining mortality rates. The following statement, made by the Statistical Bureau of the Metropolitan Life Insurance Company and based on an exhaustive investigation of 185,835 deaths from cancer in the twenty-year period from 1911 to 1930, is significant: "In interpreting these data on cancer mortality, consideration must be given to the actuality of the indicated death rates and trends, and certain facts must be borne in mind. First, most cancers affect internal organs, making more difficult a diagnosis which is, at best, not simple. Second, diagnostic procedures and the knowledge of medical men concerning cancer have improved tremendously in the period covered by this review. Third, hospitalization, operation, and autopsy—all of which contribute toward the more accurate diagnosis of cancer—have greatly increased in frequency. We believe that by far the largest part of the individual increase in the cancer death rate is spurious and may be attributed to improvement in diagnostic technique and to the more widespread use of improved methods."

OCCURRENCE

The segments of the gastro-intestinal tract in which carcinoma commonly is found are those which are subjected to the greatest trauma, either intrinsic or extrinsic. The usual sites for cancer to occur, therefore, are the lower portion of the esophagus, the lesser curvature of the stomach, the rectosigmoid, and the rectum. In 833 consecutive cases encountered in the Mayo Clinic in a period of twelve months, in which a diagnosis was made of carcinoma of the alimentary tract, the site of the lesion was that given in Table 1.

TABLE 1

SITUATION OF CARCINOMA OF THE ALIMENTARY TRACT (BALFOUR)

Patients	Situation	Per Cent
97	Esophagus	11.6
419	Stomach	50.3
10	Small intestine	1.2
91	Large intestine	10.9
216	Rectum	25.9
833	Total	99.9

All available statistical data attest the relative immunity of the small intestine to primary carcinoma. Brill reported 2.5 per cent in the small intestine in a series of 3,562 cases of carcinoma. Rankin and C. W. Mayo, in a series of 8,932 cases of malignancy of the gastro-intestinal tract, found only fifty-five, or 0.62 per cent in the small intestine, which represented an incidence of 1.2 per cent of all carcinomas in the intestinal tract alone.

Site of growth.—The various authors fail to agree on the relative incidence of occurrence of growths in different parts of the colon, but it is generally conceded that the two mobile, terminal segments, the cecum and the sigmoid, are most frequently invaded. Pemberton and Dixon, in 1934, reporting a series of carcinomas of the large intestine, which include a part of our series, gave the situation as follows: colon, 1,293 cases; rectum and rectosigmoid, 2,249 cases (Fig. 22). Jackman, Neibling and Waugh, in 1947, reporting a series of 825 carcinomas of the colon and rectum observed at the Mayo Clinic in 1944, found the situation of the lesions to be almost identical with those shown in figure 22. The incidence by segments was as follows: cecum, 3.2 per cent, ascending colon, 3.7 per cent, hepatic flexure, 2.3 per cent, transverse colon, 4.1 per cent, splenic flexure, 2.8 per cent, descending colon, 5.4 per cent, sigmoid, 17.1 per cent, rectosigmoid, 10.6 per cent, rectum, 17.1 per cent, rectum, 46.2 per cent and anorectal, 3.7 per cent. This report has been further discussed under "Symptoms and Diagnosis."

There is even greater variation in statistics of the relative involvement of the different portions of the rectum. Carcinomas situated at the rectosigmoid juncture have a tendency in many instances to prolapse into the ampulla of the rectum. When on proctoscopic examination a growth is visualized in this situation it is likely to be called a high rectal lesion, whereas the surgeon, on examination, is able to show that the growth is at the peritoneal fold or above it. Edwards stated that about 80 per cent of the lesions occur 5 to 7.5 cm. from the anus; whereas Gant, in 100 cases, found 50 per cent in the ampulla and 15 per cent in the rectosigmoid region. Kraske likewise believed the rectosigmoid was the commonest site of carcinoma. As regards the situation of the growth on the circumference of the bowel, Cole asserts that the sites of predilection are the anterior and lateral walls. Rawlings, however, believes that the posterior wall is more often affected, and Oehler says that they occur as often on the anterior as on the posterior wall. Pennington, in a study of 926 specimens of the nonannular type, found

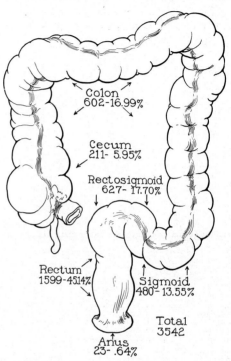

FIG. 22. Situation and relative frequency of occurrence of malignant growths of the colon and rectum (Pemberton and Dixon).

that 547 were on the anterior wall, 280 on the posterior, and only 99 on the lateral.

TABLE 2

SITUATION OF MALIGNANT GROWTHS OF THE RECTUM*
COMPARISON OF SERIES OF BACON AND OF PEMBERTON AND DIXON

Patients		Situation	Per Cent	
(Bacon)	(P. and D.)		(Bacon)	(P. and D.)
231	627	Rectosigmoid	21.2	27.8
787	1599	Rectum	72.5	71.0
68	23	Anus	6.2	1.0
1086	2249	Total	99.9	99.8

* See also Fig. 22.

Age, race, and sex.—Very little significance can be placed on the race distribution of carcinoma of the large intestine, because of the marked disparity in the literature regarding the relative incidence in the white and negro races. Raiford reported that at the Johns Hopkins Hospital the whites outnumbered the blacks about eight to one, while Gant, in 1923, stated he had never heard of or treated a case of carcinoma of the rectum in a negro, although he had maintained several large negro clinics. Actually, in 1944, of 9,342 deaths in the United States from carcinoma of the rectum and anus 510, or 5.4 per cent, were in negroes.

The sex of the patient influences somewhat the operability, mortality, and prognosis, as has been discussed elsewhere. Most authors state that men are affected more commonly than women. In the colon we have noted that the condition occurs in the male in the ratio of approximately 2 to 1. In the group of 300 cases of carcinoma of the rectum reviewed by Rankin and Jones the proportion of men to women was 3 to 2; Raiford, Pfeiffer, Gabriel, and others report a ratio of about 2 to 1.

Age is no barrier to the occurrence of malignant lesions of the colon and rectum. In a large series of cases of carcinoma of the large intestine one is struck with the number of persons aged thirty or less. The incidence of carcinoma of the colon and rectum in these young persons is probably proportionately higher than the incidence of carcinoma invading all organs of the body and occurring in persons of the same age. Williams, reviewing the reports of 1,934 cases of carcinoma in general found 0.99 per cent in persons aged thirty years or less. Yet Rankin and Comfort, in a review of 1,452 patients with carcinoma of the rectum, found the incidence in the same age period to be 3.85 per cent. In these youthful cases they found a short duration of symptoms, greater incidence of metastasis and non-resectable growths, decreased percentage of ultimate good results of three-year and five-year survivals, as well as the increased percentage of higher grades of malignancy, according to Broders' method of classification. Pennington, in a study of 7,313 collected cases reported an incident in persons aged not more than thirty years almost identical with that reported by Rankin and Comfort, i.e., 3.7 per cent.

Carcinoma of the colon and rectum in children under eighteen years of age is of very infrequent occurrence. Walker and Daly reviewed the literature in 1934 and found only ten proven cases of carcinoma of the colon in children under fifteen years of age. Subsequently, Pfeiffer and Wood (1935), Ogilvie (1936), and Warthen (1937), each added a case. Johnston in 1947 reviewed the literature and reported a case of carcinoma of the transverse colon in a thirteen year old negro boy. Altogether, 48 instances of carcinoma of the large intestine, excluding the rectosigmoid, have been noted in persons aged less than seventeen years; 31 were between the ages of twelve and fifteen and nine were aged less than ten. As to the situation of the lesion, 32.6 per cent were in the cecum and ascending colon, 30.4 per cent in the flextures and transverse colon, 2.2 per cent in the descending colon, and 34.8 per cent in the sigmoid. The longest reported survival was four years. In 43 per cent of 39 cases in which accurate microscopic diagnosis was given, the diagnosis was colloid carcinoma. (Rankin and Chumley noted an incidence of only 4.93 per cent in a series of 3,202 cases of carcinoma of the colon and rectum, which were resected, or a frequency only one-tenth that found in children.)

The recorded age incidence according to decade, in Pennington's series of 7,313 cases is as follows: under twenty, 40 cases; twenty-one to thirty, 235 cases; thirty-one to forty, 690; forty-one to fifty, 1,462; fifty-one to sixty, 2,120; sixty-one to seventy, 1,836; and above the age of seventy, 930. In our own group, the average age was fifty-seven years; most of the patients were between forty and seventy years of age.

ETIOLOGY

The origin of carcinoma of the large intestine, like carcinoma elsewhere, remains obscure, although some progress has been made in respect to its predisposing and contributing causes. It is frequently stated positively that carcinoma of the rectum does not develop in such benign rectal lesions as anal fissure, ulcerative proctitis, hemorrhoids, and strictures. The incidence of such occurrences is undoubtedly low yet are reported often enough to make their consideration important in any contemplation of the origin of rectal carcinoma. Ewing believes that sufficient evidence is lacking to prove that carcinoma develops in tissues altered by hemorrhoids, fistulas, and so forth; Pennington stated his belief that hemorrhoids, when present, are a coincidence, and Jones, although he admitted the frequent association of carcinoma of the rectum with fistula, stated that in his experience the fistulas had always started in the carcinomatous area and extended to the surface and had not been carcinomas starting about fistulas. Rosser has emphasized the significance of the benign lesions of the anus as precursors of carcinoma and in 1931 reported 12 cases of carcinoma of the anus in which benign lesions of the anus were believed to have been present prior to the onset of malignancy. These benign conditions were as follows: fistulas, 7 cases; hemorrhoids, 4 cases; chronic cryptitis, 1 case. In addition to these cases he found in the literature 18 cases since 1915. The pre-existing benign lesion is given as hemorrhoids in 7 cases, fistulas in 7 cases and leukoplakia in 3 cases.

Evidently constipation plays little or no rôle in the development of carcinoma of the left half of the colon and the rectum for as Pennington has aptly observed, constipation is decidedly more common among women, yet the incidence of carcinoma of the rectum in this sex is less than in men. And as DuPan has pointed out, the anal canal, which is the portion of the bowel most likely to be-

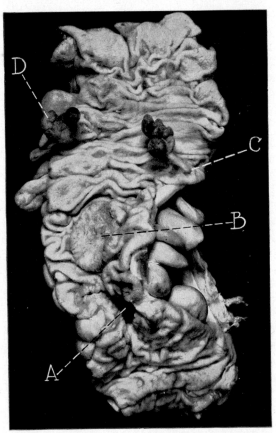

FIG. 23. Specimen from rectosigmoid. *A*, adenocarcinoma, graded 2. *B*, adenocarcinoma, graded 2. *C* and *D*, polyps of group 2, extensively involved in adenocarcinoma, graded 2. See also Figures 28 and 48.

come irritated by the passage of inspissated feces is the most infrequent site of carcinoma.

Adenomatosis (polyposis).—Proof is lacking that all carcinomas of the large intestine originate in polyps, but there is considerable evidence to support the belief that most of them arise in just such manner. The potentially malignant nature of these adenomatous polyps warrants their detailed consideration because it is in the early detection of their existence, prior to malignant degeneration and in their prompt removal, that we may best expect to reduce both the incidence and mortality of cancer of the large intestine (Fig. 23).

Dukes, of St. Mark's Hospital, London, in a most comprehensive review of the subject, published in 1930, noted the following facts which have been learned about the disease since Cripps, in 1882, recognized its familial predisposition: First that "these polypoid growths are composed of adenomatous proliferations of the intestinal mucosa"; second, that "they are the result of an inherited constitutional predisposition to epithelial tumors of the intestine"; third, that "the disease runs in certain families, being inherited as a Mendelian dominant"; and fourth, that "it almost invariably ends in cancer of the intestine."

Hitherto intestinal polypi have been described under many different terms, most frequently being designated "multiple polyposis." Other names have been "disseminated polypi" (Cripps); "multiple adenomas" (Whitehead); "diffuse adenomatosis" (Erdman and Morris); "polyadenomes en nappe" (Menetrier), and "polypoidosis" (Broders). Dukes advocates the term "polyposis" for the reason that it is a short and easily pronounceable name, that it was used as early as any, and because it is an accurate description of the condition.

Polyps of the large intestine generally have been treated as a single genus of tumor and have been described anatomically as pedunculated or sessile growths, varying in size, shape, and consistency, with an underlying papillary or adenomatous structure. Much confusion has resulted from the fact that many authors have classified these growths according to some etiologic factor, such as dysentery, chronic ulcerative colitis, hyperplastic tuberculosis, or non-specific affections of the colon. As Dukes points out, none of these are examples of true adenomatosis, but would be better described by the original name "colitis polyposa" first used by Virchow, or pseudo-polyposis as suggested by Woodward, in 1881. Again, the clinical manifestations, particularly as regards diffuse adenomatous types of polyps, have caused them to be classified as of the adult or acquired type, and of the congenital or adolescent type. Erdman and Morris suggested that the distinction between these different types be made on a clinical basis of classification rather than a pathologic one, such as (1) the adult or acquired type, manifested by the papilloma or adenoma, and (2) the adolescent, or congenital disseminated type, manifested by polyposis. This classification is a logical and very useful one.

Menzel is credited by Warwick as having first called attention to the disease, as such, in 1721, but it is highly probable that his case was of the secondary type, for the patient died of chronic dysentery. Rokitansky, in 1839, added other observations on a similar type of pathology, and in 1861 Lebert described what was probably a true case of polyposis, as did Richert in 1873. Dukes states that the condition was not accepted as a disease entity until Boas, in 1901, differentiated polyposis from isolated papillomas and adenomas.

Cripps, in 1882, was first to recognise the familial predisposition, reporting the cases of brother and sister, both afflicted with adenomatosis. Then, in 1890, Handford, in a paper entitled "Disseminated polypi of the large intestine becoming malignant," first established the significance of polyposis in the genesis of colon and rectal cancer. Bardenheuer, in the following year, and later Quénu and Landel, were the first to bring forward histologic evidence of the malignant transformations of adenomatous cells. It was their belief that approximately 50 per cent of these cases underwent malignant changes. Subsequent investigations were made by Hauser, Wechselmann, Schmieden and Westheus, and many others. Fitz-Gibbon and Rankin, in 1931, in reviewing the histopathologic characteristics of thirteen cases of adenomatosis of the large bowel, were able to show that the polyps were not all of one type and that they definitely proceed from benignancy to malignancy. They attempted to establish for polyps a histological classification. On examination of the tumors it was observed that they fell readily into three major histological divisions as follows:

Polyps of group 1. In this group are included only those growths in which the epithelium retains its normal characteristics. The tumors are usually roughly nodular, although in some of the specimens the surface is smooth and regular. The epithelium covering the growth and lining the crypts is unchanged from the standard regarded as normal, nevertheless there may be in scattered areas some evidence of slight hyperplasia. Such areas are the sites of more or less active inflammation secondary to the constant trauma to which the tumors in their exposed positions are constantly subjected. Polyps of this group vary in size from tiny clubs about 3 millimeters in diameter to masses 1 or 2 centimeters in cross section (Fig. 24). Loose connective tissue derived from the submucosa forms the matrix of the stalk and expands to sustain the nodular polyp. There is no tendency in growths of group 1 to branching or papillary forms. Polyps of this group are invariably pedunculated.

It must be recognized that peristalsis, evoked in the intestinal musculature by the irritation of what is virtually a foreign body, can attain in this region great force. Instances are recorded in which polyps of this type have been amputated from the tips of their pedicles not by ulceration but by outright avulsion by peristaltic action. Then, too, numerous cases of intussusception have resulted from the peristaltic pull on the tumors. The patient from whom was taken the polyp shown in Figure 24, had to submit three times to operative intervention for the relief of acute intestinal obstruction. Each time, intussusception of some degree was found, and each time a polyp of this type was at the bottom of the trouble.

It is conceivable that whatever initiates carcinomatous change in polyps could likewise find its expression in the epithelium of this group. There is, however, nothing about the tumors of group 1 to indicate that they are any more liable to malignant development than is normal intestinal mucous membrane. It can, therefore, be said that the polyps of this group are destined to a long and benign

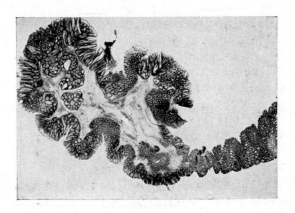

Fig. 24. Polyp of group 1. Nodular,
pedunculated tumor.

course. No such pronouncement can be made, however, for the polyps of group 2.

Polyps of group 2.—The polyps of this group are easily distinguished from those of group 1 by the abrupt and striking structural changes in both the epithelium and in the connective tissue elements (Fig. 25). The epithelium is characterized by widespread failure of the proliferating cells to differentiate completely into the units of normal intestinal mucosa. In the polyp epithelium the cells are hypertrophied, elongated, and by their increased bulk compressed from side to side. They may stay arranged in single rows, but in numerous places the press of overgrowth piles them into multilayered buds that project usually into the lumen of tubules and frequently into the connective tissue matrix as well. The nuclei, like the cells, are elongated. They are stained more deeply by all the routinely used dyes and thus give to the proliferation a darker and easily recognized color. In the cellular protoplasm, the production of mucus is sharply diminished.

These epithelial changes do not appear equally advanced over the whole of the group. Usually there is a peripheral dark zone of greater cellular activity where this changed epithelium will first be found, particularly in the early forms of this group. As the polyp ages, the changed epithelium will have displaced entirely the more

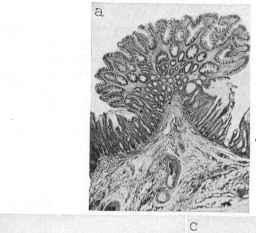

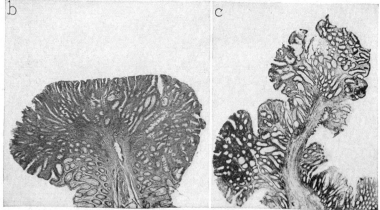

Fig. 25. Early growth of polyps of group 2. *a*, tiny bud of enlarged and deformed glandular tubules; *b*, drift of connective tissue is to left side of the tumor; *c*, mature polyps (6 millimeters). There are two dark areas of active proliferation still within it (FitzGibbon and Rankin).

differentiated structure which it has infiltrated, overgrown, and choked.

The peripheral dark zone so characteristic of growing polyps is composed almost entirely of complexes of glandular tubules. These tubules, increased both in diameter and length by the hypertrophy of the component cells, crowd and press one another into a tangled mass. One frequently finds cellular activity at its height at those points where the epithelium of the tubule debouches onto the surface of the tumor and spreads out over it to form its investing membrane. In places one can see the tubules of the polyps projecting down between the more normal glands at the base of the tumor. Nearly every polyp of this type reveals cystic enclosures which have been formed by the accumulation of secretion in the deformed and obstructed glands.

As this process of epithelial proliferation goes on there is a complementary response in the connective tissues of the submucosa. The tug of the tumor soon pulls the muscularis mucosae and some fibrils of the underlying looser areolar tissue upward to form a tiny stalk. If the tempo of growth is not too brisk, the connective tissue elements are drawn out into ever-branching divisions which form a tree-like supporting scaffolding for the epithelial complexes. At irregular places, however, in polyps of this group, the epithelium may grow out in long, tender tendrils that give to these areas a shaggy, papillary structure. It is these tendrils that are readily injured by intestinal action and are thus the source of the hemorrhages that so mark the course of these tumors.

The polyps of group 2 are also invariably pedunculated. Two massive, egg-sized tumors (6 by 4 centimeters) of this group in our specimens swung from pedicles fully 6 centimeters in length, a pattern which other and smaller polyps followed in their own ways. It is true that one frequently sees flattened, hemispherical excrescences set apparently in or on the intestinal mucosa like a plush or velvet-covered button in overstuffed upholstery. These tumors are called sessile tumors. The overhanging edges of the growth have concealed the stalk. A cross section through the tumor will reveal the short, stubby pedicle and the true cauliflower structure of the polyp. Many of these sessile growths are in fact, congeries of innumerable smaller growths, each organized in this cauliflower-like fashion. In the accompanying illustrations, the development of the polyps of each group 2 can be traced from the earliest buds to matured proliferation. The polyps of group 2, with their connective tissue foundations laid out to follow a well-considered plan of tree-like formation, attain to the largest size in these tumors. All the large tumors of our specimens, and all the larger tumors of which there is adequate pathological description in the literature, fall at once into this group. This group then will embrace most of the polyp formation developing in the large intestine. That the growths are not, however, consistently benign, is well known. Figure 26 reveals the fate that so often overtakes these tumors. The area of outright carcinoma (adenocarcinoma graded 2), is microscopic in dimensions. Had not the section luckily gone through this tiny carcinoma, the character of the growth surely would have been misjudged. In fact, this particular polyp, like many others in the series, was sectioned as a routine and pronounced benign. How many of these tumors are mislabeled, no one can know. Certainly, it is out of the question, in everyday laboratory practice, to submit all of them to serial sectioning.

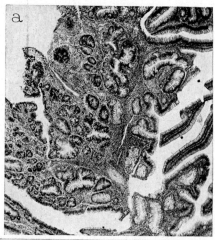

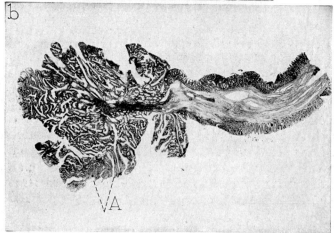

Fig. 26. *a*, Enlargement of area A, the site of a microscopic (2 mm.) adenocarcinoma, grade 2; *b*, Longstemmed, aged polyp of group 2 from splenic flexure of colon resected for generalized adenomatosis.

It would seem that the development of carcinoma in polyps depends on the rate at which the tumor is driven to grow. In the slow-paced formation of group 1 there is little, if any, likelihood of cancerous change. In the relatively more rapid growths of the polyps of group 2 it is a question only of time until carcinoma appears. Apparently, intestinal epithelium cannot proliferate indefinitely, even at a moderate rate, without ultimately losing its bearings. This matter of rate of development is strikingly illustrated in the polyps of group 3.

Polyps of group 3. In the polyps of this group, as in those of group 2, there has been failure of epithelium to differentiate. But in

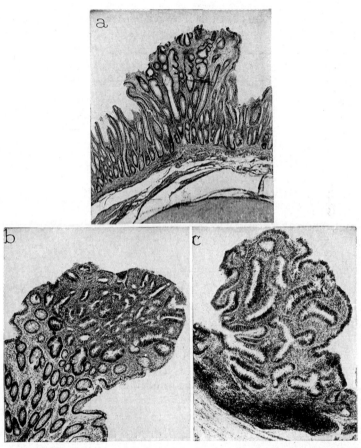

FIG. 27. The growth of polyps of group 3. *a*, sprout of enlarged tubules lined by typical polyp epithelium initiating the growth; *b*, continued proliferation of polyp epithelium. No evidence of stalk formation, such as occurs in group 2 can be seen; *c*, the polyp epithelium has completely suppressed the growth of normal tubules and has already reached the muscularis mucosae.

this group are only those tumors in the epithelium of which the processes of differentiation have been arrested at so early a stage that the cells have attained only the most rudimentary characteristics of the normal units of intestinal mucosa. There is thus no sharp line in separation between polyps of groups 2 and 3, as there is between polyps of groups 1 and 2. Polyps of group 3 are but accentuated forms of the growths of group 2, in which cellular activity reaches its height for such tumors. And thus, too, there is formed a twilight zone into which may fall tumors bearing the characteristics of both groups. Although in this border zone there are not always clear-cut distinctions between polyps of the two groups, yet it is useful to maintain this three-phase classification. In the older polyps of group 3, the cellular changes are advanced and unmistakable; in the younger polyps, other and secondary features of the tumors help to identify them for grouping.

Polyps of group 3, like those of the other groups, must start in an overgrowth of glandular tubules in the mucosa (Fig. 27). At first there is prolongation and enlargement of the tubules. These regions of incipient proliferation are so small that they will escape observation unless they are sought for with a sufficiently powerful lens. Certain authors, endeavoring to show that polyps are the result of primary injury inflicted on the intestinal mucosa at points of increased friction, and on the flexures and the mucosal folds, maintain that these early proliferations are situated on the tops of the folds, where secondary traumatic inflammatory reaction would most commonly occur. We found the sites of these tiny growths to be not so much on the tops of the folds as scattered haphazard over the mucous membrane.

Polyps of this group attain ordinarily only the size of a split pea (6 and 9 millimeters). This uniformly restricted size of growth can be interpreted in but one way. The elementary epithelium proliferates so rapidly that the nodule approaches cancerous change before the tumor has become large enough to be played on by the forces of peristaltic action or before the more temperate connective tissues have a chance to respond to such demands for growth. Figure 27c shows this changed epithelium already in actual contact with the submucosa.

It is this lag in the connective tissue stroma that gives to polyps of group 3 their characteristic appearance of rank confusion in the epithelial overgrowths. Cellular activity at the points where the tubules open on the surface must result in a disorganized nodule if there is no connective tissue to support an orderly papillary projection. And a similar course must be followed in the buds in the tubules themselves. Here the enlarging tubules must grow downward, as there is no structure to sustain an upward proliferation; and, in fact, tubules are to be seen proceeding into the normal mucosa from which they have developed and which they will ultimately infiltrate, compress and destroy. As in group 2, the irregular tubules become so convoluted that they are frequently obstructed, and numerous cysts are formed behind them. All in all, in the polyps of this group no recognizable attempt is made at organoid formations. In addition, cells of these epithelial complexes can no longer be distinguished morphologically from those seen in outright carcinoma. It apparently is but a matter of relatively short time until polyp proliferations of this type burst the barriers of the muscularis mucosae and become actually deeply infiltrating, that is, carcinomatous.

In considering the sites of the proliferations of group 3, it was mentioned that they have been found scattered throughout the intestinal mucous membrane. Similar areas of this same type of proliferation are to be seen also on the surface of some polyps of group

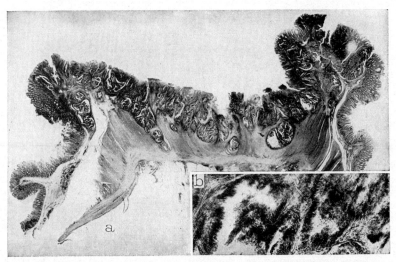

Fig. 28. *a*, Section of adenocarcinoma, graded 2, marked B in Figure 23. The carcinoma has advanced to the serosa and there remain in it only scattered traces of a former polyp epithelium, but confirmatory evidence that this carcinoma had its origin in polyps was contained in the neighboring growths, one of which is pictured in Figure 48; *b*, enlargement of this carcinoma.

2 (Fig. 28). In these buds of solid cords of epithelium, the cells, no longer moored to the glandular structure of the tubule, have thrown off their columnar cell characteristics and have become one-eyed vesicles, the form for the repeatedly described and so-called carcinoma cell.

We are convinced that the site of origin of deep seated destructive carcinomata of the colon is in these proliferations of the mucous membranes of group 3. The finding of such an order of proliferation in polyps of group 2, polyps which in themselves in time become carcinomatous, points directly to the conclusion that carcinoma of the colon is mediated through proliferations of group 3 wherever their situation (Fig. 29).

It may be well to repeat here that the nodular polyps of group

1 pursue ordinarily a benign career, that the orderly but more rapidly growing polyps of group 2 tend in time to malignant changes, and that formation of the order of group 3 are outrightly precancerous.

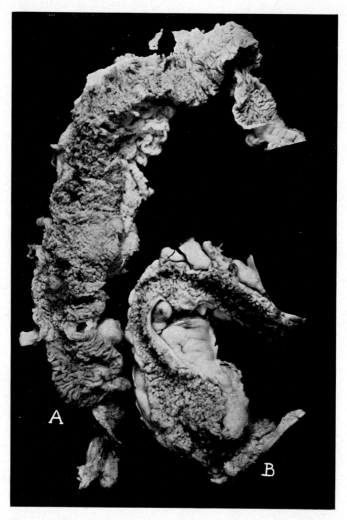

Fig. 29. Colon (*A*) and rectum (*B*) resected in two stages for adenomatosis. The dense growth of innumerable polyps of border-line group 2–3 is strikingly shown.

Helwig, on the other hand, states that such a degree of faith in the interpretation of a histologic section does not seem warranted. He also doubts that the age of an adenoma can be determined by the microscopic appearance. In his recent (1947) exhaustive study of 1,460 consecutive autopsies in which the entire large intestine, in the fresh state, was examined, he was unable to adduce evidence that any particular group of adenomas would maintain a constant benign course. Moreover, no distinguishing morphologic and histologic characteristics which would seem to warrant a complex classification of adenomas were noted.

Helwig found the establishment of the transition from simple adenoma to carcinoma to be relatively difficult. Some carcinomas, he stated, simulated the cell arrangement of an adenoma so closely the diagnosis of a malignant tumor depends on the invasion of the wall of the intestine. A factor of primary importance in the histologic diagnosis, he emphasized, is the site involved in the transition

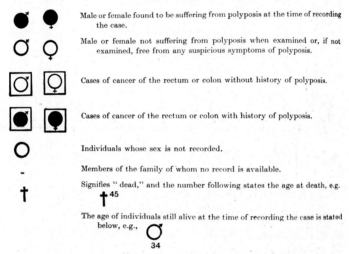

FIG. 30. Key to conventions used in pedigree charts of cases of adenomatosis (Figures 31, 32, and 33)—Dukes.

from adenoma to carcinoma. Some authors believe that this site appears first at the tip of the adenoma and others believe it occurs first at the base. In his study no definite pattern could be established for the occurrence of foci of carcinoma. In several instances the malignant changes occurred at the periphery of the adenoma, either at the tip or at the margins. In other specimens the transition occurred deep within the polyp near the stalk and at the base. The precision of the diagnosis, therefore, will be proportionate to the care taken in the selection of representative sections.

The actual incidence of malignant transformation of polyps is not known and only can be roughly estimated. Estimates have ranged from 34.6 per cent (Hullsiek), 40 per cent (Erdman and Morris), 48 per cent (Quénu and Landel) to 60 per cent (Wechselmann). In the series of 50 cases reviewed by Doering the cause of death was known in 36, and in 21 this was cancer of the bowel. In this connection Lockhart-Mummery says: "The most important factor in connection with simple adenomata, whether of the single or multiple variety, is that they show a marked tendency sooner or later to become malignant, i.e., for the cells to penetrate the basement membrane and invade the surrounding structures. We are of the opinion that all adenomata of the rectum eventually take on malignant change, and in the great majority of cases in which large adenomata have been removed, malignant change has been found to have already occurred in some part or other of the tumor. So marked is this tendency for simple adenomata to become malignant, that personally we look upon adenomata as merely a stage

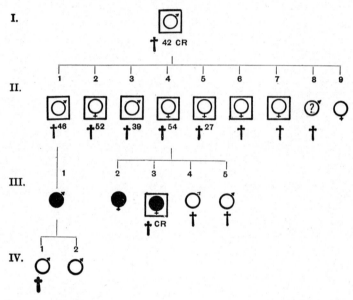

Fig. 31. Lockhart-Mummery's case No. 1, 1925. Amplified by Dukes, 1929. The only surviving members of this family who can be traced are III 1 and 2 and IV 2; III 1 is at present under treatment and III 2 has been treated by colectomy—Dukes.

in the development of malignant disease, and regard simple adenomata of the rectum as a definitely precancerous condition. It follows from this that on no account should a single adenoma of the rectum be allowed to remain, even if it is causing no troublesome symptoms; it should be freely removed as soon as possible." With this statement we are in complete agreement.

To Lockhart-Mummery chiefly must go credit for working out the pedigree of such cases. In a masterly review of the subject Dukes recently brought the pedigree charts of Lockhart-Mummery up to date, and suggested that from his study of the cases the risks of cancer of the rectum are far higher in families afflicted with polyposis than in the population at large. He further asserts that the disease is transmitted by both males and females, that both males and females suffer from the disease, and that the inheritance can be traced through several generations. If members of these families survive the other complications of polyposis and ordinary risks of life, they develop cancer of the rectum or colon, usually in the early thirties or forties.

The key to conventions used in the pedigree charts prepared by Dukes is shown in Figure 30. In Figure 31 is shown the pedigree of Lockhart-Mummery's first case, published in 1925 and ampli-

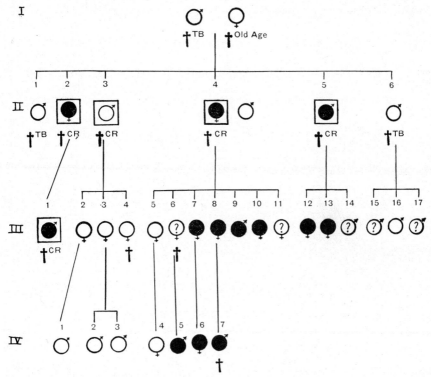

Fig. 32. Jüngling's case, 1928. (No. 6 in generation III was either a case of tuberculosis of the colon or cancer of the colon)—Dukes.

fied by Dukes in 1929. Figure 32 illustrates Jüngling's case which shows a larger number of cases of polyposis than in most of the other charts. According to Dukes, this is due to the fact that the author tried to get all surviving members of the family sigmoidoscoped. Zahlmann's case is shown in Figure 33. Figure 34 represents the family tree of one of our own patients in whom a diagnosis of polyposis was made and for whom a total colectomy was performed. His history is as follows:

A man, thirty years of age, sought relief because of a long history of diarrhea. His father, mother, a maternal aunt, and three brothers were said to have died of carcinoma of the large intestine; the history of the latter three was suggestive of polyposis of long standing that had probably undergone malignant degeneration. For a period of eight years the patient suffered severe attacks of "summer diarrhea" lasting several months and consisting on an average of ten daily rectal discharges of feces, mucus, and blood. During the two years prior to admission he was never completely free of diarrhea and some general abdominal discomfort which at times became moderately severe. He had undergone considerable

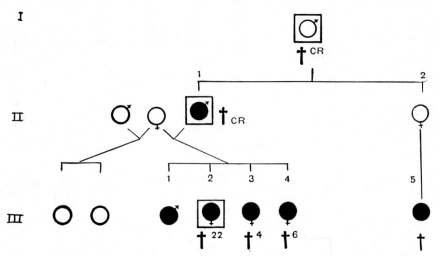

Fig. 33. Zahlmann's case, 1903. (Note that the woman who married II, had been married formerly to a man free from polyposis and had two healthy children by him. Her four children by her second husband—who suffered from polyposis and eventually died of cancer of the rectum—all developed polyposis)—Dukes.

treatment for "spastic colitis," "amebic dysentery," and "mucous colitis," and, at one time or another, took emetin, quinine, thymol, yatren, and stovarsol, without apparent relief.

The patient appeared to be undernourished, and was about 10 pounds under normal weight. The lower part of the abdomen was moderately tender. The concentration of hemoglobin was 63 per cent and erythrocytes numbered 4,380,000 in each cubic millimeter of blood. Proctoscopic and roentgenologic examinations revealed multiple polyposis.

The following operative procedures were instituted: October 7, 1930, ileostomy; February 20, 1931, partial colectomy to a point near the rectosigmoid juncture, and April 3, 1931 combined abdominoperineal resections of the rectal stump. The pathologist reported multiple polyposis of the entire colon and rectum and many pedunculated and sessile adenomatous polyps (largest 2.5 cm. in diameter). The patient recovered satisfactorily, and was living and well when last heard from in 1935.

Probably the most striking of the many pedigree charts of familial polyposis published in recent years is that worked out by Friedell and Wakefield. A diagnosis of congenital polyposis was made in 20 members of a family, seven of whom were examined at the Mayo Clinic. Three of the latter group were known to have developed cancer of the rectum. The authors state that in only about a half of the patients with disseminated polyposis of the colon is there a definite hereditary factor. The hereditary tendency does not produce any known genetic pattern. It is not sex linked and is neither a mendalian dominant nor a recessive.

The symptomatology, diagnosis, and treatment of polyposis is considered in the chapter on differential diagnosis.

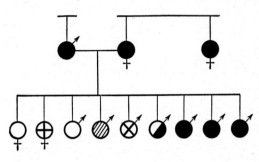

♂ Male   ♀ Female

● Death carcinoma large bowel

◐ Multiple polyposis (Patient)

◍ Death in infancy

⊕ Death carcinoma uterus

⊗ Amebic dysentery

○ Apparently well

FIG. 34. Family tree of patient with adenomatosis (Rankin's case).

REFERENCES

1. BACON, H. E.: Evolution of sphincter muscle preservation and re-establishment of continuity in the operative treatment of rectal and sigmoidal cancer. *Surg., Gynec., and Obstet.*, **81**: 113–127 (Aug.), 1945.
2. BALFOUR, D. C.: The place of surgery in the treatment of carcinoma of the alimentary tract. *Canadian Med. Assoc. Jour.*, **32**: 245–252, 1935.
3. BUREAU OF THE CENSUS (United States Department of Commerce), Annual Report (1944), U. S. Government Printing Office, Washington.
4. COLE, P. P.: The intramural spread of rectal carcinoma. *Brit. Med. Jour.*, **1**: 431–433 (March 1), 1913.
5. CRIPPS: Quoted by Dukes.
6. DUBLIN, LOUIS J.: The mortality from cancer. Monograph 1, New York, Metropolitan Life Insurance Company.
7. DUKES, C.: The hereditary factor in polyposis intesteni, or multiple adenomata. *Cancer Review*, **5**: 241–256 (April), 1930.
8. EDWARDS, F. S.: Remarks on carcinoma of the rectum. *Clin. Jour.*, **4**: 81–86 (May 30), 1894.
9. ERDMAN, J. F. and MORRIS, J. H.: Polyposis of the colon. *Surg., Gynec., and Obstet.*, **40**: 460–468 (March), 1925.

10. EWING, JAMES: Neoplastic diseases. Ed. 3. Philadelphia, W. B. Saunders Co., 1928. p. 89.

11. FITZGIBBON, G., and RANKIN, F. W.: Polyps of the large intestine. *Surg., Gynec., and Obstet.*, **52**: 1136–1150 (June), 1931.

12. GABRIEL, W. B.: The end-results of perineal excision and of radium in the treatment of cancer of the rectum. *Brit. Journ. Surg.*, **20**: 234–248 (Oct.), 1932.

13. GANT, S. G.: Diseases of the rectum, anus, and colon. Philadelphia, W. B. Saunders Co., 1923, 3 vols.

14. HANFORD: Quoted by Dukes.

15. HENDRICK, J. A.: Cancer of the colon. *New Orleans Med. and Surg. Jour.*, **87**: 150–152 (Sept.), 1934.

16. JACKMAN, R. J., NEIBLING, H. A., and WAUGH, J. M.: Carcinoma of the large intestine. *Jour. Am. Med. Assoc.*, **134**: 1287–1289 (Aug. 16), 1947.

17. JOHNSTON, J. H.: Carcinoma of the colon in childhood and adolescence. *Am. Jour. Surg.*, **73**: 703–712 (June), 1947.

18. MENETRIER, P.: Quoted by Struthers, J. E.: Multiple polyposis of the intestinal tract. *Surg., Gynec., and Obstet.*, **38**: 610–624 (May), 1924.

19. OEHLER, JOHANNES: Ueber Rectumcarcinome. *Beitr. z. klin. Chir.*, **87**: 583–630, 1923.

20. PEMBERTON, J. DE J., and DIXON, C. F.: Summary of end-results of treatment of malignancy of the thyroid gland and the colon, including the rectum and anus. *Surg., Gynec., and Obstet.*, **58**: 462–464 (Feb.), 1934.

21. PENNINGTON, J. R.: Diseases and injuries of the rectum, anus and pelvic colon. Philadelphia, P. Blakiston's Son and Co., 1923.

22. PFEIFFER, D. B.: The principles underlying the surgery of carcinoma of the rectum. *Ann. Surg.*, **86**: 374–387 (Sept.), 1927.

23. QUÉNU and LANDEL: Quoted by Rankin, Bargen, and Buie.

24. RAIFORD, T. S.: Carcinoma of the large bowel (Part II, the rectum). *Ann. Surg.*, **101**: 1042–1050 (April), 1935.

25. RANKIN, F. W., BARGEN, J. A., and BUIE, L. A.: The colon, rectum and anus. Philadelphia, W. B. Saunders Company, 1932.

26. RANKIN, F. W., and COMFORT, M. W.: Carcinoma of the rectum in young persons. *Jour. Tennessee State Med. Assn.*, **22**: 37–42 (June), 1929.

27. RANKIN, F. W., and JONES, R. D.: Carcinoma of the rectum. *West Virginia Med. Jour.*, **25**: 5–9 (Jan.), 1929.

28. RANKIN, F. W., and MAYO, CHARLES, 2nd: Carcinoma of the small bowel. *Surg., Gynec., and Obstet.*, **50**: 939–947 (June), 1930.

29. RANKIN, F. W., and SCHOLL, A. J.: Resection of the proximal colon for malignancy. *Arch. Surg.*, **7**: 258–279 (Sept.), 1923.

30. RAWLINGS, L. B.: Some points in the symptoms and treatment of rectal carcinoma. St. Bartholomew's Hosp. Rep., **42**: 135–148, 1906.

31. RICHERT, Quoted by Dukes.

32. ROKITANSKY: Quoted by Dukes.

33. ROSSER, C.: The etiology of anal cancer. *Am. Jour. Surg.*, **11**: 328–333 (Feb.), 1931.

34. SCHMIEDEN, V., and WESTHUES, H.: Quoted by FitzGibbon and Rankin.

35. VIRCHOW: Quoted by Struthers.[18]

36. WALKER and DALY: Quoted by Warthen.

37. WARTHEN, H. J.: Carcinoma of the colon in childhood—report of case. *Virginia Med. Monthly*, **64**: 140–142 (June), 1937.

38. WARWICK, M.: Intestinal polyposis and its relation to carcinoma. *Minnesota Med.*, **5**: 94–97 (Feb.), 1922.

39. WECHSELMANN, LUDWIG: Quoted by FitzGibbon and Rankin.

40. WHITEHEAD: Quoted by Dukes.

41. WOODWARD: Quoted by Dukes.

CHAPTER III

PATHOLOGY

Adenocarcinomas comprise the majority of the histologic types which are observed in the colon and rectum; squamous cell carcinomas comprise a small group common to the lower rectum and anus. Carcinomas of the large intestine and anus may, as a matter of convenience, be classified on a combined basis of their gross characteristics and microscopic anatomy, as: (1) medullary adenocarcinoma; (2) scirrhous or fibrocarcinoma; (3) mucoid (colloid) adenocarcinoma; (4) papillomatous carcinoma; (5) squamous carcinoma; and (6) melanoma. All carcinomas of the large intestine, however, originate in the crypts or glands of Lieberkühn, and those beginning in the anal canal are typical squamous carcinomas. When the latter are found above the ano-rectal line, their origin is explained on the theory that regenerative cells of the glandular epithelium have the ability to produce either a secretary (glandular) or a protective (squamous) epithelium. Certain gross forms assumed by carcinomas of the large intestine have a definite bearing on the symptomatology and roentgenologic findings. These, however, will be taken up separately in a consideration of pathologic characteristics prevalent in different segments of the large bowel.

Of considerably more significance than the classification of carcinomas of the large intestine on clinical grounds, or according to physical attributes of the invading growth, is the now well-recognized intimate relationship between adenomas and carcinomas. No one who has studied the work of Quénu and Lendel, Lockhart-Mummery, Dukes, FitzGibbon and Rankin, or any number of other investigators, can fail to be impressed with the fact that adenomas of the large intestine definitely are precancerous growths. The findings in these investigations and a consideration of malignant transformations of polyps in general are elaborated under "adenomatosis." Likewise, of inestimable practical value is a microscopic grading of neoplasms on the basis of cell differentiation as has been described by Broders.

Grading of carcinoma.—It is well known, states Broders, that pathologists for a long time have appreciated, in a general way, the possibility of detecting the varying clinical malignancy of carcinoma by microscopic examination. However, it is only in recent years, through careful study of carcinomatous cells, that concrete knowledge of practical therapeutic and prognostic value to victims of carcinoma has been obtained. Older clinicians and surgeons fully appreciated the fact that different types of carcinoma varied in clinical malignancy; for example, melanotic carcinoma was known to be more malignant than basal cell carcinoma. They were also fully aware that carcinomas of the same type in different situations differed in clinical malignancy; thus, the average squamous cell carcinoma of the uterine cervix was known to be more malignant than the same type when situated on the lip. However, when it came to carcinomas of the same type, in the same situation, there was no general appreciation of variation in clinical malignancy; a carcinoma of the lip was considered a carcinoma of the lip and a carcinoma of the stomach a carcinoma of the stomach and nothing more. Experienced physicians, however, had observed that papillary, polypoid, or elevated carcinomas were less malignant than those that were flat or infiltrating. This observation is aptly expressed in the aphorism, "A cancer that comes to you is less malignant than one that goes away from you."

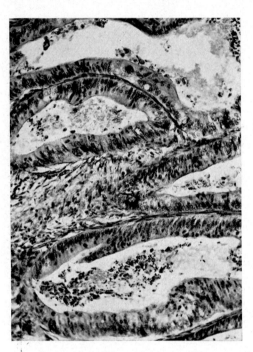

Fig. 35. Adenocarcinoma of the rectum, graded 1 (Broders).

In a study of 2,000 epitheliomas, 1,628 of which were of the squamous-cell type, Broders classified them into four groups according to differentiation and mitosis. The more nearly the cell approaches the embryonic or undifferentiated type the more malignant the tumors, and the converse is true, in that the more nearly normal the tumor cell, the lower the grade of malignancy. The results of grading are expressed in numerals from 1 to 4, and entirely independent of the clinical history. The number of mitotic figures and the number of cells with single large deeply staining nucleoli (one-eyed cells) play an important part in the grading, and an increase in the mitotic figures, especially if they are irregular, tends to raise the grade to some extent (Figs. 35 to 38). Broders states: "A carcinoma graded 1 is one in which the proportion of differentiated cells ranges from almost 100 down to 75 per cent, that of the undifferentiated cells from practically 0 up to 25 per cent; in a carcinoma graded 2, the proportion of differentiated cells ranges from 75 down to 50 per cent, that of undifferentiated cells from 25 up to 50 per cent; in a carcinoma graded 3, the proportion of differentiated cells ranges from 50 to 25 per cent, that of the undifferentiated cells from 50 up to 75 per cent, and in a carcinoma graded 4, the proportion of differentiated cells is from 25 per cent to practically 0, that of the undifferentiated cells from 75 up to 100 per cent."

This method of grading carcinomas has met with widespread approval of surgeons and pathologists alike in this country and in Great Britain. Dukes, pathologist of St. Mark's Hospital, London, in reporting a comparison of Broders' method of grading carcinoma in 120 surgically excised carcinomas of the rectum with his method of classification based on the depth of penetration of the wall of the bowel by the cancer, stated that the results confirmed the work of Broders and Rankin as regards the prac-

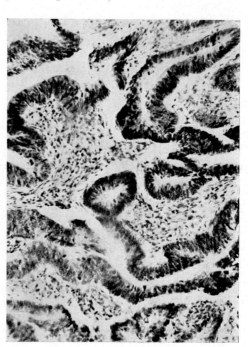

FIG. 36. Adenocarcinoma of the rectum, graded 2 (Broders).

tical application of the index of malignancy in estimating prognosis. Dukes, however, does not believe that Broders' method can be satisfactorily applied to fragments of a tumor removed for diagnosis before operation, but states that if this were practical it would provide information of great value to the surgeon, enabling him, perhaps, to adapt the method of excision to the degree of malignancy. In our own experience we have been struck with the constancy with which the grade of the preoperative biopsy has agreed with that of the section made from the excised specimen. In regard to this question Broders recently wrote:

"At this point I should like to state that as a rule there is practically the same grade of malignancy throughout a carcinoma. It is rather difficult to define the border between two grades, and if one is in doubt as to whether a carcinoma is of a lower or a higher grade, it is best to put it in the latter. It is not the rule to find characteristics of a low grade 1 carcinoma in one part of a growth, and characteristics of a high grade 2 carcinoma in another part; it is equally unlikely that the grade will be 1 in one part and 3 in another. Frater found practically no exception to the rule in carcinoma of the urinary bladder. Certain adenocarcinomas have been the exceptions, but the percentage is so small that its influence is practically negligible.

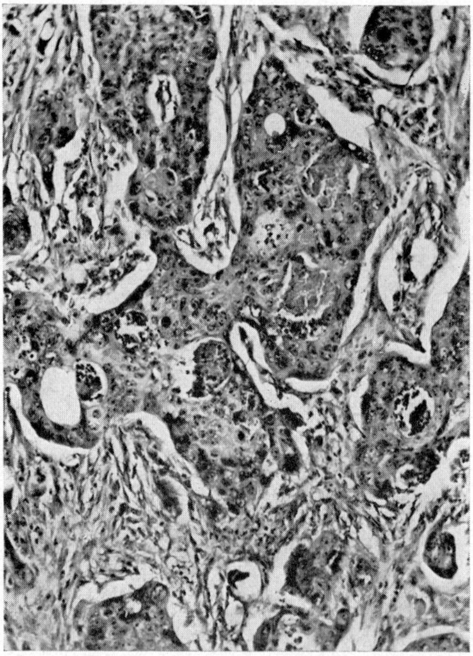

"Carcinomatous cells of a given neoplasm usually remain about the same throughout the course of the disease. Sometimes they increase in activity; then again, they may decrease in this respect. Since the grading of carcinoma is based on the fundamental principle of cellular differentiation, it is very important for the microscopist, especially in examination of early lesions, fully to appreciate the extent to which the carcinomatous cells are deviated from the normal, or in other words, the extent of differentiation or anaplasia."

FIG. 37. Adenocarcinoma of the rectum, graded 3 (Broders).

The practical application of Broders' index of malignancy, and of Dukes' classification of rectal carcinomas, are considered at length under "prognosis."

Mucoid (colloid) carcinoma.—It is generally estimated that about 5 per cent of carcinomas of the large intestine are of the mucoid variety. Parham noted that 5.5 per cent of these of the rectum and rectosigmoid were of this type, whereas Zinner found the mucoid type in 41 per cent of 123 cases of carcinoma of the rectum. In a recent report Raiford distinguished between primary mucoid carcinoma and adenocarcinoma with mucoid degeneration, stating that in a series of 128 carcinomas of the rectum, 1.6 per cent were of the former type and 24.2 per cent were of the latter type. Of 97 carcinomas of the colon, there were no mucoid growths, but of those undergoing mucoid degeneration there were 37, or 38.2 per cent. Rankin and Chumley reported on 158 cases of mucoid carcinoma of the colon and rectum in which operation was performed. These represented 4.93 per cent of 3,202 cases of carcinoma of the colon and rectum, which were resected. The following distribution was noted: Cecum and ascending colon, 42 (26.5 per cent); transverse colon, 26 (16.4 per cent); descending colon, 3 (1.8 per cent); sigmoid, 14 (8.8 per cent), and rectosigmoid and rectum, 73 (46.2 per cent). Of the 158 cases, resection was performed in 122 (77.2 per cent), palliative operations were performed on 12 (7.5 per cent) and exploration only in 24 (15.3 per cent). The average of life of the inoperable group was seven and one half months; the longest period of life was twenty-four months. In this group of cases were 115 men (72.7 per cent) and 43 women (27.2 per cent). The average age was fifty and two-tenths years; the oldest patient was aged seventy-five years and the youngest sixteen.

The genesis and significance of the material found in growths designated mucoid, colloid, or gelatinous carcinoma have long been

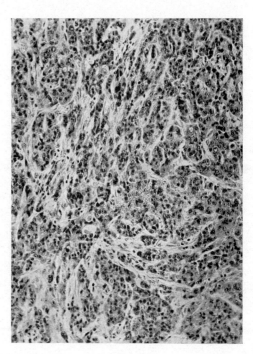

Fig. 38. Adenocarcinoma of the cecum, graded 4 (Broders).

a subject of controversy. It has been described as a product of degeneration, but most investigators now agree that it is secretory in origin and derived from the epithelial cells of carcinoma originating from any of the epithelial structures of the gland. Broders stated that adenocarcinomas tend to control themselves by differentiating into gland or gland-like structures, sometimes with the production of colloid or mucoid material. A distinction between mucus and colloid is no longer maintained, for they are considered identical.

Miles, Boyd, and a majority of investigators are of the opinion that these carcinomas are degenerative stages of the other varieties. McFarland, on the other hand, suggested that one proof that colloid carcinoma is a distinct entity and not a degenerated type is the regularity with which the mucoid structure appears in the metastatic growths.

From the study of a large series of mucoid carcinomas Parham came to the following conclusions: "(1) The epithelial cells possess an uncontrolled function of secreting a mucinous substance and its accumulation is often destructive to the carcinoma cells; (2) the formation of mucus is a sign of functional differentiation of the carcinoma cells corresponding to the morphologic differentiation in carcinoma with cells of the acinar or columnar types; (3) the mucus-forming characteristics may be possessed by cells either showing or not showing other signs of differentiation; (4) mucoid carcinoma is usually slow of growth and late in metastasizing to lymph nodes and to other organs; it often grows by permeation and may cause extensive thickening of the wall of the affected organ; (5) local lymph nodes are often involved long before metastasis has reached distant glands; although histologically less malignant on account of permeation of adjacent tissues, it is particularly difficult to eradicate; death is often delayed but the eventual mortality is greater than in other types of carcinoma, and (6) recurrence is often limited entirely to the site of origin."

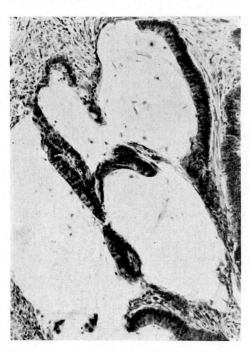

Fig. 39. Mucoid adenocarcinoma of rectum, graded 1 (Broders).

Ochsenhirt, in a study of the mucus-forming cells in carcinoma of the colon and rectum, made sections from 188 of these tumors. The sections were stained with mucicarmine which stains mucus red, in contrast to other tissues which are stained blue. These were then graded according to Broders' method of grading malignancy and a method was devised for the purpose of grading the number of mucus-forming cells present (Figs. 39 and 40). Ochsenhirt concluded that the presence of mucus in carcinoma is the result of partial differentiation of the cancer cells; the more malignant the carcinoma, or the less the extent of differentiation, the less numerous the mucus-secreting cells. In other words, the number of mucus-secreting cells in the carcinoma is inversely proportional to the grade of malignancy, as determined by Broders' method.

Multiple carcinoma.—The literature on multiple primary malignant tumors has grown to be extensive since Billroth reported the first case in 1869. At that time Billroth stipulated three postulates which should be fulfilled before multiple carcinoma can be indicated as independent growths: (1) The lesions must show such definite histologic differences as to exclude the possibility that they are of the same origin; (2) each lesion must arise from its parent epithelium, and (3) each lesion must be held accountable for its own group of metastases. To these postulates Mercanton has added: "If after removal of two carcinomas the patient remains free from disease, the two growths must have been independent, else there should have been other metastases." It is manifest that when growths from intestinal epithelium are concerned, the first of Billroth's postulates cannot be fulfilled. Ewing stated: "We do not speak of recurring

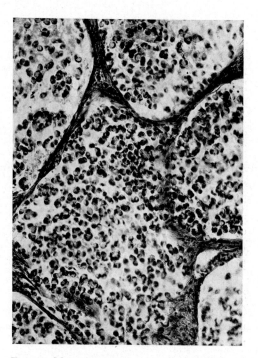

Fig. 40. Mucoid adenocarcinoma of transverse colon, graded 4. Most of the cells are of the signet ring type (Broders).

uterine myomas, for these are clearly multiple, so why not carcinoma or sarcoma?" Hanlon showed that these postulates are impossible to fulfill in a large percentage of cases of true and undisputed multiple primary malignant neoplasms. He, and later Hurt and Broders in their study of such cases, followed the criteria of Goetze, which are: (1) the tumors must have the macroscopic and microscopic appearance of the usual tumors of the organs involved; (2) exclusion of metastasis must be certain, and (3) diagnosis may be confirmed by the character of the individual metastasis.

Wells, in 1901, collected 17 cases of multiple primary tumors in general, and then followed reports by Wooley (1903), Theilhaber and Edelberg (1912), and Bartlett (1914). Major, in 1918, made an exhaustive review of the literature and presented 628 examples of multiple primary malignant tumors. In this large number of cases not a single instance of multiple malignancies in the colon was recorded. More recently the literature has been reviewed extensively by Bargen and Rankin (1930), Norbury (1930), Hanlon (1931), Warren and Gates (1932), Hurt and Broders (1933), and Felsen and Wells (1934). Hurt and Broders found the literature on this subject and the report of cases confusing, because there was no agreement as to classification of malignant growths in general, or as to what constitutes a condition of multiple primary neoplasm. They found that few reports in the literature include cases in which there were malignant tumors in paired organs or in the same organ, because of the difficulty of excluding the possibility that the second lesion was metastatic. Yet, they contend, it is known that cysts of the ovary are often bilateral, and it is also known that certain types of these cysts often become malignant, so it would seem that in cases of bilateral papillary carcinoma of the ovaries the evidence is in favor of two or more primary growths than of metastasis from one ovary to the other ovary. Moreover, it is agreed by most authorities that polyps of the intestinal tract are the forerunners of malignant tumors and in such cases, in which more than one malignant growth is found, the conclusion would be that two separate malignant growths had developed on two separate polyps.

In their study of 2,124 patients with malignant tumors treated at the Mayo Clinic in the calendar year of 1929, Hurt and Broders found 71 patients who had had one other primary malignant neoplasm or more. This shows the percentage of proved cases of multiple malignant tumors in this series to have been 3.34. These cases were reviewed in 1931, or two years after one of the malignant tumors in each case had been observed. There were 15 patients whose first malignant tumor existed more than two years before 1929; that is, in 1926 or before. Therefore, they state, it is reasonable to assume that about 15 of the 2,053 patients with single malignant tumors seen in 1929 will, at some time later than 1931, have another primary malignant tumor. This reasoning would bring the total number of persons with multiple primary malignant tumors, past and future, to a theoretic total of 86, or 4 per cent of the 2,124 cases of malignant neoplasms reviewed. It is their further belief that if this study included, also, those cases in which only clinical diagnosis was made, the percentages of cases of multiple primary tumors would have approached or exceeded those of Owens, who included such cases in arriving at the figure of 4.7 per cent of 3,000 cases studied.

In their series there were 152 separate malignant lesions among 71 patients. There were 9 primary multiple lesions of the large intestine. Six of these patients had more than one primary malignant neoplasm of the large bowel, and 5 had malignant neoplasms other than those of the bowel. There was a family history of malignant tumors in 44.4 per cent of the cases.

As regards cases of primary multiple carcinoma confined to the large intestine, they have been divided into those which developed on the basis of adenomatosis and those which do not. The occurrence of multiple carcinoma of the former type of origin is well known, although there have been instances in which it would appear that the authors have not recognized the fact that adenomatosis had preceded the carcinoma. Czerny, in 1880, was evidently the first surgeon to resect multiple malignancies of the colon; he resected two independent carcinomas in the transverse colon and the sigmoid simultaneously. The patient recovered. Fenger, eight years later, reported a similar case in which he had performed colostomy, but the patient died. Necropsy failed to reveal the existence of polyposis. In the intervening years few similar cases have been recorded. However, many cases have been reported of multiple malignant lesions of the large intestine that have developed on the basis of adenomatosis.

Bargen and Rankin, in 1930, reported 16 cases not previously recorded of multiple carcinomas of the colon and rectum, in which cases polyposis preceding the carcinomas were not included. In the same year Norbury, in an illuminating report, recorded 3 cases of his own. Berson and Berger, in 1945, collected from the literature (from 1932) 66 cases of double and six of triple cancer of the large intestine. To these they added 13 cases of double and three of triple cancer encountered among 344 cases of cancer of the large intestine, a frequency of 4.6 per cent.

The multiplicity of lesions has an important bearing on prognosis. It is not uncommon, after excision of the rectum or partial resection of the rectum for malignant disease, for the patient to die within a few years of carcinoma of the large intestine. Gabriel recorded 3 cases in which recurrence took place in the bowel below the colostomy and these, he believed, were probably carcinomas arising independently in pre-existing adenomata.

The question of the origin of these tumors and the probable reasons for their recurrence offers much food for speculation. The frequent occurrence of single adenomatous polyps throughout widely disseminated portions of the colon has been discovered at necropsy, has been revealed by roentgenograms after barium enemas, has been disclosed by proctoscope search for disease, or has been suspected because of unexplained rectal bleeding. Polyps should be considered omens of possible future malignant disease of the large intestine.

It is not known, nor is it fair to predict, whether or not a given polyp will become malignant. However, careful investigation of every case of rectal bleeding, and removal of the cause of such bleeding, offer much hope for early recognition of malignant disease of the colon and its subsequent eradication. Multiplicity of such lesions is probably much more common than is generally suspected.

COLON

The different gross forms assumed by adenocarcinomas situated in the colon bear a direct influence on the symptomatology as well as the roentgenologic findings. Growths in the proximal half of the colon differ considerably from those usually encountered in the distal half. In the proximal portion of the colon the bulky, fungating, soft, friable medullary carcinomas which tend to ulcerate seldom produce obstruction because the lumen of the colon is greater here than elsewhere, the fecal content is liquid, and the tendency is toward penetration of the bowel wall rather than encirclement of its lumen (Fig. 41). Quite to the contrary, carcinomas situated in the distal portion of the colon are scirrhotic, constricting "napkin ring" neoplasms which eventually completely encircle the lumen, producing chronic, subacute, or acute obstruction (Figs. 43 and 44). These obstructing carcinomas usually produce some degree of dilatation and hypertrophy of the intestine above the growth. One of us (Rankin) has reported three cases of megacolon secondary to stenosing carcinoma of the sigmoid. The slowly progressive, obstructing process produced a huge colon which pathologically agreed in all particulars with Hirschsprung's description of congenital megacolon. There may be, on the other hand, only dilatation with marked attenuation of the walls of the colon. The normal mucosa on such occasions is to a considerable extent re-

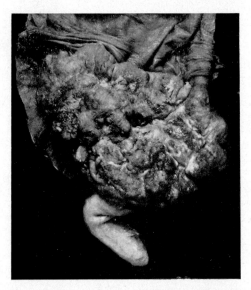

FIG. 41. Resected specimen of carcinoma of the cecum. Characteristic bulky ulcerating growth. See also Figure 42.

placed by innumerable small ulcers, and this greatly enhances the likelihood of peritonitis following manipulation at exploration of these obstructed segments of intestine. Papillomatous tumors, usually of a low grade of malignancy, may be encountered in the colon. These lesions occasionally assume large proportions and may give rise to obstruction just as in the case of the annular lesion (Fig.

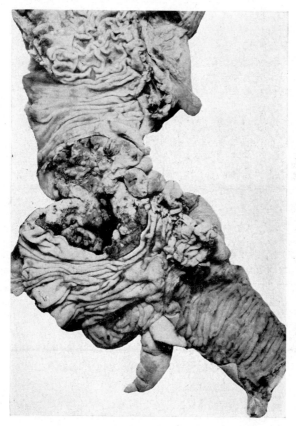

Fig. 42. Resected specimen of annular carcinoma of the ascending colon. This form is rarely encountered in the right half of the colon.

45). Bleeding is frequently noted in association with the growth of the left side, because of irritation produced by the hard feces present in this segment of the bowel.

Irrespective of the type of pathologic lesion, ulceration, invasion of the surrounding tissues, and secondary infection usually takes place. Fortunately this infection most frequently remains localized, but may terminate in extensive suppuration, peritonitis, or fistulous communications between the bowel lumen and some neighboring viscus, such as the small intestine, the stomach, or urinary bladder. Carcinomas of the transverse colon show a decided tendency toward invasion of the stomach. Raiford reported

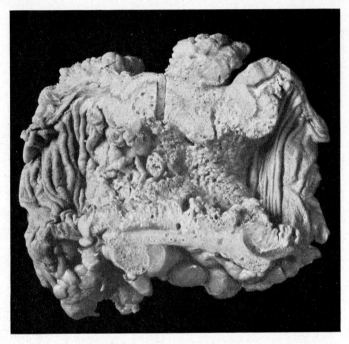

Fig. 43. Resected specimen mucoid carcinoma of transverse colon. Characteristic annular constriction of the bowel.

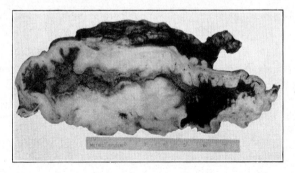

Fig. 44. Resected specimen of annular carcinoma of the transverse colon in fourteen-year-old girl (Warthen).

such occurrence in 7, or 50 per cent, of the carcinomas of the transverse colon in Johns Hopkins Hospital series. In a series of 35 vesicocolic fistulas, Rankin and Gorder recorded an incidence of 20 per cent originating in carcinomas of the sigmoid. Bargen and Cox in a study of 1,502 consecutive cases of carcinoma of the colon noted an operative diagnosis of perforation in 141 cases, an incidence of 9.3 per cent.

RECTUM

The incidence of occurrence of malignant neoplasms in the various segments of the rectum, that is, the anus, ampullary portion, and the rectosigmoid, has been discussed in the chapter on general considerations. Most carcinomas of the rectum are adenocarcinomas (Figs. 46 to 48). Secondary mucoid degeneration occurred in about one-fourth of 128 cases reported by Raiford, in exactly one-third of Zinner's cases, and in only about a twentieth of the cases studied by Rankin and Chumley. Mucoid carcinoma is considered in detail, elsewhere. The scirrhous type of carcinoma which probably represents a defense mechanism on the part of the body, is more commonly noted at the rectosigmoid. Here, because of the small calibre of the bowel in this segment these lesions give rise to early signs of obstruction. The epithelioma, which are comparatively rare, are

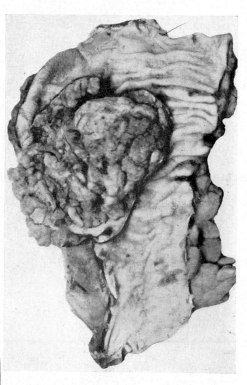

Fig. 45. Resected specimen of large obstructing carcinomatous adenoma of the sigmoid flexure showing proximal dilatation and hypertrophy. Adenocarcinoma, graded 2 (see Figure 57).

confined almost entirely to the anal canal. They originate in the anal epidermis and are comparable to neoplasms arising from squamous epithelial cells situated elsewhere. These growths are usually highly malignant and are seldom amendable to surgery. Metastasis occurs early and this by way of the inguinal nodes. Melanoma occurs with even less frequency than epithelioma. They have been classified as carcinoma and sarcoma.

Rankin and Chumley, in 1929, reported that a search of the records at the Mayo Clinic revealed only 18 proved cases of lym-

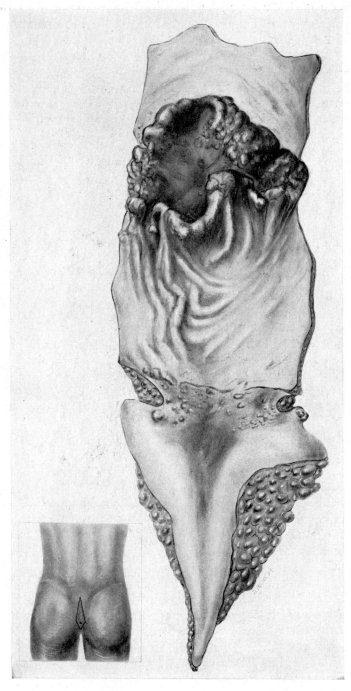

FIG. 46. Ulcerating adenocarcinoma of the rectum, graded 3. Characteristic crater formation with indurated and nodular edges.

phosarcoma of the colon and rectum; 3 of these were situated in the rectum. In 3 cases the tumor resected consisted of a large polypoid mass projecting into the lumen of the bowel. Two of these were rectal growths and in one of them two lymphosarcomatous polyps were found. The regional lymph nodes were involved in 11 of the 15 cases in which operation was performed.

In the earliest stages of its development, carcinoma of the rectum is confined to the mucosa and submucosa. Beginning with a

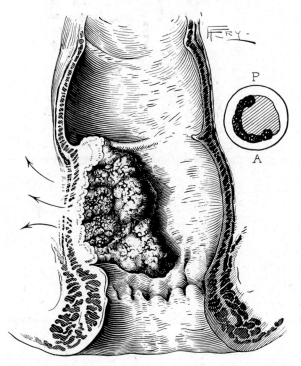

Fig. 47. Ulcerating adenocarcinoma of the lower rectum which has extended to the extra rectal tissues causing fixation of the growth and metastasis to the regional lymph glands.

small flattened surface, its growth is progressive in all directions; at the rectosigmoid, this occurs chiefly in an annular manner to produce the stenosis which is noted in well over 50 per cent of cases. In the ampullary portion the surface is more likely to become ulcerated, the edges indurated and nodular, and finally the ulceration deepens toward the muscularis and a typical crater is formed. However, the growth may be of the proliferative type and fill the entire lumen of the bowel. The significance from the standpoint of prognosis of the ulcerative (penetrating) and proliferative types of growths has been studied by McVay, Dukes, and Rankin and Olson (see "Prognosis").

Growths that tend to penetrate rather than to grow into the lumen of the bowel eventually, by infiltration and extension, affix themselves to the fascia propria of the rectum. The extension may then progress until either the bladder, prostate, uterus, vagina, or

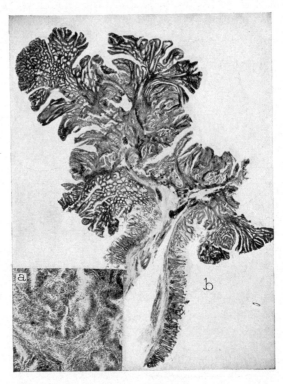

FIG. 48. *a*, Microscopic appearance and, *b*, cross section through a polyp of group 2 (Fig. 23, *C*). The polyp is practically destroyed by the advancing carcinoma graded 2. Had not the growth of this carcinoma been cut short by extirpation the picture shown in Figure 28 undoubtedly would have been produced.

sacrum is involved. Direct extension of carcinoma of the rectum is comparatively slow, and, according to Miles, invasion of the surrounding tissues and organs does not take place until the greater part of the circumference of the bowel has become involved. From observations of tumors in the ampulla of the rectum, he infers that by the time three-quarters of the circumference of the bowel is involved the growth is more than one year old.

METASTASIS

Metastasis in carcinoma of the large intestine is relatively late when other portions of the gastro-intestinal tract are taken into consideration. It has been clearly demonstrated by Broders, Rankin and Olson, Gabriel, Raiford, and others, in large series of cases, that the grade of malignancy has a direct bearing on the percentage of metastasis and absence of metastasis, since the percentage of cases showing metastasis increases in proportion to the grade, and absence of metastasis increases in inverse proportion to it. The findings in these studies are considered in detail in the chapter on prognosis. The following tabulation reveals the incident of glandular involvement according to the grade:

Grade 1 .... 27 per cent
Grade 2 .... 35 per cent
Grade 3 .... 50 per cent
Grade 4 .... 56 per cent

Broders observed that once the mucoid type of carcinoma metastasized the prognosis is poor, and Hayes found the highest incidence of lymphatic involvement and recurrence in the whole intestine to be in the group of mucoid carcinomas.

Lymph nodes and tissue should be invariably subjected to microscopic examination during operation in order to determine if one is working in an invaded area. Grossly, a lymph node may appear normal, and yet microscopic study will disclose malignancy. The commonest source of error, however, consists in presuming nodes to be involved which are enlarged as a result of inflammation.

The possibility of determining grossly whether lymph nodes were involved by the tumor or not was studied by Gabriel, Dukes and Bussey in a series of 1,242 nodes removed from perineo-abdominal specimens. Of these, 905 were considered from gross appearance to be free of metastases; subsequent microscopic examination showed 18 to contain metastatic tumor, an error of 2 per cent. On the other hand, in 337 nodes which were thought, from their gross characteristics, to contain cancer, metastases were present actually in only 132. An error was therefore made in 205 cases or 61 per cent of the total. The commonest source of error consists in presuming nodes to be involved which are enlarged as a result of inflammation.

Raiford states that although involvement of the skeletal system was rare in his series of cases it is frequently described and when present shows a predilection for the skull, ribs and vertebrae.

Colon.—The regional lymph nodes are usually the first sites of secondary growth. Sherrill, however, observed that occasionally hepatic metastasis occurred without involvement of local nodes. Hayes also reported one such case and in another adjacent nodes were inflamed but not malignant, yet there was distant metastasis. Ordinarily, though, the lymphatic vessels serve as an index to the extensiveness of the malignancy and their involvement influences prognosis considerably. A detailed anatomic consideration of the lymphatic system has been considered in the chapter on anatomy.

Hayes determined the frequency of metastasis from the various segments of the colon excluding the cecum, as follows: the sigmoid, descending and transverse colon, hepatic flexure, splenic flexure, and ascending colon. One of us (Rankin), in 1933, reported on a study of 753 cases of carcinoma of the colon and rectum, which were subjected to radical surgery. There were 187 cases of cancer of the right colon, 266 cases of the left colon, and 300 cases of cancer of the rectosigmoid and rectum. The incidence of glandular involvement, as determined in this study, was as follows: right colon, 34 per cent; left colon, 31 per cent; and rectum, 46 per cent.

Coller, Kay and MacIntyre, in 1941, reported on studies of 46 specimens of carcinoma of the colon removed at operation and which had been cleared by the Spalteholtz method. They found regional lymph nodes involved in 60.87 per cent of instances. Of the carcinomas of the right colon, 62.50 per cent showed metastasis in comparison with 60 per cent of those of the left colon. An average of 52 nodes were isolated per specimen as compared with 14.06 nodes per specimen reported by Hayes who employed the usual mode of dissection. Mayo and Schlicke, in 1942, in a clinicopathologic study of 334 cases of carcinoma of the colon and rectum found the ability of the surgeon to detect metastasis at the time of operation to be good. Table 3 compares operative observations with necropsy findings in the 95 cases in which abdominal exploration was undertaken. The material employed in this study was obtained

TABLE 3

A STUDY OF METASTASIS AND RECURRENCE (MAYO AND SCHLICKE)
Cases in which Abdominal Exploration Was Carried Out

Operative Procedure	Cases	Findings	Per Cent of Cases in Which No Metastasis Was Found	Per Cent of Cases in Which Metastasis Was Found	Per Cent of Cases with Regional Nodes Involved	Per Cent of Cases with Hepatic Metastasis	Per Cent of Cases with other Metastasis	Per Cent of Cases with Local Invasion
Exploration only.....	13	Operation	30.8	69.2	0	53.8	38.5	0
		Necropsy	15.4	84.6	69.2	69.2	61.5	46.2
Palliative operation.	38	Operation	26.3	73.7	23.7	42.1	42.1	68.4
		Necropsy	5.3	94.7	60.5	57.9	68.4	71.1
Preliminary operation.	44	Operation	81.8	18.2	2.3	(4.5?)	11.4	(38.6?)
		Necropsy	47.7	52.3	34.1	11.4	27.3	36.4
Total..	95	Operation	52.6	47.4	10.5	26.3	27.4	45.3
		Necropsy	26.3	73.7	49.5	37.9	48.4	51.6

TABLE 4

A STUDY OF METASTASIS AND RECURRENCE (Mayo and Schlicke)
Incidence and Distribution of Metastatic Growths

Site of Primary Tumor	Rectum	Recto-Sigmoid	Sigmoid	Descending Colon	Splenic Flexure	Transverse Colon	Hepatic Flexure	Ascending Colon	Cecum	Multiple Tumors	Total
Cases	83	41	77	18	10	13	11	24	29	28	334
Per cent without metastasis	44.6	29.3	37.7	44.4	30.0	23.1	54.5	41.7	41.4	42.9	39.5
Per cent with metastasis	55.4	70.7	62.3	55.6	70.0	76.9	45.5	58.3	58.6	57.1	60.5
Per cent of total											
Regional nodes	42.2	58.5	44.1	38.9	30.0	53.8	36.4	50.0	55.2	53.6	47.0
Distant nodes	6.0	2.4	6.5	0	10.0	7.7	0	8.3	3.4	3.6	5.1
Liver	21.7	31.7	26.0	11.1	20.0	15.4	27.3	20.8	13.8	17.9	22.2
Lungs and pleura	16.9	7.3	7.8	5.6	0	0	9.1	12.5	10.3	10.7	10.2
Other	18.1	24.4	36.4	5.6	50.0	53.8	27.3	37.5	31.0	10.7	26.9
Per cent showing local invasion	28.9	43.9	44.2	50.0	70.0	61.5	36.4	33.3	48.3	17.9	39.2

from the clinical records and protocols of the necropsies of 334 patients who died at the Mayo Clinic during the five year period ending December 31, 1939. Table 4 reveals the incident and distribution of metastatic growths in the 334 cases. The highest incidence of metastasis in this series occurred in cases of carcinoma of the transverse colon, followed by those of the rectosigmoid and splenic flexure, while the lowest incidence occurred in the hepatic flexure. When lesions of the transverse colon and multiple lesions are excluded, the incidence of metastasis is found to be 4.9 per cent higher for the left portion of the colon than for the right portion.

Somewhat different findings were reported by Gilchrist and David, in 1947. They studied 200 patients operated on more than five years previously for carcinoma of the large bowel. Specimens of the right colon obtained by resection averaged 54 nodes each; specimens of the left colon averaged 41 nodes. The incidence of metastasis respectively in these two segments was 86.6 per cent and 44.4 per cent.

Rectum.—Malignant lesions of the rectum may spread by any of four distinct ways: (1) extension through continuity of tissue; (2) by invasion of nerves; (3) by invasion of venous system, or; (4) through the lymphatic system.

(1) Direct Extension.—Local extension through continuity is discussed in the preceeding section.

(2) Invasion of Nerves.—The spread of neoplastic cells through perineural invasion recently has been studied by Seefeld and Bargen. In 100 cases of rectal carcinoma, lymph nodes were involved in 47 per cent, nerves in 30 per cent, and veins in 20 per cent. Invasion of all three increased with the degree of malignancy of the carcinoma.

(3) Invasion of Venous System.—Venous invasion in rectal

carcinoma has been observed by Mayo, McArthur, Smith, Monsarrat and Williams, Miles, and more recently by Coller, Kay, and MacIntyre, Dukes and Bussey, Grinnell, and Seefeld and Bargen. Its incidence of occurrence is approximately 20 per cent of all cases of malignant lesions of the lower rectum. Recent studies by Dukes and Bussey confirm the earlier (1904) impressions of Clogg that when dissemination was by way of the blood stream it frequently did so before the disease had spread to the lymph nodes. The vascular invasion was shown to originate within the involved intestinal wall itself and not from distant extension. As a consequence, a small, relatively innocuous-appearing lesion may be the seat of widespread hepatic metastasis. The explanation of why in such cases the rate of cure declines in direct proportion to the degree of penetration or the bowel wall, even in the absence of lymphatic involvement, is discussed in the chapter on prognosis in connection with the studies of Dukes and Bussey.

(4) Invasion of the Lymphatic System.—Decidedly more important than the other avenues of spread is the dissemination of cancer cells through the lymphatic channels, so that an intimate knowledge of the lymphatic system of the rectum is essential to the proper performance of an adequate radical resection. The detailed anatomy of these structures have been described by Delamare, Villemin, Huard and Montagne and more recently by Nesselrod.

There is an abundance of evidence that metastasis of cancer of the rectum by means of the extramural lymphatic system is more widespread and of infinitely greater consequences than that which takes place in the intramural lymphatic channels.

Intramural Channel.—Miles states that a continuous subcutaneous plexus of lymphatic ducts as has been described anatomically does not exist and that the spread of cancer cells in the submucosa of a carcinomatous rectum for a distance of several inches above the growth, as described by Handley, could not occur. Leitch believes that the cells noted by Handley, and considered malignant owing to the fact that they took up mucicarmine stain, actually were cells of Auerback's plexus, which occasionally stain diffusely with mucicarmine. All investigators are in agreement that spread of cancer in the submucosa is limited to a few lines beyond the microscopic margin of the growth. Leitch is of the opinion that the lymphatics of the mucosa do not exist as a continuous plexus, but are arranged in a decussating arborescent pattern from the collecting stems which pierce the muscular coat. Spread in the intramural lymphatic channels is just as limited (Fig. 49). We may conclude from these observations, states Miles, that from clinical as well as from histological findings the intramural spread of cancer of the rectum is always of comparatively trivial extent. Black and

Waugh (1948) from a study of 103 specimens of bowel removed at
operation at the Mayo Clinic concluded that (1) there is no appreciable difference in the intramural spread of carcinoma above or below the lesion; (2) the grade of malignancy of the lesion has no relation to the degree of intramural spread; and (3) for resections of
the left half of the colon for carcinoma, only 2 centimeters of

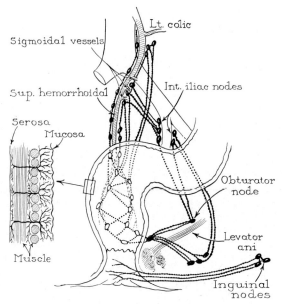

Fig. 49. The extramural and intramural lymphatic sys-
tems of the rectum (intramural system after Leitch).
(Glover and Waugh: courtesy of *Surgery, Gynecology and
Obstetrics.*)

normal bowel need be allowed above and below the lesion in order to
remove the whole of the primary lesion.

Extramural Channels.—These channels (Figs. 49 and 50) are
described by Miles as follows:

"The collecting stems from the intermediary lymphatic system
form an extensive plexus from which, and also from the ano-rectal
glands, efferents pass to their ultimate destination in three directions, namely, downward, laterally, and upward. Cancer cells derived from a growth in the rectum, wherever situated, after
entering the extramural lymphatic system may traverse the lymphatics in a downward, lateral, or upward direction or in all of them
simultaneously. During the transit the progress of these cells may
be arrested at any point in the region traversed by the lymphatics
and so lead to the formation of nodules. The various tissues
through which the extramural lymphatics pass, therefore, are liable

to be the seat of metastatic deposit, which may either be recognizable to the naked eye or may exist in a microscopical state. When
estimating the possible extent of the spread of cancer it may be regarded as an axiom whenever a visible metastasis exists, other
metastases which cannot be recognized without the aid of the mi-
croscope also exist along the course of the lymphatics at points

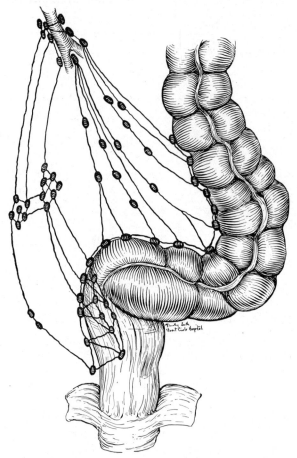

Fig. 50. Extramural lymphatic structures of rectum,
rectosigmoid, and colon (after Miles).

more distant from the site of the primary growth. Although cancer
cells may spread downwards and laterally, the chief and most constant path by which the spread takes place is in an upward direction, first of all invading the retrorectal glands, and then extending
along the superior hemorrhoidal and the inferior mesenteric vessels
towards the median aortic glands. From this main line of invasion
spread takes place in the substance of the pelvic mesocolon towards
the paracolic glands.

"The pelvic mesocolon is therefore highly dangerous tissue and is practically always the seat of metastatic deposits, although perhaps only in a microscopical state unless the primary growth is extensive. Accordingly unless the whole of this structure is removed during the operation for cancer of the rectum, existing metastases, however minute and indiscernible to the naked eye they may be, will continue to grow and will eventually give rise to symptoms indicative of so-called recurrence."

Gabriel, Dukes and Bussey, in 1935, disagreed with Miles as regards the frequency of metastatic deposits in the paracolic glands, situated along the mesenteric border of the pelvic colon. They found metastasis to the paracolic glands only in one of 100 cases studied in which more than 2000 lymph glands were investigated. This was a very advanced carcinoma. They summarized the normal course of lymphatic dissemination as follows: "The first glands to be affected are those in immediate vicinity of the growth, after which a continuous spread takes place along the glands accompanying the superior hemorrhoidal vessels. Until these lymphatic channels are all blocked, no downward or lateral spread is found but when carcinomatous metastases are present in all the hemorrhoidal glands then there may be extension in other directions."

Although in a majority of instances extension is continuous from lymph node to lymph node, it is of practical significance to recognize the possibility of intervening uninvolved nodes between the rectal growth and highly situated, involved nodes. Wood and Wilkie reported six cases in which glands near lesions in the lower rectum were free of involvement whereas those situated near the upper end of the rectum contained metastases. Gilchrist and David, in 1947, reemphasized the importance of the widest possible resection of the mesentery of the sigmoid in low lying carcinomas of the rectum owing to the frequency of small, high lying lymph nodes containing metastasis in such cases. They cited three instances in which at necropsy it was observed that complete removal of all node metastasis would have been accomplished if the field of resection had been 1 cm. wider.

Lateral dissemination along the levator ani muscles, the coccygei, base of the bladder, cervix or base of the broad ligament and finally into the internal iliac nodes has been noted in several instances by Miles. Similarly, Gilchrist and David observed such involvement in four cases, Coller, Kay and MacIntyre in six, and Gordon-Watson and Dukes, in one each. This lateral spread through the lymphatic system is an important consideration in low-lying lesions and will be dwelt upon in more detail in the chapter on prognosis.

Determination of the incidence of retrograde nodal metastasis in carcinoma of the rectum and rectosigmoid has been the object of painstaking studies by a number of investigators. Glover and Waugh have stated that even in far advanced cases of carcinoma in this region, retrograde spread occurs in only 1 per cent. Gilchrist and David, in 1947, reported an incidence of 4.6 per cent. The prognostic significance of these studies is discussed in the chapters on prognosis and choice of operation.

REFERENCES

1. BARGEN, J. A., and RANKIN, F. W.: Multiple carcinomata of the large intestine. *Ann. Surg.*, **91**: 583–593 (April), 1930.
2. BERSON, H. L., and BERGER, LOUIS: Multiple carcinoma of the large intestine. *Surg., Gynec., and Obstet.*, **80**: 75–84 (Jan.), 1945.
3. BLACK, W. A., and WAUGH, J. M.: The intramural extension of carcinoma of the descending colon, sigmoid and rectosigmoid. *Surg., Gynec., and Obstet.*, **87**: 457–464 (Oct.) 1948.
4. BRODERS, A. C.: The grading of carcinoma. *Minnesota Med.*, **8**: 726–730 (Dec.), 1925.
5. BRODERS, A. C.: Practical points on the microscopic grading of carcinoma. *New York State Jour. of Med.*, **32**: 667–671 (June), 1932.
6. COLLER, F. A., KAY, E. B., and MACINTYRE, R. S.: Regional lymphatic metastasis of carcinoma of the rectum. *Surgery*, **8**: 294–311 (Aug.), 1940.
7. DUKES, C. E.: Cancer of the rectum: analysis of 1000 cases. *Jour. Path. and Bacteriol.*, **50**: 527–539 (May), 1940.
8. DUKES, C. E.: The classification of cancer of the rectum. *Jour. Path. and Bacteriol.*, **35**: 323–332 (May), 1932.
9. GABRIEL, W. B.: The end-results of perineal excision and of radium in the treatment of cancer of the rectum. *Brit. Jour. Surg.*, **20**: 234–248 (Oct.), 1932.
10. GABRIEL, W. B., DUKES, C. E., and BUSSEY, H. J. R.: Lymphatic spread in cancer of the rectum. *Brit. Jour. Surg.*, **23**: 395–413 (Feb.), 1935.
11. GILCHRIST, R. K., and DAVID, V. C.: Lymphatic spread of carcinoma of the rectum. *Ann. Surg.*, **108**: 621–642 (Oct.), 1938.
12. GILCHRIST, R. K., and DAVID, V. C.: A consideration of pathologic factors influencing five-year survival in radiresection of the large bowel and rectum for carcinoma. *Ann. Surg.*, **126**: 421–438 (Oct.), 1947.
13. GLOVER, R. P., and WAUGH, JOHN M.: The retrograde lymphatic spread of carcinoma of the "rectosigmoid region." *Surg., Gynec., and Obstet.*, **80**: 434–448 (April), 1945.
14. GRINNELL, R. S.: The lymphatic and venous spread of carcinoma of the rectum. *Ann. Surg.*, **116**: 200–215 (Aug.), 1942.
15. HAYES, J. M.: The involvement of the lymph glands in carcinoma of the large intestine. *Minnesota Med.*, **4**: 653–663 (Nov.), 1921.
16. HURT, H. H., and BRODERS, A. C.: Multiple primary malignant neoplasms. *Jour. Lab. and Clinical Med.*, **18**: 765–787 (May), 1933.
17. LEITCH, ARCHIBALD: Quoted by Miles, W. E. (18).
18. MILES, W. E.: Cancer of the rectum. London, Harrison, and Sons, Ltd., 1926, 72 pp.
19. MONSARRAT, K. W., and WILLIAMS, I. J.: Intramural extension in rectal cancer. *Brit. Jour. Surg.*, **1**: 173–182, 1913–1914.

20. McVay, J. R.: Involvement of the lymph-nodes in carcinoma of the rectum. *Ann. Surg.*, **76**: 755–767 (Dec.), 1922.
21. Norbury, L. E. C.: Multiple primary malignant growths. With special reference to the colon and rectum. *Proc. Roy. Soc. Med.*, **24**: 6–23 (Dec.), 1930 (Section of Surgery: Subsection of Proctology).
22. Ochsenhirt: Quoted by Rankin and Chumley.
23. Parham: Quoted by Rankin and Chumley.
24. Raiford, T. S.: Carcinoma of the large bowel (Part II, the rectum). *Ann. Surg.*, **101**: 1042–1050 (April), 1935.
25. Rankin, F. W.: Megacolon secondary to carcinoma of the sigmoid. *Surg. Clin. N. Amer.*, **1**: 863–874, 1921.
26. Rankin, F. W.: The curability of cancer of the colon, rectosigmoid, and rectum. *Jour. Am. Med. Assn.*, **101**: 491–495 (Aug. 12), 1933.
27. Rankin, F. W., and Broders, A. C.: Factors influencing prognosis in carcinoma of the rectum. *Surg., Gynec., and Obst.*, **46**: 660–667 (May), 1928.
28. Rankin, F. W., and Chumley, C. L.: Colloid carcinoma of the colon and rectum. *Arch. Surg.*, **18**: 129–139 (Jan.), 1929.
29. Rankin, F. W., and Gorder, A. C.: Unpublished data.
30. Rankin, F. W., and Olson, Paul F.: The hopeful prognosis in cases of carcinoma of the colon. *Surg., Gynec., and Obst.*, **56**: 366–374 (Feb.), 1933.
31. Seefeld, P. H., and Bargen, J. A.: The spread of carcinoma of the rectum: invasion of lymphatics, veins, and nerves. *Ann. Surg.*, **118**: 76–90 (July), 1943.
32. Sherrill, J. G.: Cancer of the intestine. *New York Med. Jour.*, **91**: 331–334 (Feb. 12), 1910.
33. Wood, W. Q., and Wilkie, D. P. D.: Carcinoma of the rectum: an anatomico-pathological study. *Edinburgh Med. Jour.*, **40**: 321–343, 1933.

CHAPTER IV

SYMPTOMS AND DIAGNOSIS

SYMPTOMS

There are no symptoms that one might designate as being distinctive of malignant disease of the large intestine. Although certain combinations of well-known symptoms and signs are definitely suggestive diagnostically, careful proctoscopic and roentgenologic examinations are virtually indispensable for decisive determination of both the nature and the location of the lesion. It is quite evident to those clinicians and surgeons whose special interest in diseases of the large intestine bring them in frequent contact with late cases that as routine examination of the gastro-intestinal tract is undertaken more and more widely for vague symptoms referable to this tract, earlier diagnosis of malignant lesions will be affected, and there will be a concomitant increase in the number of favorable end-results following extirpation. Sight cannot be lost of the fact that almost a year has elapsed before the average patient with cancer of the colon or rectum has an accurate diagnosis made.

The difficulty of accurate diagnosis is enhanced by the fact that the colon is so frequently the site of other pathologic processes which resemble carcinoma in their clinical manifestations; moreover, the clinical features of carcinoma will often be found to vary widely in different cases, depending largely on the situation and gross form of the tumor, and on the presence or absence of such complicating factors as ulceration, perforation, obstruction, secondary infection, metastasis, and so forth.

Since it is impossible to correlate the symptoms and signs of the entire colon as a single organ because of the differences in its two halves, the two parts should be considered as separate and distinct organs for the particular purpose in hand. The right half of the of the colon, to the middle of the transverse segment, develops with and parallels functionally the portion of the small bowel which is distal to the papilla of Vater; that is, its function is absorptive, and symptoms referable to it are indicated by disturbances of physiologic function. The left half of the large bowel, which develops with the rectum from the hind-gut, is a storehouse, absorbing perhaps less than 10 per cent of the fluid content of the gastro-intestinal tract, and symptoms referable to it revolve around obstructive phenomena.

Right half of the colon.—A number of outstanding conditions influence the production of symptoms in the right half of the colon, namely (1) the liquid content of this segment; (2) the types of pathological growths in this portion, which are large, ulcerating, are covered with stubby protuberances, and are inclined to occupy the lateral wall of the bowel, without producing obstruction; and (3) the anatomic consideration of the size of the bowel which here is twice that of its fellow on the opposite side, with thinner musculature. On this basis of symptomatology, cases of carcinoma of the right half of the colon may be divided into three distinct groups, which should be considered separately: (1) the dyspeptic group, usually diagnosed chronic appendicitis or cholecystitis; (2) the group characterized by anemia and weakness of unexplained origin; and (3) the group in which the tumefaction is frequently discovered accidentally or in the course of a routine examination, without having previously produced symptoms.

Group 1, or the dyspeptic group, represents a large number of cases which because of the uncertainty and indefiniteness of the clinical manifestations, frequently is far advanced on being presented for examination. Epigastric discomfort and local tenderness, subcostally or in the right side of the abdomen, without a tendency to disappear, frequently are early signs of cecal carcinoma. Almost as many of these patients are operated on for subacute appendicitis and chronic cholecystitis as patients with carcinoma of the rectum are operated on for hemorrhoids. Browne, 1936, in a study of 209 carcinomas of the large intestine noted that in 26 per cent of the cases a diagnosis of appendicitis had been made; 90 per cent of these patients complained of pain and soreness in the right lower portion of the abdomen from two to nine months, and 44 per cent complained of nausea, eructation, fullness after meals and lower abdominal distention. Rosser, also in 1936, reviewed 100 cases from the standpoint of diagnostic criteria and noted localized pain and indigestion as symptoms in 78 per cent of the cases in which the lesion was situated on the right side. The traditional alternating constipation and diarrhea was conspicuous by its absence in both series. Rosser failed to encounter a single instance of colic, obstipation, or obstruction, and in only 6 per cent of the cases was there a history of diarrhea. In his series 50 per cent of the cases on the right side died after exploration under incorrect or indefinite diagnosis. A tumor was palpated in 56 per cent of the cases.

In the second group, characterized by weakness and by anemia without visible loss of blood and without pulmonary symptoms, one finds a considerable number of right colonic carcinomas. This anemia is nearly always unassociated with visible loss of blood and frequently is called to attention by attacks of unexplained weakness or inability to carry on work. The anemia may be noted in the course of a routine examination. The exact explanation of this type of anemia is not clear, but it seems definitely related to some perverted function of the mucous membrane of the large intestine, which is impaired to such extent that absorption of toxins results. Sometimes the concentration of hemoglobin is as low as 25 or 30 per cent before the patient is forced to undergo a physical examination. Usually when such depletion of the blood has occurred, however, localizing signs are present, and the disease is readily diagnosed by the characteristic roentgenogram. So often does this picture of anemia occur that we are of the opinion that no patient should receive a diagnosis of primary or secondary anemia until a thorough examination of the entire colon has precluded the possibility of malignancy in its right half. It is axiomatic among clinicians that pernicious anemia should always be differentiated from gastric malignancy, but we are confident from our own experience that more often it is necessary to exclude carcinoma of the right half of the colon. The differential diagnosis is in no wise difficult because, of course, the blood picture of pernicious anemia does not resemble secondary anemia, but the distinction between the two forms of anemia is so important that it must always be made.

Koons reviewed a series of cases in an effort to explain this anemia, and found that the average reading for hemoglobin of 70 patients who came to operation for carcinoma of the right side of the colon was 60 per cent. In this series, however, there were 19 cases of operable carcinoma of the cecum in which the hemoglobin was less than 50 per cent, and the average color index was 55 plus. He asserted that the size of the growth usually was in direct ratio to the degree of anemia. Koons, Whipple, Smith and Murphy, Stiles and Schmit all attribute the anemia, in great part, to a toxic process. Raiford reported a decided tendency toward increasing anemia at the proximal end of the colon and stated that it was obvious that bleeding, which is seldom perceptible in the gross, could not account in full for the low value of hemoglobin.

In Rosser's series, blood was noted by the patient in 14 per cent of the proximal colon carcinomas as against 78 per cent for lesions in the left half of the colon. Moderate anemia was recorded in 66 per cent of cases and severe anemia in 38 per cent.

The third group comprises those cases in which there is an unsuspected and accidentally found tumor in the right iliac fossa. In approximately 10 per cent of lesions of the cecum observed by us, either a tumor is discovered by the patient when he least expects it, or, in the course of a routine health examination a mass is palpated which on further examination proves to be carcinoma.

If patients are obese and palpation is difficult, these cases are not discovered until complications develop, such as perforation or generalized metastasis. These cases do not just represent the earlier stages of the two other types as has been frequently suggested: in certain instances this doubtless is the case, but many of these silent carcinomas have been found inoperable because of hepatic metastasis.

The predominant symptoms of the relatively small number of carcinomas encountered at the hepatic flexure are similar to those produced by lesions arising in the cecum and ascending colon. Obstruction is slightly more frequent, due to angulation of the bowel at this point and because of its slightly smaller diameter; but the character of the fecal current is unchanged and consequently stenosis occurs late. In view of the close proximity of this segment and the proximal transverse colon to the gallbladder and duodenum, lesions situated here frequently become attached to and mimic disease of these structures.

Left half of the colon.—In the left half of the colon, obstructive phenomena dominate the clinical picture. There are obvious reasons for this: (1) pathological growths of this side of the large bowel are inclined to be of an encircling type, frequently incorporating the whole lumen of the bowel, and causing progressive stenosis; (2) the fecal content of the left half of the colon is hard and formed, and with difficulty can be forced through a closing segment. According to Burgess, obstructions occur six times as often on the left side of the colon as in the right half—87 per cent as against 13 per cent. Clinical symptoms depend on the amount of obstruction present when symptoms manifest themselves to the patient. Obstruction is of two types, acute or chronic.

With the exception of a small group of cases, which vary according to the concentration of the population in any given area, acute intestinal obstruction is rarely produced by carcinoma of the large intestine. In our own experience the incidence has been less than 5 per cent. McLanahan, in reporting his experience and that of Stone with such lesions, stated that only rarely was a patient so obstructed that operative decompression was necessary. Others, however, have noted acute obstruction in a somewhat higher percentage of cases.

There appears to exist a difference of opinion as to just what constitutes acute obstruction of the large intestine. Patients frequently admit an inability to relieve themselves by defecation and it is a common experience to find, on questioning them, that there has not been a bowel passage for a period of ten days or longer. Because of this history, and roentgenographic evidence following barium enema of advanced stenosis of the bowel lumen, many patients are diagnosed as being acutely obstructed and are subjected to an

immediate emergency procedure. Yet a careful study of such patients will usually reveal the blood chemistry to be normal, that
there is free passage of flatus, and that above all things the patient
is in need of a preoperative regimen directed toward overcoming
advanced dehydration. Cecostomy or some other decompressive
measure may or may not be required subsequently. Consistently
satisfactory results attending this conservative treatment of the
markedly obstipated patient has prevented us from often resorting
early to such measures, which, under the circumstances, carry a relatively high risk.

The symptoms of acute obstruction of the colon, as we recognize it, are not unlike those of acute small bowel obstruction: Complete blockage of the bowel even to the passage of gas, marked
abdominal distention, usually evidences of hyperactive peristalsis,
and, finally, vomiting which eventually becomes fecal in nature.
Usually this acute obstruction is ushered in without warning, the
presence of the malignant lesion being unsuspected. Occasionally,
however, we have observed an acute obstruction to become superimposed on a chronic one. The sudden plugging of the stenosed
lumen by a seed, or other foreign body, has been noted on several
occasions. More often the inciting agent has been inspissated barium, unwisely administered orally in the course of a roentgenologic
examination of the gastro-intestinal tract in instances of annular
lesions of the colon. One of us (Rankin) in reviewing 381 cases of
carcinoma of the colon and rectum which had been operated on,
recorded the performance of cecostomy only four times and enterostomy only twice. It is quite evident from these figures that the
incidence of acute large bowel obstruction in this series was very
small.

Burgess, of Manchester, England, reported that 35.6 per cent
of his cases were admitted to the hospital with complete obstruction. Roscoe R. Graham, in a study of 104 consecutive cases of
acute intestinal obstruction found the seat of obstruction to be the
colon in 24 cases or 23 per cent of instances, and of this group carcinoma was the causative agent in 19, or 79 per cent.

Haggard reported 90 per cent of instances of intestinal obstruction of the large bowel due to cancer. In other words, in a group of
persons in adult life, in whom acute intestinal obstruction is diagnosed, if one can by any means determine that the lesion is limited
to the large intestine, and at the same time can exclude the possibility of strangulated hernia, the chances are between 80 and 90
per cent in favor of the lesion causing the stenosis being a carcinoma of the left half of the colon.

Acute obstruction of the colon has been the subject of detailed
consideration by Brindley in 1945 and by Michel in 1947. The

former reported an incidence of 20.6 per cent in a series of 190 cases of cancer of the colon. Michel reported an incidence of 27 per cent in 203 such cases. There was a mortality of 32.7 per cent.

A history of progressively increasing *constipation* can be obtained in between 40 and 60 per cent of cases. Rosser reported an incidence of 52 per cent and Browne noted that 53 per cent complained of persistent and increased constipation, whereas they had previously been normal. It is difficult, however, to define the meaning exactly of the word "constipation." The direct question as to the number of stools each day may or may not elicit this information satisfactorily. These patients will often deny constipation, notwithstanding the daily intake of large doses of purgative medicine necessitated by their inability satisfactorily to relieve themselves by defecation.

As the patient becomes obstipated and complete obstruction of the bowel approaches, borborygmus and visible peristalsis, associated with flatulence and colicky pains, may be noted. Visible peristalsis is a striking phenomenon when observed in a slender individual. One may observe, and likewise feel, a peristalsis rush, representing the effort of the bowel to force its content through the intestinal lumen at the site of an annular constriction. As the wave reaches the constriction there is a sudden rebound and the proximal segment of colon may be observed to dilate considerably then slowly subside. Borborygmi may be audible at a great distance on such occasions, and pain increases as does the peristaltic activity, in crescendo fashion, until the rush has spent itself, and the markedly distended colon subsides.

Diarrhea, especially as the lumen of the bowel becomes encroached upon, either persistent or alternating with constipation, is occasionally noted, but probably less frequently in lesions of the colon than in lesion of the rectosigmoid. When diarrhea is the prevailing symptom, the history may be misleading, as the average patient is likely to consider anything diarrhea from a frequent desire to go to stool to ten or twelve large, watery stools a day. Usually it does not cause alarm until the patient has become dehydrated or weakened from the loss of fluids. Actually, diarrhea seldom occurs. These frequent motions often consist of only a minute quantity of waste matter, mucus, and probably blood, and represents the so-called compensatory or pseudodiarrhea which exists in the face of almost complete obstruction. Rosser recorded diarrhea as present in 29 per cent of his cases, whereas Browne noted it in 17 per cent, and only 13 per cent of his patients experienced alternating periods of diarrhea and constipation. Seventeen and four-tenths of the total number of patients in his series were treated for dysentery.

Blood, usually bright to dark red, and mixed with the stool, or appearing with the passages of mucus and small flakes of fecal material is, with obstipation, the cardinal sign of malignant involvement of the distal segment of colon. Little confidence is to be placed in the presence or absence of occult blood in the stool as a diagnostic measure. If tests for occult blood give positive results, the lesion may be anywhere between the buccal cavity and the anus. If the blood is red, if it is in the stool or on it, and if it persists on repeated examinations, one may expect to find, in a majority of instances, a lesion in the vicinity of, or distal to, the splenic flexure. Blood is rarely discovered when the growth is in the right side of the colon, but when it does appear it usually gives the stool a dark color and tarry consistency. Blood was observed by the patient in 61 per cent of Rosser's cases and in 58 per cent of those reviewed by Browne.

Tenesmus is noted in direct ratio to frequency as the growth approaches the rectal sphincter; that is, the lower the growth, the greater is the irregularity of the bowel and the more likely is straining at stool to develop. It is seldom noted with lesions proximal to the rectosigmoid.

TABLE 5

FREQUENCY OF SYMPTOMS IN CARCINOMA OF THE LARGE INTESTINE (POSTLETHWAIT-DUKE HOSPITAL)
First Five in Each Group

Rectum and Rectosigmoid (258)		Left Colon (99)		Right Colon (84)	
Melena	220 (85%)	Abdominal pain	71 (72%)	Abdominal pain	62 (74%)
Constipation	115 (41%)	Melena	53 (53%)	Weakness	24 (29%)
Tenesmus	77 (29%)	Constipation	42 (42%)	Melena	23 (28%)
Diarrhea	73 (28%)	Nausea	25 (25%)	Nausea	20 (24%)
Abdominal pain	68 (26%)	Vomiting	23 (23%)	Abdominal mass	19 (23%)

Pain has not been a prominent symptom in our experience. When present, it has been usually associated with ineffectual peristaltic activity and the accumulation of gas in instances of a markedly stenosed bowel lumen. Rosser obtained a history of localized pain in only 6 per cent of his cases, while Browne observed that pain was prominent when the descending colon and sigmoid were involved. In 88 per cent the patients complained of discomfort in the lower quadrant radiating across the abdomen long before actual pain was experienced.

In recent years pain as a significant symptom of operable carcinoma of the colon has been emphasized by several authors. Estes in 1943 stated that he and his associates were of the opinion that a marked improvement in their operability rate resulted from their acceptance of abdominal pain as a criterion of early carcinoma of the colon. Pfeiffer states that pain brings patients to the doctor more often than anything else and believes we may make greater progress in arriving at early diagnoses if, rather than centering our attention on the earliest but rather vague symptoms as change in bowel habits, we consider all cases of chronic abdominal pain, especially if pain is colicky in nature, as due to cancer of the large intestine until proved otherwise. It will be noted that the Duke Hospital cases (Table 5) abdominal pain was the most frequently noted symptom in cases of carcinoma of both halves of the colon.

Actual acute perforation from carcinoma of the colon is of infrequent occurrence; more often it is chronic and culminates in the formation of abscess or becomes adherent through ulceration to an adjacent viscus. Of 1,502 consecutive cases of carcinoma of the colon reviewed by Bargen and Cox, in 141 cases a diagnosis was made at operation of perforation, which is an incidence of 9.3 per cent. Clinical, preoperative, and historic data were available in 20 cases: in 13 of these pain was severe enough to be called acute, in 1 case the pain was less severe, and in the other 6 pain was not a prominent symptom; the temperature in these cases seldom rose above 101 F. The site of the lesion was as follows: sigmoid, 6 cases; cecum, 4 cases; transverse colon, 4 cases; rectosigmoid, 2 cases; and 1 each in the ascending colon, hepatic flexure, splenic flexure and descending colon. In only 8 of the cases was an abdominal mass present and palpable. A study was made at the same time of 30 cases of perforation due to diverticulitis, and the differential diagnostic features studied. This is considered in the chapter on differential diagnosis.

Rectum and rectosigmoid.—Unquestionably, carcinoma of the rectum is capable of producing early symptoms, but in a vast majority of instances the patient either disregards them or else the attending physician misinterprets them. It is not possible to determine the exact time at which a carcinoma of the rectum begins, but it is highly probable that many of them have existed one or more months before suggestive symptoms and signs were in evidence. The average duration of symptoms before diagnosis has been recorded by various authors as follows: Postlethwaite (258 cases), 9.1 months; Rankin and Jones (300 cases), 11.7 months; Brindley (167 cases), 9.4 months; Browne (94 cases), 11 months.

The signs and symptoms of carcinoma of the rectum may be different in different persons, and any of them may be produced by other rectal or intestinal disorders. The most frequently encountered symptoms are bleeding and changes in bowel habit.

Bleeding.—Bright blood which may appear mixed with the stool or may simply streak the stool, is almost universally recognized as the most significant first indication of cancer of the rectum. However, it is not necessarily always the earliest sign. Months may be required for the growth to penetrate the mucous membrane and until this occurs there is little likelihood of bleeding. The actual blood loss is usually small in amount and not associated with much anemia except in far advanced cases. Occasionally, however, the first knowledge of rectal disease is a sudden hemorrhage.

In the study of a series of 539 cases of carcinoma of the rectum, one of us (Rankin) found that bleeding had been present for several months and in nearly a third of the cases the earliest sign of carcinoma was blood in the stool; 89.5 per cent of these patients had noted blood at stool. In a similar study of 1,937 cases of carcinoma of the rectum and sigmoid, Buie obtained a history of bleeding in 84 per cent. Brindley reported 80 per cent, Rosser 78 per cent, and Browne stated that in the rectal cases of his series it was universal. The average hemoglobin reading in Rankin's series was 72 per cent.

Changes in bowel habit.—A change in bowel habit may be and frequently is the earliest symptom. Patients, however, attach less significance to such disorder than to bleeding and are prone to temporize with increasing constipation or alternating constipation and diarrhea until tenesmus and abdominal discomfort influence them to consult a physician. Miles stresses the importance of a history of intractable episodes of constipation during the latent period prior to the appearance of objective symptoms. It is due, he believes, to functional inertia of the colon which fails to respond readily to medication and is not associated with abdominal distention, as is the case during later obstructive phases of the disease.

In Rankin's series, referred to above, constipation was the predominant complaint in 332 cases, or 55 per cent, and in 20 per cent diarrhea was the principal clinical manifestation. In this connection it should be remembered that the average duration of symptoms when these data were obtained was over eleven months. In other words obstipation or evidences of partial obstruction is not an early sign. Constipation was a cardinal complaint in 61 per cent of Rosser's cases and diarrhea was reported in 22 per cent. True diarrhea is not of frequent occurrence, although patients will not infrequently speak of ten or twenty loose stools a day. This pseudodiarrhea, which consists primarily of mucus and blood with small quantities of fecal material, is more commonly observed when lesions are situated at the rectosigmoid and often lead to a diagnosis of dysentery. This occurred in 15 per cent of a series of cases reported by one of us (Graham) and in 17 per cent of the cases reviewed by Browne. The frequent stools often follow the taking of cathartics and therefore are not connected with diarrhea.

The so-called ribbon stools no longer possess significance as regards carcinoma of the rectum. They depend upon the consistency of the stools and the tonicity of the anal sphincters and are seen in cases of constipation more often than in cases of organic disease of the bowel, including carcinoma and benign stricture.

Pain.—Pain is seldom a prominent symptom of carcinoma of the rectum until the malignancy is far advanced or the anal canal, which alone is endowed with pain sensations, is involved. When the growth has become fixed, with involvement of other viscera, the pain may be severe. Sacral pain, backache, and shooting pains in the hips and thighs are common complaints and suggest metastasis to the bones or root pains resulting from pressure on the sacral nerves. Although localized pain as an early symptom is uncommon, carcinomas situated in the ampulla not infrequently give rise to a discomfort which the patient describes as a heavy sensation or feeling of fullness. Moreover, they complain of inability to obtain relief from it at stool. Rosser noted localized pain in only 6 per cent of his cases, but in 61 per cent of the rectosigmoid cases he noted evidences of some degree of obstruction and colicky pains in the abdomen.

Excessive loss of weight and strength, as has been shown by Rankin and Jones in their study of 300 cases, are worthless symptoms in the early recognition of the condition. Fifty-six per cent of their patients were normal or obese at the time of examination (average eleven and seven-tenths months after onset of symptoms).

Obviously, all or any of these symptoms are inadequate clinical signposts by which to diagnose carcinoma of the rectum, and their main use is to succeed in directing attention to some unusual condition in the bowel, bringing about its detection in the course of an examination more thorough than usual. In the presence of these suggestive phenomena it is imperative, if an early diagnosis is to be made, that one resort to the simple expedients of a digital and proctoscopic examination. By the former procedure alone a presumptive diagnosis is possible in between 90 and 95 per cent of all carcinomas of the rectum and rectosigmoid. Yet all too frequently patients with these symptoms are subjected to roentgenoscopic examinations who have not had this simplest of all procedures in the examination of the intestinal tract. It is likewise astonishing that so few of these patients are subjected to sigmoidoscopy; only 15 per cent of Browne's 209 cases had such an examination made.

To wait for the appearance of the classical textbook symptoms of abdominal malignancy such as marked loss of weight and strength, profound anemia, dehydration, palpable masses, and severe pain is merely postponing the diagnosis until generalized metastasis has occurred and there is no hope for a cure.

DIAGNOSIS

Diagnostic errors in the recognition of organic lesions of the large intestine are of both omission and commission. Failure to make a proper examination for these lesions results in more failures of diagnosis, or at least of failure to recognize them until their late stages, than any other single factor. The diagnosis of lesions of the large intestine is made by a painstaking anamnesis supplemented by careful physical examination and corroborated by roentgenoscopy. In the case of the colon, certain combinations of well-known symptoms are suggestive of a lesion, either benign or malignant, but a roentgenologic examination, expertly done, is practically indispensable for decisive determination of the nature of the lesion and its situation. As regards the rectum, Daniel Fisk Jones has so truly stated "There is no disease that can be diagnosticated with more accuracy than cancer of the rectum after the patient once presents himself, and yet there are few diseases which are diagnosticated so late in their course."

Thomas Copeland might well have made this statement one hundred and thirty-eight years ago, for even at that early period he had a thorough knowledge of the symptoms of carcinoma of the rectum, the characteristic feel it imparted to the examining finger, and also the tendency of physicians to mistake such cases for piles, which they would treat. In his *Observations of Some of the Principal Diseases of the Rectum,* written in 1810, Copeland gives an excellent description of a slow, progressing stenosis from cancer of the rectum, saying:

"The first symptoms of the disease is an habitual costiveness; but this is so frequent in occurrence and produced in so many ways that it is not likely that the cause should be sought for in an organic affection of the rectum. Mild purgation is resorted to, and the symptoms being relieved, the cause is no longer sought after. When this has subsisted for some time the patient complains of what is called piles, and what is often really so, as a consequence of obstructed circulation in the parts. The remedies usually given in such cases are applied, sometimes with relief, but more frequently otherwise and then the good maxim of the inexpediency of curing piles, perhaps rescues the practitioner from the discredit of failing to relieve his patient. The piles are sometimes removed by ligature or excision and this gives temporary abatement of the most painful symptoms, while the cause of the disease is still unknown. In a short time as the gut continues to decrease in diameter the efforts to expel the feces becomes more violent and the consequent progress of the disease more rapid. The stools, which have been evacuated with difficulty, become contracted in size, appearing like earth-worms in their form, or small pellets. In this stage it is some-times, in the male, mistaken for enlarged prostate gland, but if the finger be introduced into the rectum, the gut will be found either obstructed with small tubercles or intersected with membranous filaments, or else the introduction of the finger will be opposed by a hard ring of a cartilaginous feel. The patient often lives a long time in this distressing situation, until, at last worn out with pain, the discharge, or perhaps the total obstruction of the rectum, he yields to his fate."

Every case of cancer of the rectum can be diagnosed by meas-ures available to every physician: well over 75 per cent, and prob-ably nearer 90 per cent, of all lesions of the rectum and rectosig-moid are within reach of the examining finger; the remainder may be readily visualized through the electric proctoscope. Jones states that he cannot agree with Lockhart-Mummery that this instru-ment should be used only by experts. Certainly it would seem that with a little experience the average physician should be able to maneuver the scope under direct vision, and with the aid of air in-flation, up to the rectosigmoid.

Two highly illuminating studies relative to the diagnosis of car-cinoma of the different portions of the colon and rectum were made during 1947. One is an unpublished study by Postlethwait of 441 cases observed at Duke University Hospital over a period of 15 years, ending January 1, 1946; the other is a study by Jackman, Neibling and Waugh of 817 cases observed at the Mayo Clinic dur-ing the year 1944. The results of these studies are comparable (Ta-ble 6) except for the handling of cases erroneously treated as some other disease during the course of the patient's symptoms, the car-cinoma being undiscovered. The main purpose of the Mayo Clinic study was to determine how many carcinomas of the large intestine (1) within reach of the examining finger, (2) beyond reach of finger but visible at sigmoidoscopic examination,and (3) beyond direct visualization but discernible in roentgenograms of the colon, are diagnosed and treated as some other disease during the course of their symptoms arising from unsuspected carcinoma. More than half (54.3 per cent) of all their patients with carcinoma in any part of the large intestine, or 70 per cent of those with carcinomas in the sigmoid and rectum, had lesions which could be palpated with the examining finger. About a fourth (23 per cent) of the patients of this group had received some form of treatment for disease of the color or rectum, but not for carcinoma, during the course of the pa-tient's symptoms which were produced by the carinoma. A fourth (25.8 per cent) of those patients whose lesions were not palpated but could be visualized through the sigmoidoscope, had received treatment for some disease other than carcinoma. In the third group, made up of patients whose lesions were diagnosed by roentgenologic studies, only 9.9 per cent of the patients had received treatment directed toward any other condition. All told then, 90 per cent of the 634 patients with carcinomas located in the terminal portion of the large intestine had lesions that could be felt with the finger or visualized through the sigmoidoscope, yet 23.6 per cent were treated for some disease process other than carcinoma which had remained undiscovered.

TABLE 6

DIAGNOSIS OF CARCINOMA OF THE LARGE INTESTINE

COMPARISON OF SERIES OF CASES: DUKE UNIVERSITY HOSPITAL (POSTLETHWAIT) AND MAYO CLINIC (JACKMAN, ET AL)—1947

Location of Lesions	Duke Hospital 441 Cases			Mayo Clinic 817 Cases		
	Cases	% of 441	% of 321	Cases	% of 817	% of 634
Sigmoid, rectosigmoid and rectum....	321	72.7	100	634	77.6	100
Accessible to examining finger.......	247	56.0	76.9	444	54.3	70.0
Inaccessible to finger; visible (sigmoidoscope)....................	23	5.2	7.1	132	16.2	20.8
Total lesions visible at sigmoidoscopy.	270	61.0	84.0	576	70.5	90.0
Beyond reach of sigmoidoscopy.....	171	39.0		241	29.5	
Discernible in roentgenograms of colon...........................	105	*		232	28.4	
Diagnosed only at abdominal exploration........................	**			9	1.1	

* Only 120 of the 171 lesions beyond reach of sigmoidoscope were observed roentgenographically; 105, or 87.5% of these were positive.
** This figure is not available.

Although carcinoma represents approximately 70 per cent of all lesions of the colon, the difficulty of accurate diagnosis is enhanced by the fact that the large intestine is the site of such a variety of other pathologic processes which resemble carcinoma. Then too, carcinoma mimics certain of the other conditions: in the proximal colon these are subacute appendicitis and chronic cholecystitis; in the distal colon, and rectum they are chiefly hemorrhoids and dysentery. In Browne's series of 209 cases of cancer of the large intestine 26 per cent received a diagnosis of appendicitis; in 17 per cent of the cases a diagnosis of dysentery had been made; and 18 per cent of the rectal cases had undergone treatment for hemorrhoids. One of us (Graham) in reporting on a series of carcinomas of the rectum noted that approximately 50 per cent of the cases had received originally an incorrect diagnosis of bleeding piles or colitis, yet in all but three instances the growth was within reach of the examining finger. Jones reported that at the Massachusetts General Hospital over 75 per cent of patients who eventually received a diagnosis of cancer of the rectum had been treated for hemorrhoids.

The differential diagnosis of carcinoma of the colon and rectum has been considered in detail in a separate chapter.

An adequate examination in suspected lesions of the colon and rectum should consist of (1) digital examination; (2) sigmoidoscopic examination; and (3) roentgen-ray studies of the colon after barium enema, in the order named.

Digital examination.—The digital examination is very important, but never

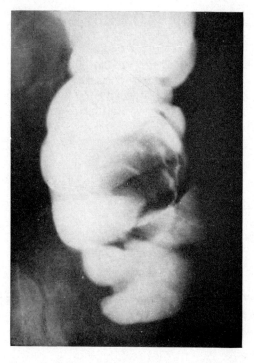

Fig. 51. Large adenomatous polyp of cecum which showed beginning malignant changes.

conclusive. In determining the fixation of a cancer and the presence of enlarged lymph nodes the finger is invaluable. However, in spite of the fact that there is a definite "cancer feel," there are instances in which inflammatory lesions with perirectal masses of induration impart an identical impression. In a majority of instances there will be felt an ulcerated area with a hard, raised, irregular border. In the annular type a hard mass is felt, in the center of which there is a ragged opening with hard edges.

The position employed in making the examination will depend very much on the training of the physician. The knee chest position is probably employed most often and there is no question but that this position tends to pull the growth out of the pelvis. It is particularly advantageous when the patient is fat or has a large gluteal region. However, the Simms position permits the patient to relax in comfort during the examination and it also permits one, as D. F. Jones has pointed out, to reach higher than any other position. This he claims is because of the position of the knuckles in relation to the ischia and also because it permits one to force the anus backwards and upwards to the tip of the coccyx without much discomfort. Terrell, Pennington, and many other experienced proctologists and surgeons prefer this position.

The examination should never be conducted in a hurried and haphazard manner, as is too often the case. Patients should be informed that a finger will be inserted into the rectum and reassured that the attending discomfort will not be considerable if they do not contract their muscles together. As Pennington stated "to gain

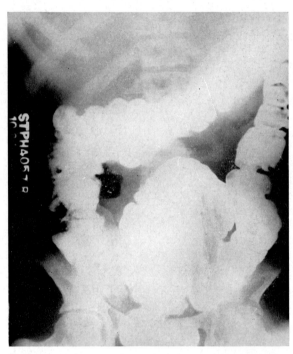

Fig. 52. Carcinoma of the ascending colon (Medical College of Virginia, Hospital Division).

the patient's confidence, assure him that you will be gentle; then make this promise good." The buttocks should be separated and a lubricant gently massaged into the anus and about its margin, so that the finger will slip through with as little friction and produce as little discomfort as possible. In the event the anus is very spastic because of a fissure or acute inflammation incident to persistent tenesmus, an anesthetic ointment should be employed and sufficient time permitted for it to take effect. In this manner co-operation of the patient can be obtained and relaxation secured, without which a satisfactory examination is impossible.

Just why there should be a hesitation on the part of the physician to consider digital examination of the rectum as essentially a part of a physical examination as the examination of the eye, ear, nose and throat, or other cavities of the body, is unexplainable. Certainly, there are few examinations which will elicite such valuable information with the expenditure of so little effort, yet there is probably no examination that is more consistently neglected.

Proctoscopic examination.—Direct visualization of the rectum and terminal sigmoid by means of the proctoscope (sigmoidoscope)

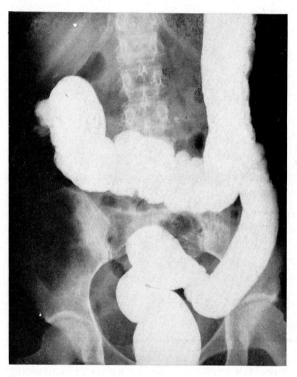

Fig. 53. Annular obstructing carcinoma of the hepatic flexure which would not permit the passage of barium.

should invariably precede radiologic examination. The proctoscope will reveal not only the characteristics of the growth, which is usually a single, semifixed, punched-out ulcer with indurated and nodular edges, or a papillary adenomatous type of lesion, but in addition it will show its size, its mobility, and the degree of obstruction to the bowel. All these factors are important, because the obstruction of the growth, fixation, and extension to the perirectal tissues influence the determination of operability. Biopsy is not so essential in the differentiation between cancer and a benign lesion as it is to estimate the grade of the lesion in accordance with Broders' index of malignancy. The grading is an important factor in estimating prognosis and assists in the selection of operation or other measures. A positive report on microscopic examination is conclusive, but a negative one is not. The latter may mean that the specimen was not taken deeply enough or from the proper site; a second section may prove the error.

Proctoscopic examination of the rectum is not a difficult maneuver, nor is it a particularly dangerous one if reasonable care is

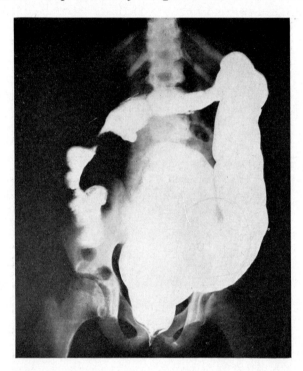

Fig. 54. Carcinoma of the hepatic flexure of the colon.

exercised in its performance. However, if carried out carelessly and with haste, the undertaking may prove hazardous. A few cases have been reported in which the scope was pushed through the rectal wall and into the abdominal cavity, and a much larger number of such disasters have come to our attention which were not reported. Nevertheless, we are convinced that such an occurrence can be avoided in every instance provided an electric proctoscope is employed, and the precaution is taken to advance the instrument beyond the anal canal under only direct vision in a rectum that has been inflated with air. Sigmoidoscopy is a different matter; more experience and skill is required for its successful accomplishment.

Persistence of symptoms suggestive of carcinoma of the rectum or sigmoid, particularly bright blood at stool, following a negative proctoscopic examination and roentgenologic studies, not infrequently signifies that the examinations have been inadequate. If on repeated rectal examination, the cause of such symptoms is not found, or in the event the examinations have been unsatisfactory, every effort should be made to have the patient examined by a physician trained in proctoscopic methods. It has been our experience on a number of occasions to encounter growths that were missed at the initial examination.

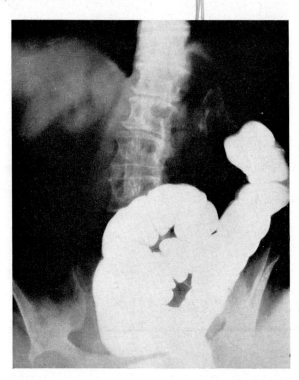

Fig. 55. Annular obstructing carcinoma of the descending colon. This case and the one illustrated in Figure 52 demonstrate the danger of employment of the barium meal for the diagnosis of lesions of the colon.

Roentgenology.—Of greatest importance in the diagnosis of colonic malignancy has been the advancement of roentgenologic technic to the present point of accuracy; it is now possible to parallel the information that has been obtainable for a decade or more in lesions of the stomach and duodenum. The characteristic roentgenologic evidence of malignant disease in the large bowel is so accurate that Weber in 102 cases of carcinoma of the colon above the middle of the sigmoid flexure, proved at operation, error in examination was made in only 3 cases. A filling defect or visualized interference with the integrity of the lumen of the bowel is so pronounced in the majority of instances in which accurate preparation has been made that experience with the fluoroscope promises to continue this accuracy. The barium clysma, roentgenologically controlled, aided by palpatory manipulation, and vertification of the results by roentgenography, is the method of choice for accurate

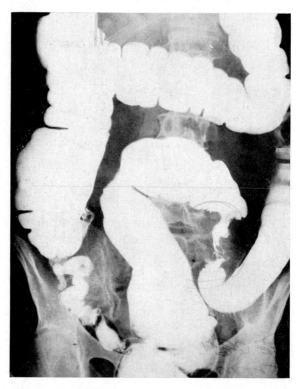

Fig. 56. Extensive annular carcinoma involving the sigmoid flexure.

localization of the filling defect and for precise interpretation of its pathognomonic characteristics (Figs. 51 to 57).

The opaque enema is urged in contradistinction to the oral meal for two reasons: first, the oral meal is a positive menace in the presence of an obstructing lesion, since not infrequently it produces acute obstruction superimposed on a chronic process (Figs. 53 and 55) and, second, the oral meal is of considerable less practical value in diagnosing carcinoma of the colon because of the irregular distribution of the barium throughout the lumen.

Weber, by modification and elaboration of Fischer's technic (inflation with air after partial evacuation of the opaque enema) has been able to depict the topography of carcinoma in minute detail and thus enhance diagnostic accuracy. It was failure of ordinary roentgenologic methods (Fig. 58) precisely and consistently to demonstrate the presence of polypoid lesions, whether single or multiple, that first prompted Weber to develop and employ this method which has produced such excellent results (Fig. 64).

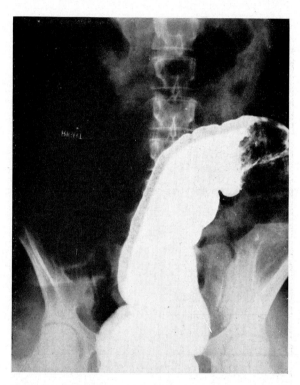

Fig. 57. Extensive carcinomatous adenoma of the sigmoid flexure. Resected specimen shown in Figure 45.

Weber described his technic as follows:

"I have applied the 'combined method' of Fischer, modified along the lines indicated, to the demonstration of polyps and polyposis of the colon. Diagnostic results have been gratifying. In the application of this technique it is essential that all residues and fecal remnants be entirely removed, and that the walls of the colon be collapsed. On the day before the examination, the evening meal is withheld, and 2 ounces (60 c.c.) of castor oil is administered. On the following morning, the distal part of the colon and rectum are cleansed by one or two plain, low enemas. Saline purgatives, and cathartics which depend on the property of activating the bowel by irritation, are to be avoided. The patient then presents himself at the roentgenologic laboratory, and the opaque enema is administered under roentgenoscopic control. The opaque material in the enema should be minutely divided, uniformly suspended, and the suspension should be well sustained. Several commercial preparations of the opaque salt are available which are satisfactory, or a suspending agent, such as gum acacia, may be added to the enema when it is prepared in the laboratory. The consistence of the enema should approximate that of heavy cream.

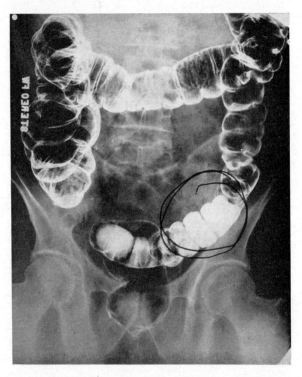

Fig. 58. Roentgenogram after Weber's modification of the combined method of Fischer. Polypoid tumor situated in the sigmoid (from Weber).

"Roentgenoscopic and roentgenographic study should be completed with dispatch because the opaque salt sometimes goes out of suspension rapidly, owing perhaps to the dehydrating function of the colon. It is not always easy to obtain ideal distribution and concentration of opaque material on the mucosal surface of the colon. No more than a uniform thin coat is desirable. The patient is told to evacuate the enema as completely as possible, and it will usually be found that a sufficient amount of the material remains in the lumen after evacuation. If large collections of the material are still seen after the attempt at evacuation, the rectum can be insufflated with a volume of air sufficient to induce a desire to defecation, whereupon the patient usually will return with as near the ideal distribution and concentration of opaque material as is possible in his case. The colon is inflated, under roentgenoscopic control, and care is exercised not to overdistend any of the segments. The procedure is facilitated by frequent rotation of the patient on the roentgenoscopic table, and by manipulation of the bowel through the abdominal wall. Insufflation carried out in this way has not been in any way more distressing to the patient in any case than administration of the opaque enema. The fluoroscopic image of the air-filled colon lacks sufficient detail to be of diagnostic value. The enema tip is removed from the rectum as soon as the cecum has been moderately distended, and stereroentgenograms are made with the patient lying on the abdomen. The grid diaphragm is of distinct advantage in educing the fine detail requisite for precise demonstration of the character of the lesion."

Carcinoma of the colon must be distinguished roentgenographically from various other pathologic processes. This has been considered in the chapter on differential diagnosis.

REFERENCES

1. BARGEN, J. A., and COX, F. W.: Perforating lesions of the large intestine. *Minnesota Med.*, **15**: 466–469 (July), 1932.
2. BRINDLY, G. V.: Carcinoma of the rectum; factors affecting its cure. *Jour. Am. Med. Assn.*, **108**: 37–43 (Jan. 2), 1937.
3. BRINDLEY, G. V.: Acute obstruction of the colon. *Texas State Jour. Med.*, **40**: 571–577 (Mar.), 1945.
4. BROWNE, D. C.: Early recognition of carcinoma of the colon and rectum. *New Orleans Med. and Surg. Jour.*, **88**: 495–500 (Feb.), 1936.
5. BUIE, L. A.: Carcinoma of the rectum, rectosigmoid, and sigmoid. *Surg. Clin. N. Am.*, **4**: 361–367 (April), 1924.
6. BURGESS, A. H.: Treatment of obstruction of colon. *Brit. Med. Jour.*, **2**: 547–556 (Sept.), 1923.
7. COPELAND, THOMAS: Observations on some of the principal diseases of the rectum and anus. Kingstreet, Seven Dials, W. Smith and Co., 1810.
8. ESTES, W. L. JR.: Early diagnosis of cancer of the colon. *Penn. Med. Jour.* (Aug.), 1943.
9. GRAHAM, A. STEPHENS: Carcinoma of the sigmoid and rectum: common diagnostic errors which are readily avoidable; case reports. *Virginia Med. Monthly*, **64**: 143–146 (June), 1937.
10. GRAHAM, ROSCOE R.: Carcinoma of the colon. *Am. Jour. Digest. Diseas. and Nutrit.*, **1** (no. 8): 584–588 (Oct.), 1934.
11. HAGGARD, W. D.: Intestinal obstruction from carcinoma of the colon. *Ann. Surg.*, **94**: 717–721 (Nov.), 1931.
12. JACKMAN, R. J., NEIBLING, H. A., WAUGH, J. M.: Carcinoma of the large intestine. *Jour. Am. Med. Assoc.*, **134**: 1287–1289 (Aug. 16), 1947.
13. JONES, D. F.: Malignant disease of the rectum. Thomas Nelson and Sons' *Loose Leaf Living Surgery*, **5**: 219–241, 1929.
14. MICHEL, M. L.: Acute malignant obstruction of the large bowel. *South. Surgeon*, **23**: 299–320 (May), 1947.

15. MILES, W. E.: Cancer of the rectum. London, Harrison and Sons, Ltd., 1926, 72 pp.
16. McLANAHAN, SAMUEL: One stage abdominoperineal resection for carcinoma of the rectum. *South. Med. Jour.*, **30:** 382–386 (April), 1937.
17. NEWMAN, GEORGE: Great Britain Ministry of Health Report on Public Health and Medical Subjects, London, Bulletin, 46, 1927.
18. PENNINGTON, J. R.: Diseases and injuries of the rectum, anus, and pelvic colon. Philadelphia, P. Blakiston's Son and Co., 1923, 933 pp.
19. PFEIFFER: In discussion of Estes.[8]
20. POSTLETHWAIT, R. W.: Personal communication.
21. POSTLETHWAIT, R. W.: Malignant tumors of the colon and rectum. *Ann. Surg.*, **129:** 34–46 (Jan.), 1949.
22. RAIFORD, T. S.: Carcinoma of the large bowel, Part I: The colon. *Ann. Surg.*, **101:** 863–885 (March), 1935.
23. RAIFORD, T. S.: Carcinoma of the large bowel, Part II: The rectum. *Ann. Surg.*, **101:** 1042–1050 (April), 1935.
24. RANKIN, F. W.: Colostomy and posterior resection for carcinoma of the rectum. *Jour. Am. Med. Assn.*, **89:** 1961–1966 (Dec.), 1927.
25. RANKIN, F. W.: The recognition, surgical treatment, and prognosis of organic lesion of the large bowel. *South. Surgeon*, **3:** 227–234 (Sept.), 1934.
26. RANKIN, F. W.: Common errors in the diagnosis and treatment of cancer of the colon and rectum. *South. Med. Jour.*, **30:** 386–392 (April), 1937.
27. RANKIN, F. W., and JONES, R. D.: Carcinoma of the rectum. *West Virginia Med. Jour.* **25:** 5–9 (Jan.), 1929.
28. ROSSER, C.: Neoplasms of rectum; incidence, interrelationship, and diagnostic criteria. *South. Surgeon*, **5:** 290–297 (Aug.), 1936.
29. WEBER, HARRY M.: The roentgenologic demonstration of polypoid lesions and polyposis of the large intestine. *Am. Jour. Roentg., and Rad. Therap.*, **25:** 577–589 (May), 1931.

CHAPTER V

DIFFERENTIAL DIAGNOSIS

Unfortunately, early diagnosis of carcinoma of the large intestine may not be made from any group of symptoms, and the evidences which one may call suggestive are not uniform; moreover, they may mimic various other lesions. Differential diagnosis in the colon must be made, in the main, from hyperplastic tuberculosis, segmental chronic ulcerative colitis, diverticulitis, nonspecific granuloma, abscess of the appendix, single benign tumors, polyposis, and occasionally from megacolon, actinomycosis and syphilis; in the rectum and rectosigmoid from bleeding hemorrhoids, polyposis, and chronic constipation.

Since cases of carcinoma make up approximately 70 per cent of the total in which operations on the large intestine are required, it would seem advisable when the presumptive evidence points to a malignant lesion that it be so considered until conclusively proved otherwise. One of us (Rankin) in 1931 reviewed the work of the section on colonic and rectal (exclusive of proctology) surgery at the Mayo Clinic. Of 542 patients observed in this section in 1930, 369 (or 68 per cent) were admitted for carcinoma (Table 7).

TABLE 7

DIAGNOSIS OF SURGICAL DISEASES OF THE LARGE INTESTINE AND RECTUM (1930)

	Cases
Carcinoma	369
Internal obstruction (acute and subacute)	70
Fecal fistula	32
Diverticulitis	12
Benign lesions (not classified elsewhere)	12
Tuberculosis	9
Ulcerative colitis	7
Stricture (benign)	6
Imperforate anus	5
Lane's kink and adhesions	2
Diverticulum (Meckel's)	4
Polyposis	3
Prolapse of rectum	3
Rectovaginal fistula	2
Intussusception	2
Sarcoma	1
Megacolon	3
Total	542

Although certain combinations of frequently observed symptoms and signs are very suggestive diagnostically, careful roentgenologic examination is virtually indispensable for determination of the exact nature and situation of the growth; moreover, it will often disclose carcinomas that have not been suspected. The importance of the examining finger and the proctoscope cannot be overestimated as differential diagnostic aids in an investigation of diseases both of the colon and the rectum. However, even when the lesion can be visualized by the proctoscope, roentgenography is still often advisable since multiple lesions are not infrequently encountered.

Although occasionally it is impossible to distinguish roentgenologically a non-malignant lesion from carcinoma, the roentgenologist well trained in the interpretation of colonic pathology is capable of making an accurate diagnosis in a very high percentage of cases. Weber, in 1929, made a correct diagnosis in 99 of 102 organic lesions of the large bowel, proximal to the middle of the sigmoid flexure, as was proved by subsequent exploration.

Carcinoma, diverticulitis, and the chronic ulcerative non-malignant diseases, such as chronic ulcerative colitis, tuberculosis, and non-specific granuloma, all are manifested roentgenologically by lumenal deformity, and it is often possible to distinguish these diseases from one another by the character of the change in contour which the particular pathologic process has produced. It has been found that the opaque enema, studied roentgenoscopically and roentgenographically, is the most reliable method of demonstrating the lumen of the colon.

The filling defect produced by carcinoma is annular, polypoid, or obstructing. Some colonic spasm usually attends a given lesion, but in general the carcinomatous filling defect is characterized by the jagged irregularity of the canal through the malignant tissue, by its constancy of situation, and by the association of a palpable indurated mass at the site of the defect (Figs. 51 to 57).

The filling defect produced by diverticulitis simulates that of carcinoma more closely than that of any other disease. It is spindle shaped, its contours tend to be serrated in a regular fashion rather than roughly jagged, and many or few of the extraluminal shadows of diverticula are seen in other parts of the colon.

Chronic ulcerative colitis, when it involves only a short segment of the colon, may simulate carcinoma in its roentgenologic aspects. Even so, the filling defect produced by this type of lesion is usually comparatively long in extent, the margins of the canal tend to be smooth rather than irregular, and the wall of the involved segment, although obviously thickened, remains relatively pliable. Hyperirritability is usually a prominent factor (Figs. 62 and 63).

The hyperplastic type of tuberculous colitis usually affects the proximal segments of the colon, and this disease too, in its roentgenologic aspects, may resemble carcinoma closely. The filling defect is irregular in outline, has a corrugated appearance, and is associated with a palpable mass of a peculiar, boggy consistence. Usually part of the terminal portion of the ileum can be shown to be involved in the process. It is, however, only when an unusually short segment of the right half of the colon is involved with a tuberculoma that the roentgenologic differential diagnosis from carcinoma becomes difficult. Tuberculous enterocolitis is commonly secondary to chronic pulmonary tuberculosis, and this association may be of value in making the differential diagnosis.

Polypoid lesions of the colon, when they are large, produce a central defect in the colon which is characterized by its smoothness and by absence of mural infiltration. Smaller polypi may escape roentgenologic detection entirely unless the roentgenologist will resort to special technical methods. It has been found that a modification of Fischer's combined method is of special value in demonstration of such lesions. Very small polyps can be brought to light with this technic, and it has become difficult to realize how any lesion which has attained sufficient size to be recognized by gross pathologic investigation should escape roentgenologic detection (Fig. 58).

Roentgenographically, nonspecific infectious granuloma may mimic carcinoma or hyperplastic tuberculosis; or the defect in the roentgenogram may often be more suggestive of an extraneous lesion than a tumor in the lumen of the bowel (Fig. 65).

The following diseases from which carcinoma must most often be distinguished are considered in detail from the standpoint not only of diagnostic features but also of etiology, pathology, and treatment, since organic diseases of the large intestines are closely interrelated and because occasionally at exploration for carcinoma one of these non-malignant lesions is encountered.

SARCOMA

Sarcomas of the large intestine are infrequently encountered. A search of the records of the Mayo Clinic by Rankin and Chumley, in 1929, revealed only 18 proved cases of lymphosarcoma of the colon and rectum. The average age in this series was forty-five years. Only three of the patients were less than thirty years and the youngest was aged eleven. Thirteen were males and five were females. Goldstein reviewed 600 cases of primary sarcoma of the digestive tract which were distributed as follows: tongue, 65; esophagus, 36; stomach, 265; gallbladder, 16; liver, 59; pancreas, 19; appendix, 18; and, large and small intestine, 135. The distribution of the lesions in the series studied by Rankin and

Chumley was: cecum, 13; descending colon, 1; sigmoid, 1; and, rectum, 3 (Fig. 59).

The condition is seldom diagnosed except at necropsy or during exploratory operation. In none of the 18 cases was diagnosis made before tissue from the tumor had been studied microscopically.

Treatment.—Radical extirpation, roentgenray therapy, or a combination of the two are the procedures employed. The prognosis is not good. Glandular metastasis is usually noted at exploration; this had occurred in 11 of the 15 cases in Rankin and Chumley's series in which resection was made. Four of their patients died in the hospital and four died from recurrence within a year of operation. Six patients were living at the time of the report but only two had survived a period of three years.

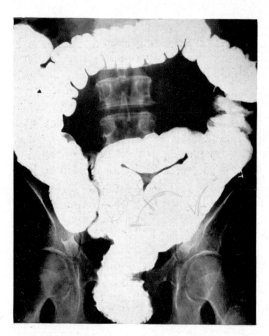

FIG. 59. Lymphosarcoma involving entire rectum; diagnosis confirmed microscopically (F. M. Hodges).

TUBERCULOSIS

Tuberculosis of the colon easily divides itself into two types; first, the diffuse ulcerative type, the lesions of which are usually scattered throughout the large and the small bowel, and which follows advanced pulmonary lesions; and second, the hyperplastic type, the lesion of which is almost habitually localized to the ileocecal coil and may be resected satisfactorily with the hope ultimately of an extremely good end-result. The relative infrequency of this latter lesion, however, is emphasized in Table 7 by the fact that only 9 cases occurred among the 542 patients with organic colonic lesions. Rarely is hyperplastic tuberculosis of the large bowel secondary to a demonstrable lesion elsewhere in the body. Pathologically it is characterized by proliferation of the connective tissue in all of the coats of the bowel, the walls of which become vastly thickened but seldom ulcerated. The symptoms and early signs of hyperplastic tuberculosis of the

ileocecal coil are so slight and indefinite that they readily and frequently escape attention. Like other organic lesions in this situation, hyperplastic tuberculosis manifests itself in a dyspeptic syndrome which may be of slight significance and give few localizing
signs save an occasional attack of tenderness over McBurney's
point, or some irregularity of the bowel, such as may be described
in the sequence of events accompanying any organic colonic lesion.
Here, as in carcinoma, one is frequently confronted with the wrong
diagnosis of chronic appendicitis, and it is almost as frequent an
occurrence to obtain a
history that appendec-
tomy has been performed
a few weeks or months
previous to recognition
of the true condition as
it is to find that a patient
with carcinoma of the
rectum has been oper-
ated on previously for
hemorrhoids. In certain
cases a tumor is palpable,
and the accidental dis-
covery of a mass by the
patient himself is the
first warning of the
trouble. The differential
diagnosis rests between
carcinoma and a chron-
ically inflamed, retroce-
cal thickened appendix
which is palpable and
which may be not in-

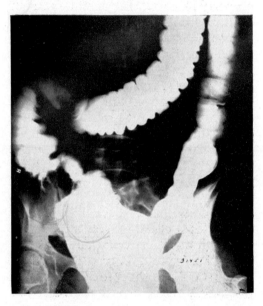

FIG. 60. Hyperplastic tuberculosis of the cecum
and terminal ileum. Subsequently resected and
diagnosis confirmed microscopically.

frequently mistaken for either of the other lesions. The diagnosis is
usually established roentgenologically, and there is small reason for
an experienced roentgenologist's failing to establish the differential
diagnosis between carcinoma and tuberculosis in this region. Fluoroscopic examination, aided by palpatory manipulation, will elicit
characteristic signs and symptoms which confirm the diagnosis.
These signs have to do with an irregular filling defect of corrugated
appearance almost always associated with a palpable mass in the
ileocecal coil. Two of the most characteristic roentgenologic phenomena associated with tuberculosis in this region are involvement
of the terminal portion of the ileum and irritability around the
affected segment of bowel. The difference in the filling defect from
that of carcinoma is mainly that it is larger and longer, less irregu-

lar, and more often associated with a concomitant small intestinal lesion (Fig. 60).

Hyperplastic tuberculosis is rarely seen proctoscopically and when it is seen one is likely to confuse it with malignancy of the rectum. A study of the microscopic section of such a lesion is the only certain way of making a definite diagnosis, and discovery of malignant characteristics rules out the existence of tuberculosis. One should be on guard, however, if malignant cells are not found on the first examination; possibly the specimen has been improperly removed. In general, one should be able to identify a carcinoma grossly on proctoscopic examination. Our efforts to discover the bacillus of tuberculosis in the tissues have not met with the success which has been reported by some.

Treatment.—Satisfactory extirpation of hyperplastic lesions of the ileocecal coil is advisable when the disease is localized to this segment and when the general condition of the patient is compatible with such a procedure. Rankin and Major reported four deaths, or a mortality of 8 per cent, in a series of 50 patients who underwent resection of the diseased bowel. Ordinarily, the prognosis is extremely satisfactory following removal of this type of growth, and although subsequent treatment and observation are necessary over a long period of time after the operation, there is small question of the desirability of surgical attack.

Our own preference is to do this type of resection in one stage, although one must recognize that circumstances not infrequently make it safer to do a graded operation and here, as in carcinoma, safety should be the foremost consideration which tempers surgical judgment. We believe that an end-to-side ileocolostomy should be carried out as the first step of the maneuver. Having implanted the ileum into the transverse colon and having left about 30 to 45 cm. of the terminal portion of the ileum to be extirpated with the colon, because of the intimate association of the lymphatic supply and blood supply of the terminal portion of the ileum and the cecum, one may either abandon the operation at this point or proceed to resect the terminal portion of the ileum and the right half of the colon, using the same steps for mobilization and exeresis as in malignancy, except that division of the mesentery may be made closer to the bowel since removal of the contiguous lymphatic structures is unnecessary in the case of hyperplastic tuberculosis. The details of technic are considered in the chapter on operative procedure.

DIVERTICULITIS

One of the most interesting, but by no means uncommon, lesions of the large bowel is diverticulum, which is noted in approximately 5 per cent of all patients who are sent for roentgenologic examination of the colon. These diverticula, which occur either singularly or in numbers, and perhaps are scattered throughout the colon, but usually are limited to the sigmoid segment, are without significance save when inflammatory changes—diverticulitis—take place. The manner of production of these diverticula is controversial, and many theories, substantiated by experimental evidence, have been advocated by different authors as to the method and factors in their formation. Whether intracolonic pressure, the constant association of diverticula with the opening in the mesentery between the blood vessels, the "pull" on the bowel by the mesentery, constipation, or some other anatomic type is the vital factor we do not know. Probably no one factor produces them constantly, but the outstanding features of their formation have to do with inherent weakness of the intestinal wall, which, with increased intracolonic pressure and some environmental or constitutional factor, may be responsible for them.

The production of diverticulitis is a simple mechanical process. The sacs, which are in reality hernias through the musculature of the bowel, become filled with dejecta and fail to empty. The neck of the sac is the narrowest portion; it becomes constricted with advancing edema, round-cell infiltration, and hyperemia, and its failure to empty results in the so-called "left-sided appendicitis," which may go on to formation of abscess. In advanced cases the inflammatory change extends to the mesentery, produces marked thickening, and frequently affixes the diverticula to an adjacent viscus or to the lateral parietal peritoneum, at times even resulting in perforation and formation of abscess or in formation of fistula, such as is sometimes seen between the bladder and sigmoid or between the sigmoid and coils of small intestine.

A convenient classification of diverticula is as follows:

I. Diverticulosis, which includes that group of cases in which evidence of diverticula is found on roentgenologic examination, or at necropsy, and in which, from all available data, the diverticula bear no relation to the patient's complaints.

II. Diverticulitis.
    1. Acute.
    2. Chronic.
    3. Complicated by
        (a) abscess.
        (b) fistula
             external $\left.\begin{array}{l}\text{external}\\\text{internal}\\\text{multiple}\end{array}\right\}\begin{array}{l}\text{vesicocolic}\\\text{enterocolic}\end{array}$
        (c) malignancy

In the division of diverticulitis (Fig. 61) are found practically all types and complications of this lesion. The symptoms are not pathognomonic, but pain is the most common symptom of any kind, ranging, as it does, from sharp pain, probably secondary to formation of gas, to a slow, boring type of discomfort. Its usual situation is in the lower left abdominal quadrant, or in the lower left mid-abdominal section, and its reference depends on the accompanying complication, which usually is attachment to or perforation of another viscus. Constipation is a common accompaniment of diverticulitis, particularly when it is advanced to the stage of complication, or when tumefaction or stenosis of the lumen of the bowel is present. In nearly two-thirds of cases reported by Rankin and Brown, constipation only, or constipation alternating with diarrhea, which was atypical, was the most outstanding symptom. Diarrhea only was present in 11 per cent of the cases, although it was not true diarrhea; it was usually more of a rectal tenesmus associated with the passage of a small amount of pus, mucus, or fecal material. In two of the cases passage of unmixed pus by bowel occurred, signifying the presence of an abscess which had ruptured into the lumen of the bowel, a very satisfactory termination of a

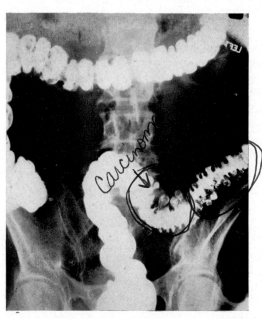

Fig. 61. Colon after barium enema. Diverticulitis of the proximal sigmoid; note also carcinoma rectosigmoid, graded 2 by Broders (F. M. Hodges).

complicated and difficult situation. Tumefaction occurred in 31 per cent of the cases; in 26 per cent of the cases there were vesical symptoms, signifying attachment of the diverticulum to the bladder, and resulting in inflammatory cystitis. In seven cases of this 26 per cent the attachment to the bladder resulted in formation of fistula between the bladder and the sigmoid, with the resulting passage of gas and feces by urethra, a pathognomonic sign of the development of an ostium between the two viscera. This complication is a serious one when it requires surgical intervention, and special observation should be made of the renal infection in deciding on the type and extent of surgical intervention.

Blood in the stool is of little significance in diverticulitis, from a diagnostic standpoint, and although it is present in a number of cases, usually proctoscopic examination will reveal that the presence of the diverticulitis had little, if anything, to do with the presence of the blood. It is important, however, when blood occurs in the presence of diverticulitis, to rule out associated carcinoma. The coexistence of carcinoma and diverticulitis is naturally a possibility and is occasionally observed, but the development of carcinoma at the site of diverticulitis is an exceedingly rare and bizarre condition, the occurrence of which has been grossly exaggerated. In the series of 227 cases of diverticulitis studied by Rankin and Brown a malignant condition was found accompanying it in only 4 cases, evidencing the fact that diverticulitis as a precursory or producing agent of carcinoma is so rare as to be unique. Morton in reporting (1946) on 111 cases of diverticulitis stated that bleeding was present in almost 20 per cent. Stone agrees with him that bleeding is not a rare symptom of diverticulitis. David, on the other hand, believes as we do that there is little reliable evidence to prove diverticulitis is a common source of hemorrhage. "Until definite pathologic evidence is forthcoming," he states, "I feel that we should be reluctant to place too much emphasis on diverticulitis as a source of hemorrhage, as it engenders a sense of complacency which might well lead to overlooking a small carcinoma or a bleeding polypus."

The diagnosis of diverticulosis is readily made by barium enema observed roentgenoscopically. The diverticula manifest themselves as rounded, knob-like projections along the lumen of the bowel, showing considerable variation in size, and usually occurring most numerous in the sigmoid portion of the colon. Roentgenologic evidence of the presence of diverticulosis consists principally of the signs of extreme irritability that always are present with inflammation of a hollow viscus (Fig. 61). All degrees of spasms are seen, from the mild type manifested by a sharp, serrated appearance of the haustra in a somewhat narrower segment of bowel to almost complete occlusion of the lumen. The filling defect almost universally encountered is either of one type or a combination of two types: a false filling defect resulting from spastic narrowing of the affected segment which may be so marked as to produce complete occlusion, or a true filling defect resulting from encroachment of pericolic inflammatory tissue on the lumen of the bowel. Antispasmodic drugs, administered until the physiologic effect is obtained, will modify the appearance at least of the former, but will have little effect on the latter except to relieve concomitant spasm. These filling defects make roentgenologic differential diagnosis of diverticulitis and carcinoma confusing, but it can usually be accomplished by careful and painstaking observation. Differential points are the somewhat concentric contours of the segment noted in diverticulitis, contrasted with the sharp irregular contours in carcinoma, the maintenance of mobility in the former, compared with the stark immobility of the latter, and the relatively long segment of colon involved with diverticulitis, whereas carcinoma usually involves a much shorter segment.

Treatment.—The treatment of diverticulitis is largely medical, and it is our feeling that surgical intervention should be reserved for such complications as (1) acute perforation, (2) formation of abscess, (3) fistula, (4) inflammatory obstruction, and (5) malignancy. The type of operation indicated depends on the complication present, and in general it may be said that a procedure for drainage is more desirable than radical resection. It has been our experience, in dealing with diverticulitis which is causing obstruction and tumefaction, and which is uncomplicated by abscess and fistula, that prolonged diversion of the fecal current by colostomy results in recession of the inflammatory process in a high percentage of cases, permitting subsequent re-establishment of the lumen of the bowel. Resection must be undertaken only for urgent reasons, and its performance is more hazardous than resection in the presence of carcinoma.

Surgical intervention in vesico-enteric fistula should be by a graded procedure. The mortality rate is very high following resection in a single stage, the operation is difficult, and we believe it should be almost a routine to perform colostomy first, clear up the infection in the urinary tract, increase the patient's resistance, subsequently divide the bladder from the sigmoid, close the openings in both viscera, and at a later stage close the colonic stoma.

CHRONIC ULCERATIVE COLITIS

Chronic ulcerative colitis has been recognized as a desperate condition when it necessitates surgical intervention. Until recently, it has been attacked by perhaps more different types of therapeutic agents than one can readily describe. The etiology of this disease, although still somewhat controversial is ascribed by Bargen to an organism of the diplostreptococcus variety found in the ulcers in the rectum of patients with the disease, in the wall of the diseased colon after death, in distant foci of infection, or in the blood stream of some of the animals with the more severe type of the disease. Bargen has been able to reproduce similar characteristic lesions in rabbits and dogs by injection of this organism. Finally, the clinical evidence of improvement of patients after administration of a specific serum and vaccine prepared from these diplostreptococci strongly suggests that the organism is a probable factor in the disease, whether or not it is the sole agent. It is a severely debilitating infectious disease of insidious onset, the course of which is characterized by passage of blood, mucus, and pus in the stool or on the stool. Abdominal cramps and tenesmus mark the passage of these stools, which may or may not be increased in number at all times throughout the course of the disease. It is not unusual to find chronic ulcerative colitis beginning as a severe, fulminating illness, with many bloody rectal passages accompanied by gruelling cramps, fever, and prostration. The failure to recognize the fact that between these two extremes are all gradations of seriousness in symptoms, depending, in large measure, on the extent of intestinal involvement, has complicated and clouded the clinical picture, as well as the diagnosis.

It is an established fact that the disease affects various portions or all portions of the large bowel, usually by a diffuse type of lesion but occasionally by one that is localized in some one segment. Rarely is the terminal portion of the ileum attacked, although it is occasionally. There is strong reason to believe, supported by clinical, proctologic, and roentgenologic signs and symptoms, that chronic ulcerative colitis almost invariably begins in the rectum. When a large portion of the colon is invaded, liquid, mushy stools, mixed with pus and blood, are noted. Distress from gas, griping, and various sensations along the course of the colon are often noticed. It is almost always observed that the patient has a peculiar, grayish pallor, and anemia in consonance with this picture is the rule. In the more severe cases a morbid body odor prevails; an anxious, rather characteristic, sometimes described as hopeless facial expression is not uncommon and much loss of weight is customary. Lack of intestinal control usually causes the patient to feel that he must remain near a toilet room. Septic fever may occur in the complicated, severe, or fulminating cases, due to absorption from the colon, or from formation of abscesses and other complications, but in the chronic, usual case, a slight elevation of temperature also is noted. Mild leukocytosis may be present, and chronic invalidism occurs early in the disease.

Proctoscopic examination gives the most important data for diagnosis. The picture of the mucosa of the rectum and lower part of the sigmoid is described as having four phases in the active period of the disease; namely, hyperemia, edema, miliary abscesses, and miliary ulcers. The condition is not easily confused by an experienced proctologist with that of any other known lesion in this situation. When the disease enters the state of remission, and healing begins, the glazed, contracted scars and pitted mucosa are rarely difficult to distinguish from other lesions. Granular ulceration, punched scars, and contraction of the lumen of the bowel are pathognomonic proctoscopic signs. Myriads of miliary abscesses and ulcers pepper the highly inflamed walls of the bowel; intense spasm, and later scarring contractions, produce the characteristic deformity, shown in the roentgenograms of a narrowed, shortened, and non-haustrated colon (Figs. 62 and 63).

Failure to perform sigmoidoscopic examination routinely when a complaint referable to the colon presents itself is very apt to permit a diagnosis of chronic ulcerative colitis or dysentery when actually carcinoma is responsible for the symptoms. One of us (Graham), in 1937, reported a number of such cases in which so-called compensatory diarrhea that exists in the face of almost complete obstruction of the large intestine prompted the diagnosis of chronic ulcerative colitis, amebic dysentery, spastic colon, and so forth. The following case is typical:

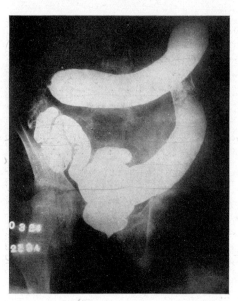

FIG. 62. Early chronic ulcerative colitis.

A woman, aged 51 years, was admitted to the hospital, with a diagnosis of chronic ulcerative colitis. Eleven months previously she commenced to have many small loose stools each day, consisting of fecal material, mucus, and blood, and this had persisted more or less up to the time of admission. During the same period she suffered intermittent abdominal cramps, the severity of which commenced to increase considerably about the ninth month of her illness. The other symptoms were gradual loss of weight (21 pounds) and strength; she had been bedridden for six weeks prior to admission to the hospital. Seven months previously, during a short stay in her local hospital, practically every laboratory test that could be desired had been made, including a complete gastrointestinal roentgenological study. The significant findings were, hemoglobin 68 per cent and a radiologic diagnosis of probable regional chronic ulcerative colitis of the descending colon. As for treatment, various regimes for chronic ulcerative colitis, including Bargen's specific serum, were employed, but without evidences of improvement in the patient's condition. The one examination which had not previously been made, namely, a sigmoidoscopic study, permitted a diagnosis of an annular ulcerating carcinoma situated at the rectosigmoid, a biopsy of which revealed adenocarcinoma, graded 3.

Treatment.—Without hesitation we would urge that these patients first be given medical treatment, whether according to the regimen established by Bargen, or by a satisfactory method used by others, or by a combination of the two, and that patients with the more severe cases, or one should say, the more complicated cases, who have failed to respond to medical treatment, be subjected to operation. In that group of cases in which the colon is isolated by ileostomy one must look forward to resection of the entire colon in most cases because of the presence of a focus for systemic disease, or the development of multiple polypi which subsequently may become malignant.

The spectacular results hopefully anticipated from the administration of chemotherapeutic agents and antibiotics have not materialized. Cave, in his recent (1946) valuable report on late results in the treatment of non-specific chronic ulcerative

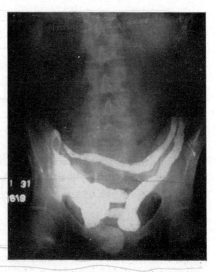

FIG. 63. Advanced chronic ulcerative colitis.

colitis, stated that the sulfonamides, except perhaps sulfathalidine, have been disappointing; penicillin has proved of no value; and in a personal communication from Dr. Charles Keefer, he learned that streptomycin which was tried in a considerable number of patients in the Army had proved valueless. These have also been our own personal experiences. Cave critically analyzed results in 50 of the 80 survivors of 101 patients operated upon for intractable ulcerative colitis. The 50 patients represent those who could be reached for a personal interview and examination. Twenty-four had been operated on five or more years previously. The average patient had gained 45 pounds. There was found to be surprising adaptability in the care of the ileostomy. Forty were at work. They included laborers, a bank clerk, insurance agents, a detective, dentist, a college professor, and a number of housewives who had resumed all of their household activities. Many of the younger patients played golf, baseball and tennis. In four of Cave's patients therapeutic abortions were undertaken owing to the fear of what would happen to the ileal stoma and to the mucous fistula of the divided lower sigmoid segment, if pregnancies were allowed to proceed. Peterson, however, states that three of his patients who had colectomies have delivered normal babies without difficulty.

Elsom and Ferguson also reported favorably on end results of surgery in their appraisal of the medical versus the surgical treatment in a series of 50 cases, of which 23 were treated medically and 27 by surgical measures.

ADENOMATOSIS (POLYPOSIS)

Adenomatosis, which probably is the more accurate term, is one of the most potentially serious lesions found in the colon. Because there is a marked tendency of these polyps to undergo malignant degeneration this condition has been considered in detail in the chapter on etiology.

There is usually little difficulty in establishing the diagnosis if the condition is kept in mind and the patient is subjected to a thorough gastro-intestinal investigation. The patients are usually young adults of an average age of 30 years. However, the extreme ages do not escape, for there are reported cases of occurrence of the disease in children of $2\frac{1}{2}$ years and adults past 70 years of age. The chief complaint usually is concerned with some alteration in the bowel habitus, particularly diarrhea. A history of continuous, intermittent or recurring diarrhea existing for months or years may not alone suggest a specific influence, but, if the irregularity occurs in a young adult in whose family other members have been similarly affected, the search should be directed toward adenomatosis. The age incidence and the hereditary or familial factor have been repeatedly emphasized by several observers and in our own series these influences have been frequently noted. The stools may contain blood or mucus, which are in no way characteristic of this particular entity.

A story of recurrent cramps may imply intermittent obstruction. It is a common complaint and is often due to intussusception. The polyps stimulate the bowel activity to abnormal proportions, which induces various degrees of invagination in the bowel. The infectious processes, such as amebiasis, chronic ulcerative colitis, and the dysenteries, can usually be eliminated as causative factors by bacteriologic and cultural studies of the stools.

Weight loss, a secondary anemia, debility, and general weakness parallel the intensity of involvement and infection, which at times are so marked as to create grave suspicion of malignancy. Quite often the diagnosis is made by the simple procedure of placing an examining finger into the rectum, where open nodular polyps are felt. This portion of the gastro-intestinal tract, so easily accessible to investigation, is more frequently the site of adenomatosis. Schmieden and Westhues quoted the statistics of Thorbecke, who found the rectum involved in 54 of 70 cases in which polypoid tumors were found. Similarly, Soper found the rectum involved 95 per cent of 61 cases of polyposis of the colon. The examination should not rest at this point, but should be supplemented by sigmoidoscopic search and roentgenologic studies of the barium-filled colon if one would deny oneself the embarrassment of subsequent exposure of unsuspected polyps at higher levels when they may prolapse through a colostomy stoma. Polyposis will often elude detection by the usual roentgenologic methods for visualizing colonic lesions, consequently when in doubt, it is well to employ the "combined double contrast" method described by Fischer and modified by Weber. The technic has been described in the chapter on diagnosis. The lacy net-work of shadows produced after expulsion of the barium and injection of air into the rectum is said to be pathognomonic of generalized polyposis (Fig. 64).

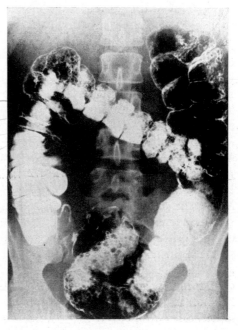

Fig. 64. Combined method. Generalized polyposis. The lacy network of shadows is pathognomonic of the condition. See also Fig. 66 (H. M. Weber).

Treatment.—The debilitation resulting from prolonged diarrhea, blood loss, and chronic infection, and the pathologic knowledge of the high incidence of malignant change occurring in diffuse adenomatosis of the colon are the factors that have made radical surgical treatment imperative. To remove a part of the involved bowel, leaving diseased segments, has proved of temporizing benefit at the best. Obviously, then, to be permanently free from the process, treatment had to be designed to remove the whole colon.

Colectomy when first performed was a formidable procedure and, when undertaken in one stage without considerable preparation and rehabilitation, carried a high mortality. A temporary ileostomy was soon devised and its value or necessity was immediately appreciated. By sidetracking the fecal current in this way the associated infection subsided and the rectal discharges of blood and mucus were greatly reduced to allow for marked general improvement. The patient's weight usually registered an appreciable increase, the secondary anemia was frequently overcome without transfusion, and the patient's general health was more sturdy and able to withstand the shock of a major surgical procedure.

With the colon at rest and peristalsis at low ebb, the infection and some of the polyps readily subside and make the colon more easily manageable when resection is undertaken. An optional period of about six months is desirable for an ileostomy. In addition to allowing for favorable changes in the colon, the ileum is given time for necessary adjustments vital to restoration of fluid balance. At first the substance issuing from the ileostomy is liquid and more or less continuous, but in time it is altered in consistency to a semi-solid state. Whitaker's recent (1937) studies on the physiology of permanent ileostomy are discussed in the chapter on physiology. Whether the ileum dilates sufficiently to take over some of the functions of the colon or whether, as Wakefield suggested, the kidneys compensate in maintaining the electrolytic balance of the body, the benefits of the procedure preceding total colectomy or subtotal colectomy are definitely established. Any artificial stoma of the gastro-intestinal tract will meet with objection from the patients; but when the benefits of such a procedure are enumerated their sanction is readily secured, particularly when the inconvenience is temporary. With recent improvement and modification in the surgical attack on diffuse adenomatosis, the rectum is more frequently saved than destroyed and provides a site for subsequent anastomosis of the ileum, which dispenses with the ileostomy as a permanent fixture. One of us (Rankin), in 1937, reported a personal series of 13 cases operated on, in 6 of which only a total colectomy was done, and in the remaining 7 the rectum was removed as well, but as a multiple-stage procedure; there was one operative death. The details of technic are considered in the chapter on operative procedures.

ACTINOMYCOSIS

Actinomycosis is a chronic disease caused by the fungus actinomyces hominis. The mode of infection is uncertain, although the prevailing view is that the disease reaches man through diseased cattle. Good, in 1931, in reporting 62 cases of actinomycosis of the abdomen, stated that the source of the disease was evident in only a few cases. Thirty-six per cent of the patients were farmers.

The site of the lesion is predominantly primary in the ileocecal region (77.5 per cent according to Good).

The early symptoms of the disease are those usually associated with acute or subacute appendicitis, together with the presence of a mass in the region of the cecum which is in most cases fixed to the anterior abdominal wall. The pain and tenderness referable to the mass is less prominent than will ordinarily be encountered in appendiceal masses of similar size. The disease is usually characterized by the formation of abscesses, sinuses, granulation tissue and brawny, leathery infiltration of the surrounding tissues. Until sinuses appear, identification is seldom possible, and depends on the roentgenologic studies. A positive diagnosis is made by demonstrating the sulphur granules after the formation of sinuses, or by demonstrating the actinomycetic lesion in tissue, microscopically.

Treatment.—This consists of: (1) radical extirpation as for a malignant lesion when possible; (2) free drainage; (3) the administration of massive doses of potassium or sodium iodide; (4) the application of roentgen rays and radium; and (5) general restorative measures. Satisfactory results in the treatment of actinomycosis are dependent in large measure on its early recognition. The prognosis in the abdominal form of the disease is grave and extensive lesions seldom are cured. Of Good's 62 cases, follow-up reports could not be obtained in 20. In the remaining 42, however, 29 patients are dead, the average length of life is twenty-one months from the beginning of the disease.

NONSPECIFIC GRANULOMA

Nonspecific infectious granuloma of the colon has been recognized as a disease entity since about the turn of the present century. In one of the earlier publications on this condition, Moynihan, under the heading "The mimicry of malignant disease in the large intestines" reported six cases in which the clinical manifestation and gross appearance of the lesion at operation were those of malignancy. Rankin, in 1926, reviewed the literature and reported a case operated on by him. Since then we have encountered many such tumors, principally in the ascending colon. The most comprehensive résumé of this entire subject was made by Mock in 1931.

Often the right-sided tumors are diagnosed acute or subacute appendicitis and they present two clinical pictures: (1) the fulminating inflammatory variety; and (2) the subacute or stenotic type. In the first type, the attack is ushered in with pain, usually accompanied by nausea and vomiting and local tenderness over the cecal region. Some reaction in temperature is noted and the slight rise in leukocytosis and pulse rate warrant a diagnosis of acute appendicitis. In the second type, however, the symptoms are not urgent and extend over a period of from several days to several weeks, during which time there may be distinct recessing of symptoms followed by exacerbation and the appearance of a tumor mass over the outline of the colon. The great difficulty in diagnosis, even with the aid of the roentgenoscope, is illustrated in a series of cases reported by Bargen and Jacobs. Of 9 cases operated on, there was

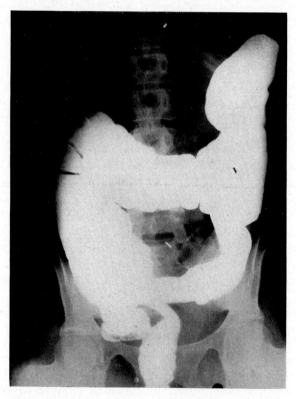

FIG. 65. Deformity of rectum and distal sigmoid due to an infective granuloma; diagnosis confirmed microscopically (Medical College of Virginia).

a clinical diagnosis of carcinoma or "tumor" in 8, and of hyperplastic tuberculosis in one instance. The roentgenologic examination in most of these cases revealed evidence suggestive of malignancy. Eventually, in every instance, the lesion proved to be an inflammatory cecal tumor. However, study of the resected tumor was necessary on two occasions in order to establish the diagnosis. Bargen states that in these cases the history is the important clue. The usual absence of anemia and the patient's general sense of well-being offer important differential suggestions. Moreover, the appearance of the patient is not that of the usual one presenting a malignant lesion in the proximal half of the colon. Finally, studied roentgenograms should permit a differentiation in most instances: the filling defect typical of a malignant condition is rarely present in such cases (Fig. 65).

MEGACOLON

There are two types of megacolon. The first is the acquired type which may be the result of any slowly stenosing process in the lower portion of the bowel, and which, gradually obstructing the lumen, is followed by dilatation and hypertrophy above, affecting first the bowel in immediate justaposition to it, and subsequently the entire colon. We have observed three cases of this type secondary to slowly stenosing annular carcinoma of the rectosigmoid, and many other observers have reported similar conditions. The second, and perhaps the more common lesion with which giant colon is associated, is so-called Hirschsprung's disease, or congenital idiopathic megacolon, the classical description of which Hirschsprung gave as follows: "A condition of congenital high-grade dilatation of the colon with thickening of all of its tunics, but particularly the tunics muscularis, and retention of large quantities of fecal matter." The pathologic picture is a constant one in Hirschsprung's disease, and unquestionably there are gradations of this hypertrophy and dilatation; a bowel may be dilated and slightly thickened, or there may be the huge, distended colon of the pot-bellied, constipated youth, who presents a clinical picture that is unmistakable. The cause of this condition remains obscure, and a search of the literature reveals numerous hypotheses advanced in explanation of it which may be classified under five headings: (1) congenital defect (Hirschsprung's); (2) obstructive process; (3) anatomic conditions such as malformation, aplasia of the musculature immediately above the rectum, mechanical obstruction, congenital stricture, general systemic conditions; (4) nervous mechanisms, such as segmental neuromuscular defects; (5) effect of the sympathetic nervous system; and (6) infectious process.

The clinical picture of true megacolon which occur in infancy is so characteristic that there is little difficulty in distinguishing it from other conditions, particularly when roentgenologic evidence is available in conjunction with a carefully taken clinical history. Usually the onset of symptoms is immediately after birth and difficulty in moving the bowels increases with growth. Distention, which is the result of retention of great quantities of gas and fecal matter, is little influenced by catharsis, and long periods of constipation, despite treatment, are the rule. Sometimes the patients go for weeks, and in some instances for months, without a movement of the bowels. The appearance of the patient is characteristic; the dry skin, the dull facies, the emaciation, are almost invariably present. The sphincter ani is generally normal, but the condition usually begins immediately above it. The characteristic roentgenologic picture of the colon completes the diagnosis.

Treatment.—Certain types of megacolon still are satisfactorily treated by resection and anastomosis. However, recent discoveries of the influence of surgical interruption of the nerve supply to the large bowel are convincing that this type of attack in certain cases and in perhaps the majority of instances is more nearly the ideal treatment than any other. Certainly, our experience with operations on the sympathetic nervous system in recent years has convinced us of its efficacy. One of us (Rankin), in 1935, reported 10 such operations; 7 were for congenital idiopathia (Hirschsprung's disease) and 3 for constipation of the obstinate variety. The general results were found to be superior to other surgical measures formerly instituted for megacolon and with a lower mortality and shorter hospitalization.

Penick in 1945 reported the results in 11 patients on whom left lumbar sympathectomy was performed by the staff of Tulane University and the Ochsner Clinic. In seven the results were highly satisfactory. All but one of the remaining four were greatly benefited. One case was a complete failure, but this result was not unexpected since the therapeutic test with spinal anesthesia had had little effect preoperatively.

The sympathetic nerves to the distal part of the colon and the rectum have their immediate origin in the intermesentric plexuses, descend on the anterolateral aspects of the abdominal aorta, from the level of origin of the superior mesenteric artery downward. On each side there are two or three large trunks, made of non-myelinated fibers arising from (1) the semilunar ganglia of the celiac plexus; (2) an anastomotic loop which crosses the aorta transversely below the origin of the superior mesenteric artery, and (3) the aorticorenal ganglion, or the renal periarterial plexus. Branches from the first and second lumbar ganglia join the intermesenteric plexus on each side. There is a difference of opinion among anatomists concerning the extent to which the lumbar mingle with those of the intermesenteric plexus proper. Some hold that the mesially directed lumbar communicating branches constituting the pelvic splanchnic nerves remain distinct in the outer portion of the plexus and ultimately form the lateral roots of the presacral nerve of Latarjet. Hovelacque, on the other hand, holds that the lumbar communicating branches actually contribute to the intermesenteric plexus. The point is one of not a little significance, for if the former view is correct, lumbar ramisectomy and ganglionectomy would affect only that portion of the bowel innervated through the presacral nerve, namely the lower portion of the rectum and sphincter ani. If the latter view is correct, the operation would affect, but only partly, the descending and sigmoid portions of the colon, as well as the rectum and internal sphincter ani. The beneficial results of lumbar ramisectomy in cases of Hirschsprung's disease strongly favor the view that the branches which join the intermesenteric plexus from the first and second lumbar ganglia do have a share in the innervation of the colon. It is generally accepted that the fibers of the inferior mesenteric plexus, which end in the musculature of the colon and rectum, carry impulses which inhibit its activity. Further, it would appear probable that these nerves keep up a continuous influence on the tonus of the bowel. In the dog, section of the corresponding nerves always leads to immediate increase in intracolonic pressure.

With reference to control of the internal sphincter of the anus, it has been found in experimental animals and in man that the thoracicolumbar outflow provides the motor supply of this muscle. Neuromuscular dysfunction, then, seems a reasonable explanation in a large number of cases of Hirschsprung's disease, and the essential pathologic anatomy of the lesion, which is dilatation with hypertrophy of the muscular coat, makes it impossible for the intestine to transmit its content. Consequently, by interrupting the sympathetic nerve supply, the surgeon may attempt (1) to diminish the dilatation of the colon, (2) to leave its motor nerves under less disputed control, and (3) to relieve any opposition to the expulsion of the content of the bowel by the sphincteric mechanism. If the anatomic and physiologic reasoning is correct, the first and second objects are accomplished by division of the inferior mesenteric nerve, and the third by division of the presacral nerve. The details of technic, which have been described by Learmonth and Rankin, are considered in the chapter on operative procedure.

BENIGN TUMORS*

These tumors are of surgical interest mainly because occasionally they produce obstruction, either chronic or acute. They do not produce characteristic symptoms and until Fischer introduced a method whereby such tumors could be readily visualized roentgenoscopically they were seldom diagnosed except at necropsy or during exploration of the abdomen. Such tumors comprise adenomas, fibromas, myomas, lipomas, angiomas, hemangiomas, and cholesteatomas. Adenomas and lipomas are by far the most frequently encountered benign tumors of the colon. The chief signifi-

---

* Polyposis is considered separately.

cance of adenoma is its potential malignant nature, and of lipoma its tendency to cause intussusception. Buie reported 19,103 proctoscopic examinations over a period of four years at which 455 benign tumors were found, almost half of which did not produce symptoms.

Pack and Booher, in 1947, collected from the literature 153 cases of submucous lipoma of the large intestine. In 1949, Mayo and Griess added 19 cases which together with 24 cases previously reported by Comfort (1931) and Pemberton and McCormack (1937), make 43 cases in which operation has been performed for this condition at the Mayo Clinic up to the year 1948. The occur-

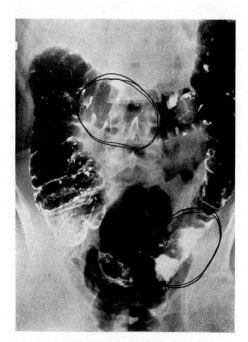

FIG. 66. Combined method. Large polypoid mass in the proximal part of sigmoid. Pedunculated polypoid mass in the distal part of the transverse colon (H. M. Weber).

rence in patients who are within the so-called cancer age, of 72 per cent of the lipomas which produce symptoms, as well as the often short duration of symptoms of loss of weight and blood in the stools may readily, states Comfort, suggest the presence of a malignant process. The preponderance of malignant lesions of the large intestines over benign lesions renders the differentiation increasingly difficult, especially since ulceration of a benign tumor not only produces, roentgenologically, a picture simulating malignancy, but the clinical course, because of anemia and obstruction, may be strikingly similar to that of a malignant condition.

In 1947, Helvig, and also Swinton and Haug, made valuable contributions to the literature of adenomas of the colon and rectum, based on exhaustive studies respectively of 1460 and 1843 consecutive autopsies in which the entire large bowel was investigated. Helwig found an incidence of benign colon and rectal polyps of 139, or 9.5 per cent and Swinton and Haug an incidence of 130, or 7 per cent. Both reports reveal an increasing incidence of benign adenomas with age, particularly after the third decade. In Helwig's series the peak incidence was reached in the eighth decade when 25.8 per cent of the men and 20.5 per cent of the women showed adenomas. Also in this series, after one case of familial polyposis was excluded, the remaining 138 specimens contained 272 adenomas. The incidence of adenomas in the 1,279 white patients was 10.4 per cent and in the 181 negro patients it was 2.7 per cent. The contrast becomes even greater when only those patients aged over 30 years are considered, for then the negro patients are 3 per cent and the white patients are 16 per cent. The incidence of a single lesion in the two reports were respectively 57 and 59 per cent. Helwig showed that adenomas of the colon are more frequent than adenomas of the rectum and that the sigmoid is the most common site of these growths in the large intestine.

Helwig made some interesting observations concerning the relation of adenoma and carcinoma (see also "Etiology"). In his study of the ten carcinomas arising in adenomas no definite pattern could be established for the occurrence of the foci of carcinoma. In several instances the malignant change occurred at the periphery of the adenoma, either at the tip or at the margin. In other specimens the transition occurred deep within the adenoma near the stalk at its base. With these facts it becomes obvious that an accurate histologic diagnosis demands that an adequate number of sections be observed. In eight of the ten intestines the transition to carcinoma occurred in only a single adenoma. In the other two intestines, carcinomatous change was present in two and three adenomas, respectively. In the 25 large intestines containing a manifest carcinoma, observed in this series, there were associated adenomas in 13 instances. In the ten intestines containing an adenoma with carcinomatous transition there were associated benign adenomas in eight instances. Swinton and Haug noted that 50, or 25.1 per cent of the patients in their series with carcinoma of the colon and rectum had associated benign polyps.

The two most important diagnostic aids which we possess are the proctoscopic examination and the roentgenologic method of Fischer (Fig. 66). Swinton has recently stressed that even with careful preparation by means of castor oil purgation, a low residue diet, colonic irrigations and double contrast method of roentgenologic examination by an experienced radiologist, the number of benign adenomas discovered in this manner is much less than the known incidence of such lesions in this region. Nevertheless, it is the best method now available. Although when the abdomen is opened careful palpation of the entire colon is indicated, exploratory operations for suspected adenomas are, as a rule, not justified since detection of adenomas of the large bowel by palpation is very difficult unless they are large or a limited area is under suspicion.

Treatment.—The treatment of these tumors varies according to its indication for some complications. When a tumor that does not produce symptoms is discovered accidentally simple colotomy with excision is sufficient (see "Palliative and Miscellaneous Procedures").

BLEEDING HEMORRHOIDS

The most constant sign of a carcinoma of the left half of the colon and rectum, in our experience, has been bright blood which may appear mixed with the stool or may simply streak the stool. If on the appearance of this danger sign every patient was subjected to the two simple procedures of digital and proctoscopic examinations, even in the presence of actually bleeding hemorrhoids, there would be few inoperable carcinomas of the rectum. Of 3,542 cases of malignancy of the large intestine, observed at the Mayo Clinic, 2,259, or roughly two-thirds of the cases occurred in the anus, rectum, and rectosigmoid. And between 90 and 95 per cent of these growths were in position to be palpated by the index finger if a careful rectal examination was made (Wheeler, Bargen). Of the remaining cases approximately a third were situated in the sigmoid, well within reach of the sigmoidoscope; in other words, not more than 25 per cent of all lesions encountered in the large bowel are so situated as to require diagnostic measures not available to every physician. Nevertheless, about 25 per cent of the patients in the foregoing series, and as high as 65 per cent in other series, were operated on for hemorrhoids before the lesion producing symptoms was identified. One of us (Graham) recently reported a series of cases of carcinoma of the rectum and rectosigmoid in which 31 per cent of the patients were so treated, yet all but one could be palpated with the finger. Fifty per cent of these cases treated first by hemorrhoidectomy were inoperable, while less than 25 per cent of the remainder of the series proved inoperable.

It is gratifying to establish without exploration that the lesion is not malignant, but to be certain of this is difficult. In addition to the foregoing conditions which most frequently confuse the diagnosis in instances of pathology of the large intestine one occasionally must differentiate between malignancy and intussusception, volvulus, foreign bodies, fecaliths, renal enlargement, retroperitoneal lesions, hydrops of the gallbladder which exerts pressure on the ascending colon, and other conditions each one of which, in our experience, has led to a diagnosis of carcinoma of the colon on one or more occasions. The roentgenogram, particularly after the method of Fischer, has in a large measure done away with the former differential difficulty.

REFERENCES

1. BARGEN, J. A.: Chronic ulcerative colitis: A review of investigation on etiology. *Arch. Int. Med.*, **45**: 559–572 (March), 1930.

2. BARGEN, J. A.: Modern management of colitis. Springfield, Charles C Thomas, Publisher, 1943.

3. BUIE, L. A., and SWAN, T.: Benign tumors of the colon. *Surg. Clinics, N. Am.*, **9**: 893–910, 1929.

4. CAVE, HENRY W.: Late results in the treatment of ulcerative colitis. *Ann. Surg.*, **124**: 716–724 (Oct.), 1946.

5. COMFORT, M. W.: Submucous lipomata of the gastro-intestinal tract; report of twenty-eight cases. *Surg., Gynec., and Obst.*, **52**: 110–118 (Jan.), 1931.

6. FISCHER: Quoted by Weber (27).

7. GOOD, L. P.: Actinomycosis of the abdomen. *Arch. Surg.*, **22**: 307–313 (Feb.), 1931.

8. GOLDSTEIN: Quoted by Rankin, Bargen and Buie.

9. GRAHAM, A. STEPHENS: Carcinoma of the sigmoid and rectum: Common diagnostic errors which are readily avoidable; Case Reports. *Virginia Med. Monthly*, **64**: 143–146 (June), 1937.

10. HELWIG, E. B.: The evolution of adenomas of the large intestine and their relation to carcinoma. *Surg., Gynec., and Obstet.*, **84**: 36–49 (Jan.), 1947.

11. MAYO, C. W., and GREISS, DONALD F.: Submucous lipoma of the colon. *Surg., Gynec., and Obstet.*, **88**: 309–316 (Mar.), 1949.

12. PACK, G. T., and BOOBER, K. J.: Quoted by Mayo and Greiss (11).

13. MORTON, JOHN J.: Diverticulitis of the colon. *Ann. Surg.*, **124**: 725–745 (Oct.), 1946.

14. PEMBERTON, JOHN DE J., and DIXON, CLAUDE F.: Summary of end-results of treatment of malignancy of the colon, including the rectum and anus. *Surg., Gynec., and Obst.*, **58**: 462–464 (Feb.), 1934.

15. PENICK, R. M. JR.: Surgical treatment of congenital megacolon. *Jour. Am. Med. Assoc.*, **128**: 423–426 (June 9), 1945.

16. RANKIN, F. W.: Surgery of the Colon, New York. D. Appleton & Co., 1926. 366 pages.

17. RANKIN, F. W.: Malformations of the colon. In: Lewis, Dean: Practice of Surgery, Hagerstown, Maryland, W. F. Prior Co., Inc., **7**: 31 pp. 1929.

18. RANKIN, F. W.: "Progress in surgery of the colon." *Bulletin of the School of Medicine of Maryland*, **17**: 35 pp. (Oct.), 1931.

19. RANKIN, F. W.: Treatment of Hirschsprung's disease. *Kentucky M. J.*, **33**: 474–478 (Oct.) 1935.

20. RANKIN, F. W. and BROWN, P. W.: Diverticulitis of the colon. *Surg., Gynec., and Obst.*, **50**: 836–847 (May), 1930.

21. RANKIN, F. W., and CHUMLEY, CHARLES L.: Lymphosarcoma of the colon and rectum. *Minnesota Med.*, **12**: 247–253 (May), 1929.

22. RANKIN, F. W., and GRIMES, A. E.: Diffuse adenomatosis of the colon. *Jour. Am. Med. Assn.*, **108**: 711–715 (Feb. 27), 1937.

23. RANKIN, F. W., and LEARMONTH, J. R.: Section of the sympathetic nerve of the distal part of the colon and the rectum in the treatment of Hirschsprung's disease and certain types of constipation. *Ann. Surg.*, **92**: 710–720 (Oct.), 1930.

24. RANKIN, F. W., and MAJOR, S. G.: Surgical treatment of tuberculosis of the large bowel. *Surg., Gynec., and Obst.*, **55**: 494–501 (Oct.), 1932.

25. SCHMIEDEN and WESTHUES: Quoted by FitzGibbon and Rankin.

26. SWINTON, N. W., and HAUG, A. D.: The frequency of precancerous lesions in the rectum and colon. *Lahey Clinic Bull.*, **5**: 84–88 (Jan.), 1947.
27. WEBER, H. M: The Roentgenologic demonstration of polypoid lesions and polyposis of the large intestine. *Am. Jour. Roentgenol. and Radium Therap.*, **25**: 577–589 (May), 1931.
28. WHEELER: Quoted by Brindley.

PART II
TREATMENT

CHAPTER VI

OPERABILITY, RESECTABILITY AND PROGNOSIS

Operability, or resectability, prognosis, and mortality are closely related. Factors which influence resectability also affect prognosis, and too low a mortality figure often reflects a low resectability, the result of an overly cautious selection of cases. By making every effort to extend the horizon of resectability rather than to contract it, one finds the death rate increasing rather than receding, but by so doing more patients out of a given number are found alive at the end of periods of five and ten years after resection.

Lockhart-Mummery has said that the word "prognosis" does not lend itself very easily to definition. As generally accepted it means a prophecy as to the future history of the patient; more particularly the chances there are of his being cured of the disease from which he suffers and the chances of his survival without treatment. The assertion is frequently made that carcinoma of the large intestine is attended by favorable prognosis if the growth is radically extirpated before visceral metastasis has developed. Such has been our observation and experience. On the other hand, prognosis in an untreated patient is very unfavorable and except in rare instances, then usually in elderly individuals, the patient dies within two years of the onset of symptoms. Oettle, in 1935, studied the fate of thirty patients with carcinoma of the rectum who refused operation. Microscopic diagnosis was established in each case. The average duration of life for twenty-eight of the patients was 10.4 months, not one of these living as long as a year. Of the remaining two, one lived three and a half years and the other four years. Eighty-four per cent complained of severe pain; 24 per cent of bladder disturbances.

Daland, Welch, and Nathanson, the following year, reviewed 100 untreated cases of carcinoma of the rectum, 80 cases in which colostomy alone was performed, and 32 cases in which the only treatment was colostomy and radiotherapy. The duration of life from onset of symptoms is shown in Table 8. The operative mortality in the group with palliative colostomy was 12.5 per cent. Similarly, Ottenheimer, in 1947, demonstrated almost identical longevity curves for 430 patients who had palliative colostomies or else received no treatment.

We consider resectability rate to be of far greater significance than operability rate in comparing statistics of various surgeons and institutions. Resectability is a readily calculable figure which is based on tangible data. It is simply the percentage of patients of all those subjected to operation on whom resection of the involved segment of bowel is undertaken. The term "operability," as employed here, implies conditions favorable and unfavorable to the removal of malignant growths situated in the colon and rectum. Intangible and variable factors are considered, such as inclusion of those patients who are considered operable but who refuse operation, when actually inoperability cannot be determined until the abdomen is explored.

TABLE 8

CARCINOMA OF THE RECTUM (DALAND, WELCH, AND NATHANSON)
Untreated cases

	Cases	Duration of Life in Months From Onset of Symptoms	
		Average	Medium
Untreated cases..............	100	17.2	14.0
Colostomy, only.............	80	16.9	14.0
Colostomy and radiotherapy...	32	18.8	15.0

In reviewing the literature, one will observe that there is some difference of opinion as to that which should constitute the "rate of operability." Newman, in reporting the results of an exhaustive world-wide study of 6,000 recorded cases of cancer of the rectum for the British Ministry of Health, defined operability as follows:

"Having diagnosed cancer of the rectum the surgeon has to decide whether the disease can be extirpated by what he regards as a 'radical operation.' The condition of the patient in which, in the opinion of the surgeon, such a result can be achieved constitutes his 'operability'; the 'index of operability' for any particular surgeon should therefore be the ratio of the number of cases *recommended* for radical operation to the total number of cases observed by the surgeon. Owing, however, to the form in which the data are usually presented in the literature the numerator of the above fraction usually employed is the number of patients actually submitted to radical operation; and even this figure is not always available as the surgeon frequently fails to record the total number of cases which he has observed, thus giving an inaccurate denominator as well. It is believed, however, that the error due to the first of these causes is negligible."

Unless statistical data are reported in minute detail they have little scientific value and an accurate comparison of results in different series of cases becomes impossible. Figures such as those prepared by Postlethwait for Duke University Hospital (Tables 9,

10) are of great value, for they reveal the entire experience of the institution over a period of fifteen years from 1931 to 1945. This detailed study reveals not only the resectability but also the "curative resection rate." The latter figure is obtained by deducting from the total number of resections undertaken those cases resected for palliation in the face of distant metastasis. One of us (Rankin) has also recently reported his total experience in private practice in which a detailed analysis of the disposition of hospitalized patients is presented (Table 40).

TABLE 9

DISPOSITION OF 441 PATIENTS OBSERVED AT DUKE HOSPITAL AND CLINIC (Postlethwait—1947)

		R	RS	S	D	S	T	H	A	C	Total
Not Admitted	Went elsewhere	11	1	2					1		15
	Refused admission	10									10
	Did not return	5									5
	Inoperable	5								2	7
	No bed	3									3
	X-ray only	2								1	3
	Total	36	1	2				1		3	43
Admitted to Hospital	Inoperable Disch	20	1	1					2	2	26
	Inoperable D.I.H.	3	2	1				2	2		10
	Op. deferred	5		1							6
	Op. refused	18	3	3				1	6	2	33
	X-ray only	3								1	4
	Died pre-op	1			1			1			3
	Operated on	143	22	55	19	8	8	13	12	36	316
	Total	193	28	61	20	8	8	17	22	41	398

While the criteria of operability or resectability must be variable, they unquestionably should be broad, as they differ with the judgment, experience, and boldness of the operating surgeon. Even among surgeons of considerable experience and outstanding ability, the personal equation in estimating operability it attested by the wide variation of the percentage of operability, ranging from 30 per cent to nearly 90 per cent. However, the standard of resectability has gradually improved with refinement of surgical technic, improvement in anesthetic methods, the advent of chemotherapy and development of greater skill by individual surgeons.

The individual rates of operability or of resectability of different surgeons and institutions will be given later in a discussion of "Mortality and End-Results."

Influences which modify the outlook preliminary to and following surgical treatment of patients with carcinoma of the colon and

TABLE 10

RESECTABILITY IN 441 CASES OF CARCINOMA OF THE COLON
AND RECTUM (Duke Hospital-Postlethwait—1947)

	Entire Group			Curative Operation		
Race	White 83%		Colored 17%	White 89%		Colored 11%
Sex	Male 57%		Female 43%	Male 48%		Female 52%
Age	11–40 15.0%	41–60 44.6%	61–90 40.4%	11–40 16.9%	41–60 49.7%	61–90 33.4%

rectum group themselves into extrinsic and intrinsic elements; the former represent general conditions of the host and certain conditions local to the neoplasm, whereas the latter represent the intensity of the malignant cells:

I. EXTRINSIC INFLUENCES:

Age and sex of patient
Loss of weight and anemia
General debility
Associated chronic diseases such as diabetes and tuberculosis
Obesity
Situation and duration of growth
Fixation
Obstruction
Size and direction of growth
Glandular metastasis
Perforation

II. INTRINSIC INFLUENCES:

Activity of the neoplastic cells, especially their ability to differentiate or approach the normal state

Age and sex of patient.—In young people cancer tends to grow with extreme rapidity and to spread quickly to other structures. Lockhart-Mummery stated that he had no record of a patient under thirty years of age treated for cancer of the rectum who had not died from prompt recurrence. Rankin and Comfort reviewed a series of 38 cases of carcinoma of the rectum in individuals aged thirty years or less and found the duration of symptoms was shorter, the percentage of metastasis greater, the rate of operability lower, and the percentage of ultimately satisfactory results after periods of three and five years greatly decreased. This series, which represented 3.85 per cent of the total number of patients with rectal carcinoma operated on at The Mayo Clinic during the years 1907 to 1926 inclusive, is too small to allow a definite conclusion to be drawn from it, but when our subsequent experience and that of other surgeons is taken into consideration also, the distinct impression is that surgery in such cases is probably seldom worth while, particularly if the degree of malignancy is graded 3 or 4. Table 11 shows the greater malignancy in the group of rectal carcinoma reported by Rankin and Comfort than in patients of all ages taken together.

On the other hand, when the lymphatic structures of advanced age have undergone atrophic changes and no longer are active, carcinoma is held in check and remains local for a much longer period than if the patient is young and possesses vigor and vitality. Consequently it is doubtful whether it is worth while operating on very old persons aged eighty years and more, except to relieve obstruction, should this develop.

TABLE 11

COMPARATIVE PERCENTAGE IN INCIDENT OF VARIOUS GRADES OF MALIGNANCY IN RECTAL CARCINOMAS IN PATIENTS THIRTY YEARS OF AGE OR LESS AND OF ALL AGES TAKEN TOGETHER (RANKIN AND BRODERS' SERIES)

Age	Grade 1	Grade 2	Grade 3	Grade 4	Total Cases
Thirty years or less...	13.15%	34.21%	31.57%	21.05%	38
All ages............	17.55%	50.00%	23.57%	8.86%	598

Age *per se* is not a satisfactory criterion by which to judge a patient's ability to withstand resection of the colon or rectum. Many persons aged seventy years and more are excellent surgical risks because of the soundness of their body structures, particularly the cardiovascular system, in which atheromatous changes have been slow to develop. Until very recently it was felt that few patients over sixty years of age constituted good risks for the abdomino perineal operation in one stage, but ample statistical data attest the generally favorable outcome even in patients aged more than seventy. Prior to 1940 the two-stage procedures, including colostomy and posterior excision, were employed in most instances of carcinoma of the rectum in persons older than sixty. In recent years, however, it has been found practical to undertake the one-stage resection, whether for lesions of the right colon or of the rectum, without regard to age in most instances. The indications for multiple-stage procedures are the same for all age periods namely, obstruction, infection and marked debility.

The influence of sex on operability is quite definite. Newman reports that the rate of operability in carcinoma of the rectum is higher and the prospects of survival are better for women than for men, after radical resection. This advantage of women over men is due probably to the greater extent of the female pelvis and its increased resistance to infection. Furthermore, the close relationship of the anterior wall of the rectum to the prostate gland and seminal vesicles results in frequent involvement of these structures in growths situated on the anterior wall.

Loss of weight and anemia.—Excessive loss of weight and strength indicate metastasis to distant organs in most cases. In fact so many patients examined by us have been in such apparent health in spite of long histories and advanced lesions that we have begun to think of the robust individual as the type subject to carcinoma of the rectum. Inoperability can rarely be proven conclusively, regardless of the degree of weight loss, until the abdomen has been explored; occasionally, as we have observed, a growth is operable in spite of considerable loss of both weight and strength.

In determining operability and prognosis very little significance can be attached to reading of the hemoglobin. Illustrative of this fact is the following experience of one of us (Graham) with five consecutive cases of carcinoma of the sigmoid or rectum which were hospitalized about the same time. Case 1, weight normal, hemoglobin 96 per cent, inoperable because of marked glandular and hepatic metastasis; Case 2, twenty-four-pound weight loss, hemoglobin 72 per cent, definitely operable (these cases were operated on consecutive days, the first being considered operable and the second questionably operable); Case 3, weight normal, hemoglobin 102 per cent, distinct glandular involvement, died nine months after palliative resection; Case 4, recent gain in weight, numerous moderate rectal hemorrhages, hemoglobin 106 per cent, operable; Case 5, thirty-pound loss in weight, numerous moderate rectal hemorrhages, hemoglobin 76 per cent, definitely operable. The determinations of hemoglobin were all carried out in the same laboratory by trained technicians and by one of the more accurate methods. It is quite evident that repeated hemorrhages in one instance produce secondary anemia and in another they stimulate the production of hemoglobin.

Anemia commonly associated with lesions of the proximal colon is not a contraindication to exploration and resection even though the concentration of hemoglobin is as low as 25 or 30 per cent. Such anemia in carcinoma of the stomach or of the left half of the colon would be prohibitive for resection, but frequently we have resected the right half of the colon in the face of profound anemia without mortality. Regardless of the percentage of hemoglobin the fact is now well recognized that employment of routine blood transfusions before and immediately after the more formidable resections, particularly the Miles procedure, influences the prognosis favorably.

General debility and associated chronic disease.—It is seldom necessary to deny surgery to patients with carcinoma of the large intestine because of their physical status. Some surgeons consider age and general debility an important influence and that freedom from such diseases as tuberculosis, diabetes, cardiorenal disease, and so forth is essential. Miles and Abel, for instance, eliminate those patients whose cardiac energy is estimated to be below 25 per cent as calculated by the Moots-McKesson pressure ratio percentage test. However, we have observed many patients withstand successfully the strain of a formidable resection of the rectum whose cardiac energy was estimated to be below the minimum requirement of these surgeons. On the other hand, there are surgeons of wide experience who exclude cases only on the grounds that metastasis is present or that important structures are involved which cannot be removed. This discrepancy in opinion naturally gives rise to marked variation in the rates of resectability.

It appears unreasonable to us to eliminate arbitrarily patients as inoperable merely because they are elderly or because their less robust organs are potentially the sites of postoperative complications. Considering the advanced stage of the disease at which so many, perhaps the majority, of patients with lesions in the large intestine present themselves for examination and treatment, such decision would deprive a large percentage of these sufferers of the hope of cure. We go even further and advocate exploration for many of those who, besides harboring carcinoma, suffer from chronic diseases such as diabetes, tuberculosis, syphilis, or cardiovascular and renal disease. Although a certain number of these patients will succumb to operation, it has been our experience that a still larger number not only survive operation but return to an improved state of general health.

Naturally, with inclusion of these cases the burden of responsibility becomes decidedly increased. Nevertheless, much of this can be offset favorably by meticulous attention to preoperative preparations, the selection of anesthesia, the choice of operation, and postoperative treatment. Emergency operations are rarely demanded in lesions of the large intestine, even when partial obstruction exists; consequently these cases may be considered chronic ailments which permit of more leisurely examination and the combating of dehydration and desiccation by intravenous administration of fluids, transfusions, and adequate dietary regime. Patients suffering with diabetes or cardiorenal disease are carefully prepared by well-trained clinicians and after surgery remain under their strict surveillance and supervision. Another feature of considerable importance in dealing with the markedly debilitated individual is the matter of graded procedures.

Obesity.—Obesity, especially if acquired rapidly, signifies faulty metabolism and lowered resistance. Mechanically, it may represent a handicap to the surgeon who finds it technically difficult to operate in the presence of large amounts of fat, particularly in instances of carcinoma of the rectum in the male subject. If the resectability is already in doubt, the presence of this fat offers a most serious condition.

In the colon a factor secondary in importance only to the anatomic peculiarities and the sufficiency of the blood supply is the presence of excessive quantities of retroperitoneal and mesenteric fat and subperitoneal deposits of fat on the bowel. If patients are obese the entire wall of the colon may be surrounded by fat in such amounts as to make it difficult to isolate a satisfactory area on the peritoneal surface for anastomosis. Moreover, in stout subjects the abdominal wall is usually thick and the pelvic mesocolon is often short, so that it may be impossible to bring a loop of sigmoid to the surface in order to establish a loop colostomy without undue tension. There is subsequently a persistent tendency for the colostomy to retract.

Not only does carcinoma usually spread faster if patients are obese, but the presence of infection, even in a mild degree, materially enhances the risk. The retroperitoneal spaces once infected permit rapid spreading and the resulting cellulitis is often fatal. Given the same pathologic process in two patients of the same age and otherwise equal chances, one finds the obese patient is a greater risk and a poorer outlook from the standpoint of ultimate cure.

Situation and duration of growth.—The situation of the growth is an important factor in determining resectability and prognosis, because the pathologic types vary in different parts of the large intestine and because of the influence on the time at which symptoms and signs appear. Carcinoma of the right half of the colon, for a reason which we are not able to explain satisfactorily, permits better prognosis than carcinoma of the left half (Table 12). In case

TABLE 12

RELATIVE PERCENTAGES OF CURES IN RELATION TO SITUATION OF LESION IN THE COLON (RANKIN AND OLSON)

	Total	Dead	Five-year Cures	Per Cent Cured
Right half of colon including cecum...	187	81	106	57.6
Left half of colon including sigmoid...	266	139	127	47.7
Total......................	453	220	233	51.3

of carcinoma of certain segments of the right part of the colon, for
example the cecum, there is a higher percentage of five-year cures
or of freedom from recurrence than when other segments are involved. A subsequent discussion of the influence of the size of the
growth on prognosis will bring out the fact that lesions of the
proximal colon were larger than those of the distal segment and
that those of the cecum were of the largest average size, whereas
those of the sigmoid were smallest. This tendency of the cecal tumors to protrude into the lumen of the bowel away from the nodes
may explain the more favorable prognosis that attends lesions so
situated.

A majority of cancers of the rectum occur in its ampullary portion. The smallest percentage occur in the anal canal and around
the external anal orifice. Growths in the rectosigmoid, because of
early obstructive signs, usually are recognized earlier than growths
of the ampulla of the rectum and are more likely to be operable
than the latter. Growths in the ampulla, because of the large size
of the lumen, may exist until a late stage before symptoms develop.
In the meantime distant metastasis may have occurred. Neoplasm
of the anal canal and perianal region is usually epithelioma and can
always be recognized by superficial general examination and by
the severe pain it often causes. It seems entirely reasonable that
it should be diagnosed in its earlier stages and consequently offer
excellent prognosis. On the contrary, these growths are in most
instances highly malignant, metastasis occurs early and by way of
the inguinal nodes rather than upward toward the retroperitoneal
nodes; five-year cures are seldom noted. Once the inguinal nodes
are involved, radical operation is seldom curative.

The duration of the growth is a factor of importance in determining resectability and prognosis, but it is estimated with great
difficulty since persons do not know of the presence of carcinoma
of the left colon and rectum until it has produced obstruction or a
break in the mucous membrane which causes blood to appear in
the stool, and in the right colon until an abdominal mass is noted
or vague gastro-intestinal symptoms prompt roentgenologic studies
of the colon. The average patient having carcinoma of the colon,
rectosigmoid, or rectum will have known of symptoms on an average of ten months or more before seeking advice and many lesions
probably have existed a number of months before the initial symptom was recognized. Naturally ample opportunity is thus afforded
a rapidly growing, highly malignant tumor to dispense cells
through the lymphatic or blood channels to distant bases, yet apparently this is compensated in large measure by the low grade of
the growth in the majority of cases—perhaps an explanation also
of the well-known tendency to remain local over a relatively long
period of time.

Lymphatic involvement seldom occurs before the muscular coats of the bowel have become deeply invaded. Dukes has shown definitely that the more deeply the carcinoma has penetrated the rectal wall the greater the incidence of metastasis, the higher the mortality rate, and the lower the incidence of three-year and five-year cures. Gordon-Watson considers six months the minimum time in which lymphatic invasion can be expected; Miles believes that the fascia propria of the rectum is seldom penetrated until the disease has existed for eighteen months, and Wilkie estimates that carcinoma of the rectum remains localized in most instances at least a year. Rankin and Broders in a study of 598 cases of carcinoma of the rectum showed that when metastasis was absent, that is, when the duration of the growth was relatively short, the total good results were 57.87 per cent and when metastasis was present the total good results were only 20.68 per cent.

Attempts have been made to estimate the duration of a growth by the extent to which it has encircled the bowel. Miles is of the belief that eighteen months is required for complete encirclement of the large intestine and Cutting states that it takes approximately a year for carcinoma to progress three-fourths of the circumference.

Fixation.—Local fixation of a segment of colon or rectum which harbors carcinoma not infrequently rules out resection. We are confident, however, that immobility results more often from inflammatory reactions than from malignant extension and that it should not be regarded as too serious a deterrent to subsequent removal, particularly if this may be done at a later stage. In many cases carcinoma which was considered inoperable at primary exploration has receded to such an extent, after sidetracking the fecal current and after constant irrigation, that radical operation became justifiable and results were entirely satisfactory.

Fortunately, one may resect portions of the stomach or of the prostate gland, or a segment of bladder, or perform hysterectomy in the course of operation for extirpation of carcinoma of the colon or rectum with relatively satisfactory mortality in certain selected cases. Similarly, it is not incompatible with satisfactory end-results to excise a large portion of the anterior or parietal abdominal wall, provided there is not a better reason for excluding radical operation. Postoperative hernia and other such sequelae should be of secondary consideration in this connection. Occasionally one of these extremely radical procedures is followed by prolonged freedom from recurrence and encourages the practice of attempting to resect a large, fixed carcinoma. In the light of comparative results with other therapeutic measures, however, the suppression of carcinoma calls for extension in the scope of operability. Consequently each one of these cases demands shrewd judgment in the decision not only as to whether they are amenable to radical resection but whether palliative operation is indicated.

Thirty-five of the 200 patients recently (1947) studied by Gilchrist and David required resection of all or part of other structures because of firm fixation of the tumor (Table 13). Fourteen, or 40 per cent, of these patients were well five years. Gilchrist and David believe this figure would be higher today as seven, or 20 per cent, died postoperatively and this mortality would be favorably influenced by chemotherapy.

TABLE 13

CARCINOMAS OF LARGE BOWEL REQUIRING RESECTION OF ALL OR PART OF OTHER STRUCTURES

(35 CASES—GILCHRIST AND DAVID)

	No. Pts.	Well 5–10 Yr.	P. Op. Deaths	Recurrence			No Follow-Up
				Local	Liver	Gen.	
Pelvic fascia.........	8	3	2	3			
Abdominal wall......	4	3			1		
Ureter and bladder..	9	2	3	1	2		1
Vagina.............	6	3	1		1	1	
Uterus.............	3		1	1	1		
Bowel.............	2	2					
Urethra and prostate.	3	1		2			
	35	14	7	7	5	1	1

Obstruction.—The principles of adequate preliminary decompression and rehabilitation before exploration is undertaken may not be deviated from without considerable risk. The fact that the vast majority of cases of progressive neoplasm of the left colon, rectosigmoid, and rectum present at some time prior to their exploration some degree of obstruction is easily demonstrated. It is not necessary that obstruction be present in such a form as to cause hypertrophy and dilatation of the bowel proximal to the growth, but simple dilatation to a small degree should be considered evidence of a certain amount of obstruction. That obstruction and ulceration enormously increase the permeability of the colonic wall is well known. Given a foul, ulcerating growth bathed in a bacteria-laden fecal current, a large amount of infection is always present. When factors favorable to increasing permeability are present, the pericolonic tissues immediately adjacent to the growth are especially tender and the spread of organisms by the examining hand most frequently accounts for ensuing peritonitis.

Local conditions in the bowel secondary to obstruction become unfavorable for primary resection and anastomosis, particularly if they are in the left half of the colon. The wall of the bowel is thickened and edematous and encroachment is made on the blood supply. The blood supply of the colon, however, is much more constant than has usually been believed. Steward's work in this connection is most enlightening and instructive. Failure of resection of the distal colon in the face of slight obstruction is due perhaps in most instances more to infection in the wall of the colon than to failure of the blood supply *per se*, although unquestionably both conditions must be given consideration. Even when immediate anastomosis is not contemplated as in exteriorization procedures and resections of the rectum, preliminary decompression of the colon is essential to satisfactory prognosis because obstruction is followed by a sequence of events which rapidly produces dehydration and undermines vital processes. When one remembers that the patients, who are usually middle aged or in the late years of life, do not appear for examination until ten to twelve months have elapsed, the fact is appreciated that the malignancy has had an opportunity to effect attrition of nature's mechanism.

Decompression of the colon is accomplished either by medical measures which are favorably instituted against chronic obstruction or even against subacute obstruction, but which obviously must be supplemented by surgical drainage in the case of increasing or acute obstruction. Emergency operations are rarely demanded in obstruction from carcinoma of the large intestine. Consequently we have found it possible by medical measures to relieve practically all chronic obstruction to such a degree that the patients were in favorable condition for operation.

Size and direction of growth and glandular metastasis.—That size of the growth has little if anything to do with the prognosis has been proven by observation on every segment of the colon and rectum. There is no evidence for the conclusion that, in the main, large growths entail a poorer prognosis than small growths; in fact, the relationship is more likely to be inverse. The probable explanation lies perhaps in the fact that the highly malignant tumors metastasize early when the parent growth is still small, while the lower-grade carcinoma sometimes assumes huge proportions before dissemination to the lymph nodes begins. From the practical standpoint of operability, one sometimes resects large growths, which are frequently considered borderline cases because of their fixation, only to find no glandular involvement and to be rewarded by a satisfactory ultimate result. Such types are more likely to be discovered among cases of carcinoma of the right side of the colon rather than those of the left side, because growths in the right half are usually large, ulcerating, infected, and frequently more or less fixed from inflammatory adhesions rather than from direct extension of the malignant process.

TABLE 14

SIZE OF CARCINOMAS OF PATIENTS FREE FROM RECURRENCE AFTER FIVE YEARS AS COMPARED WITH PATIENTS WHO SUBSEQUENTLY HAD RECURRENCE (RANKIN AND OLSON)

	Cecum	Right	Left	Sigmoid
Dead (cases)............	37	44	46	93
Size (average)..........	7.7 cm.	7.1 cm.	6.2 cm.	5 cm.
Cures (cases)..........	47	59	54	73
Size (average).........	7 cm.	7.2 cm.	5.7 cm.	5.4 cm.

Rankin and Olson, from a study of 453 cases of carcinoma resected from the colon, and McVay, from a study of 100 cases of carcinoma resected from the rectum, reached the same conclusion; namely, that the size of carcinoma of the large intestine is a poor index of its curability.

Colon.—Four hundred fifty-three surgical-pathologic specimens of carcinoma of the colon were minutely studied by Rankin and Olson from five aspects: (1) size; (2) direction of the growth, that is, whether the tumor was projecting into the lumen or toward the serosa; (3) involvement of lymph nodes; (4) grade of malignancy as determined by degree of cellular differentiation; and (5) a comparison of mucoid carcinoma with the more solid form. Because of the physiologic and anatomic differences between the right and left halves of the colon, the series was divided in accordance with whether the right or left half of the colon was involved, the point of division being the middle of the transverse colon.

In Table 14 is given the average size of carcinoma of patients who subsequently had recurrence as compared with the average size of carcinoma of those who obtained "cure" for five or more years. From this table it will be seen that in no group did the patients with poor results have appreciably larger carcinoma than did those who obtained good results. The inference is that size has little to do with the prognosis of resectable carcinoma of the colon.

It has been noted frequently that those malignant growths which project into the lumen give a better result than do those of which the dominant direction of growth is toward the serosa. A lesion which projects itself into the fecal stream will give rise to symptoms of obstruction or of bleeding early, whereas a lesion

TABLE 15

DOMINANT DIRECTION OF GROWTH (RANKIN AND OLSON)

	Toward Lumen	Toward Serosa
Average postoperative life of patients with recurrence, months	22.5	21.9
Percentage of 5-year cures	62	41

which invades the serosa will reach the lymphatic structures more quickly and will be disseminated sooner than the former. As Fitz-Gibbon and Rankin have demonstrated, colonic carcinoma not infrequently arises on the basis of polyps and they found that it is the polypoid carcinoma which assumes considerable proportions while projecting into the lumen, without serosal involvement taking place. From the prognostic standpoint it is of interest to observe that of the 24 cases which FitzGibbon and Rankin reported of carcinoma which demonstrably had their origin in polyps, 22 were of the lower grades of malignancy. In Table 15 may be seen the results of the study on the direction of growth, and it is apparent that carcinoma projecting into the lumen of the colon gives a considerably higher proportion of successful results than does that with invasion of the serosa.

When dissemination of a malignant growth through the lymphatic channels begins, the first sign of the invasion is usually found in the local lymph nodes. When only these first outposts are involved, complete surgical removal is still possible, but their involvement makes the surgeon fearful that the malignancy has already become disseminated further and that undemonstrable distant metastasis has occurred. In Table 16 are presented the

TABLE 16

NODAL INVOLVEMENT (RANKIN AND OLSON)

	With Nodal Involvement	Without Nodal Involvement
Right half of colon, including cecum (187 cases)		
Incidence	34 per cent	
Average postoperative life of patients with recurrence, months	15.7	25.6 per cent
Percentage of 5-year cures	39	66
Left half of colon, including sigmoid (266 cases)		
Incidence	31 per cent	
Average postoperative life of patients with recurrence, months	18.5	26.5
Percentage of 5-year cures	29	56

results of prognostic studies in relation to involvement of lymph nodes in colonic lesions.

Coller and his associates, in 1941, reported a much higher incidence of nodal involvement: 62.5 per cent for lesions of the right colon and 60 per cent for those of the left half. They believe that the employment of David and Gilchrist's modification of the Spalteholtz method of dissection and study of lymphatic nodes enabled them to isolate such a high percentage of nodes (average of 52 per specimen). Gilchrist and David, in 1947, isolated an almost identical average number of nodes per specimen and reported the incidence of metastasis for the right and left halves of the colon respectively as 86.6 per cent and 44.4 per cent. The number of cases involved were too small for a significant comparison of five year cures in the two halves. It is, nevertheless, interesting to note that 18 of their 30 patients (60 per cent) with lesions of the intraperitoneal colon in which the lymph nodes were involved were alive after five years and all 18 without nodal involvement survived five or more years.

Involvement of lymph nodes, provided the nodes are in immediate juxtaposition to the growth, should not hinder resection. That it is impossible to tell by palpation alone whether or not a node is involved has been a recognized fact for a long time, and microscopic section is necessary for this decision. Also, the study of Rankin and Olson's series of cases proves that many patients with growths which were shown at resection to have invaded the nodes have lived long and useful lives without recurrence.

The relationship between the grade of malignancy, as determined by cellular differentiation, and prognosis is discussed later under a separate heading, as is a comparison of mucoid carcinoma with the more solid type.

Rectum.—McVay, in 1922, studied 100 specimens which had been removed at operation for carcinoma of the rectum. In 47 per cent of the cases the nodes were involved. From these studies he concluded that "The size of the growth in the rectum cannot be relied on as an accurate index of the probable lymphatic involvement. The growths without lymphatic involvement tend to spread by direct extension and are slow growing. Carcinoma of the rectum with extensive lymphatic involvement tends to metastasize through the lymph stream early. Occasionally metastasis may take place by emboli breaking off into the portal veins. The size of the lymph node is not an efficient means of determining whether there is metastatic involvement. Systematic microscopic examination of all the regional lymph nodes in carcinoma of the rectum offers, as it does in carcinoma of the stomach, the best method of establishing an accurate prognosis for the case."

Since this study of McVay there have been many similar investigations (Table 17) in which almost identical conclusions were reached. Gabriel, Duke, and Bussey emphasized the unreliability of attempting to determine grossly whether lymph nodes are involved (see "Metastasis," p. 83). Gilchrist and David, in their 1938 report, urged wide resection of the levati ani muscle when the tumor is near the level of these structures since metastasis along them seemed to be common and they also advised radical resection of the rectum for squamous cell carcinoma of the anus on the basis of me-

TABLE 17

NODAL INVOLVEMENT IN CARCINOMA OF THE RECTUM

Author	Total No. of Cases	Percentage Involved
McVay (1922)........................	100	47
Wood and Wilkie (1933).............	100	51
Gabriel, Dukes and Bussey (1935).....	100	62
Gilchrist and David (1938)...........	25	68
Coller, Kay and MacIntyre (1940)....	53	64
Grinnell 1916–1932 cases (1942)......	107	36
Grinnell 1938–1941 cases (1942)......	75	55
Seefeld and Bargen (1943)...........	100	47
Glover and Waugh (1946)............	100	100*
Gilchrist and David (1947)..........	140	55.3

* Only specimens which represented advanced disease were studied. All were of Duke's type C.

tastasis upward along the course of the superior hemorrhoidal vessels as well as laterally to the inguinal lymph nodes. Grinnell (1942) and more recently Glover and Waugh (1946), have stressed the rare occurrence of downward invasion of the lymph nodes in carcinoma of the rectum which, in their opinion, takes place only when higher nodes are blocked by metastasis and the carcinoma in all probability is beyond the realm of surgical cure. They therefore suggest that the operation of anterior abdominal resection for growths of the upper rectum and rectosigmoid offers as satisfactory a prognostic outlook as the combined abdominoperineal resection.

Notwithstanding the low incidence of involvement of lymph glands below the level of the rectal lesion, a considerable majority of American and British surgeons who have recently (1947–48) expressed themselves upon the subject (see chapter on Choice of Operation for details of survey made by authors) advocate the combined abdominoperineal operation as offering a better prognosis than the sphincter saving measures, whether of the type advocated by Babcock and Bacon or the type of anterior resection routinely employed by Waugh, Wangensteen, Mahorner, and others. In their most recent (1947) study of factors influencing five-year survival in radical resection of the rectum for carcinoma, Gilchrist and David reported that four of 11 patients on whom post mortem examinations were performed were found to have metastasis to nodes in the retroperitoneal tissues. In three of these complete removal of all node metastasis would have been accomplished if the field of resection had been 1 cm. wider. They concluded that since lesions which are partially or completely below the peritoneal reflection have a high incidence of local and liver recurrence "pull-through or sleeve resections are not much better than local resections. The Miles operation seems to give the best chance of a cure here [rectosigmoid]."

TABLE 18

RESULTS OF PERINEAL EXCISION ON A FIVE-YEAR BASIS
(ST. MARK'S HOSPITAL 1936)

Classification of Growth	Operation Survivals	Untraced and Died of Other Causes	Alive at 5 Years	Per Cent of 5-year Survivals
Group A...............	30	2	26	93
Group B...............	50	7	28	65
Group C...............	62	5	13	23
Total............	142	14	67	52

In 1932, a method of pathologic classification of resected carcinoma of the rectum according to depth of invasion was described by Dukes. Microscopic examination of fixed sections of that part of the rectum which had been removed at the point of maximum penetration of the wall of the bowel by the growth enables the cases to be grouped in the following way:

"A cases are those in which the carcinoma is limited to the wall of the rectum, there being no extension into the extrarectal tissues and no metastases in the lymph nodes.

"B cases are those in which the carcinoma has spread by direct continuity to the extrarectal tissues, but has not yet invaded the regional lymph nodes.

"C cases are those in which metastases are present in the regional lymph nodes."

The results of surgical excision of the rectum for carcinoma in "A," "B," and "C" cases are shown in Table 18, which presents in three sections the period of survival of 129 patients operated on during the years 1927 to 1930, all by approximately the same surgical technic.

Intrinsic influences (histologic grading of malignancy by Broders' method).—Consideration of the two types of influence on prognosis, extrinsic and intrinsic, has led us to the definite conviction that the intrinsic malignancy of the carcinomatous cell affects in direct ratio all of the other factors which modify it. We do not feel that clinical observations and general conditions which influence the prognosis should be excluded from grave consideration, but we feel that the activity of the neoplastic cell is the primary factor in the decision between longevity and early recurrence. Unquestionably such factors as involvement of lymph nodes and distant or hepatic metastasis affect the length of life after operation in direct proportion to their presence or absence. We show later that involvement of nodes is directly dependent on and that its extent is proportional to the grade of malignancy. Such local conditions as fixation of the growth, perforation, penetration, and formation of abscess affect operability of the growth, but they are merely local influencing factors which are usually the result either of intense activity of the carcinomatous cell or of prolonged neglect in the absence of symptoms.

Broders has called attention to the great difference in carcinomas, the cells of which are undifferentiated as compared with those which consist of differentiated cells. He has provided a system of grading the degree of malignancy on the basis of differentiation of the cells and the ultimate outlook after treatment. By cellular differentiation is meant the structural changes which take place in the development of the adult tissue cell. The principle of grading by differentiation is based on the biologic law that the higher the degree of differentiation the less the power of reproduction, and it might be anticipated that well-differentiated carcinomatous cells would proliferate at a slower pace than those which are comparatively undifferentiated. A more detailed consideration of the technical factors which are involved in Broders' method has been taken up under "Pathology."

The scientific criteria laid down by Broders estimates the prognosis of carcinoma of the colon, rectosigmoid, and rectum more accurately, we believe, than any other yardstick that is available. Moreover, the index of malignancy applied to biopsy obtained from rectal neoplasm is of inestimable value in judging inoperability in certain cases. Studies of large series of cases of carcinoma of the colon, rectum, and anus by Rankin and Broders (1928), Dukes (1932), Rankin and Olson (1933), and Rankin (1933), and smaller series of many others, have all led to the same conclusion, which is, given the microscopic grading of the degree of malignancy in a case of carcinoma of the colon or rectum and the information as to whether the glands in the specimen were or were not involved by malignant extension, one should be able to estimate with considerable accuracy the ultimate end-results.

Colon.—Rankin and Olson, in 1933, studied 453 cases of carcinoma of the colon (down to the rectosigmoid) in which operation was performed between 1907 and 1927. In order to estimate to best advantage the influences on prognosis of the pathologic variations, all other variable factors were eliminated as largely as possible. The time that has elapsed between the appearance of the tumor and the date of its removal is, of course, a very important variant in the matter of prognosis. An attempt to control this factor was made

TABLE 19

GRADING OF MALIGNANCY IN RELATION TO POSTOPERATIVE LENGTH OF LIFE (RANKIN AND OLSON)

Grade	1	2	3	4
Right half of colon (187 cases)				
Incidence, per cent	16	53	21	10
Average postoperative life of patients with recurrence, months	25.8	22.8	17.4	14.8
Percentage of 5-year cures	68	60	48	37
Left half of colon (266 cases)				
Incidence, per cent	13	67	16	4
Average postoperative life of patients with recurrence, months	33.7	26.5	16.2	14.6
Percentage of 5-year cures	63	51	30	18

by rigid selection of cases, only those cases being considered in which the malignant growth was resectable, in which there was no demonstrable hepatic metastasis, and in which, therefore, closure was made at the end of operation with a hopeful prognosis. For the same reason, cases in which death occurred immediately after operation were excluded.

From the statistical standpoint only those cases were considered in which patients were known to have died of recurrence or to have been living more than five years free from recurrence. In each case of recurrence the exact number of months of postoperative life was known. Thus the series ranges from patients who died in the second month after operation to patients who were living twenty-four years after operation.

It is apparent from Table 19 how close the correlation is between the grade of malignancy and the prognosis, not only as concerns ultimate cure but also in the rapidity with which recurrences are fatal. The group labeled "right" includes the ascending colon, the hepatic flexure, and the right half of the transverse colon. The group labeled "left" includes the left half of the transverse colon, the splenic flexure, the descending colon, and the sigmoid flexure.

The relationship between grading and involvement of lymph nodes was also investigated. It is noted in Table 20 that grades 1 and 2 were relatively more frequent among the specimens obtained from patients who had no nodal involvement and that grades 3 and 4, on the contrary, were relatively more common among the specimens from patients with involvement of nodes. In view of this observation, comparison of the percentage of nodal involvement within the individual grades is enlightening. In grade 1, 28 per

TABLE 20

GRADE OF MALIGNANCY IN RELATION TO INVOLVEMENT
OF LYMPH NODES (RANKIN AND OLSON)

Grade	1	2	3	4
With nodal involvement (147 specimens)				
Incidence, per cent	11	55	23	11
Average postoperative life of patients with recurrence, months	24.6	19	14.1	14
Percentage of 5-year cures	47	41	15	25
Without nodal involvement (306 specimens)				
Incidence, per cent	16	63	16	5
Average postoperative life of patients with recurrence, months	34.4	27.7	19.6	15.6
Percentage of 5-year cures	72	60	54	36

cent of the specimens were from patients with involvement of nodes; in grade 2, 30 per cent; in grade 3, 36 per cent; and in grade 4, 53 per cent. This progressive increase in the incidence of involvement of lymph nodes as one passes to the higher grades of malignancy discloses definite correlation between the microscopic grade of malignancy and involvement of the regional nodes.

Further study of the table, however, disclosed that the grade exerts as much influence on prognosis in the group in which nodes were not involved as it does in the group in which they were involved, and that nodal involvement operates prognostically quite as well in one grade as it does in any other.

Dixon and Olson recently reported 12 cases of carcinoma of the colon in which twenty-year surgical cures were obtained. It is interesting to note that in none of these cases was the malignancy graded 3 or 4. Six were grade 1 and six grade 2.

Rectum.—Rankin and Broders studied 598 cases of carcinoma of the rectum operated on between 1916 and 1925 and graded the malignancy in accordance with Broders' method. Table 21 shows the relationship between grade of malignancy, ultimate result, and

TABLE 21

GRADE OF MALIGNANCY, ULTIMATE RESULT, AND DURATION OF LIFE (RANKIN AND BRODERS)*

	Grade 1 105	Grade 2 299	Grade 3 141	Grade 4 53	All Grades
Total	105	299	141	53	
Information	103 (98+% of 105)	293 (97+% of 299)	139 (98+% of 141)	52 (98+% of 53)	
Living	58 (56+% of 103)	112 (38+% of 293)	35 (25+% of 139)	8 (15+% of 52)	
Good result	55 (94+% of 58)	101 (90+% of 112)	33 (94+% of 35)	7 (87+% of 8)	
Longest	9.50 years	11.00 years	10.50 years	10.33 years	
Shortest	1.33 years	1.20 years	1.33 years	4.00 years	
Average	5.06 years	4.79 years	4.57 years	6.73 years	
Poor result	3 (5+% of 58)	11 (9+% of 112)	2 (5+% of 35)	1 (12+% of 8)	
Longest	2.25 years	3.41 years	1.91 years	2.75 years	
Shortest	1.37 years	1.16 years	1.41 years	2.75 years	
Average	1.90 years	2.54 years	1.66 years	2.75 years	
Dead	45 (43+% of 103)	181 (61+% of 293)	104 (74+% of 139)	45 (86+% of 52)	
Good result	4 (13+% of 29)	13 (8+% of 155)		2 (5+% of 37)	
Longest	8.50 years	10.12 years	6.58 years		
Shortest	1.83 years	1.17 years	4.00 years		
Average	4.81 years	4.67 years	5.29 years		
Poor result	25 (86+% of 29)	142 (91+% of 155)	87 (100+% of 87)	35 (94+% of 37)	
Longest	7.75 years	7.66 years	6.00 years	7.75 years	
Shortest	0.41 years	0.50 years	0.08 years	0.12 years	
Average	2.42 years	2.21 years	1.76 years	1.45 years	
Total good results	59 (67+% of 87)	114 (42+% of 267)	33 (27+% of 122)	9 (20+% of 45)	215 (41+% of 521)
Total poor results	28 (32+% of 87)	153 (57+% of 267)	89 (72+% of 122)	36 (80+% of 45)	306 (58+% of 521)

* This table does not include cases in which death occurred in hospital or after the patient was dismissed if the interval after the operation was too short to determine whether or not patient would have died from the carcinoma.

TABLE 22

METASTASIS, GRADE OF MALIGNANCY, AND RESULTS (RANKIN AND BRODERS)

	Grade 1	Grade 2	Grade 3	Grade 4	All Grades
Patients with metastasis........	22 (8.46% of 260)	128 (49.23% of 260)	77 (29.61% of 260)	33 (12.69% of 260)	
Information........	22 (100% of 22)	127 (99.21% of 128)	77 (100% of 77)	33 (100% of 33)	
Living........	7 (31.81% of 22)	36 (28.34% of 127)	11 (14.28% of 77)	1 (3.03% of 33)	
Good result........	7 (100% of 7)	29 (80.55% of 36)	10 (90.90% of 11)		
Poor result........		7 (19.44% of 36)	1 (9.09% of 11)	1 (100% of 1)	
Dead........	15 (68.18% of 22)	91 (71.65% of 127)	66 (85.71% of 77)	32 (96.96% of 33)	
Good result........	1 (9.09% of 11)	1 (1.23% of 81)			
Poor result........	10 (90.90% of 11)	80 (98.76% of 81)	59 (100% of 59)	26 (100% of 26)	
Total good result...	8 (44.44% of 18)	30 (25.64% of 117)	10 (14.28% of 70)		48 (20.68% of 232)
Total poor result...	10 (55.55% of 18)	87 (74.35% of 117)	60 (85.71% of 70)	27 (100% of 27)	184 (79.31% of 232)

TABLE 23

ABSENCE OF METASTASIS, GRADE OF MALIGNANCY, AND RESULTS (RANKIN AND BRODERS)

	Grade 1	Grade 2	Grade 3	Grade 4	All Grades
Patients without metastasis......	60 (20.00% of 300)	162 (54.00% of 300)	60 (20.00% of 300)	18 (6.00% of 300)	
Information.........	58 (96.66% of 60)	158 (97.53% of 162)	58 (96.66% of 60)	17 (94.44% of 18)	
Living..............	32 (55.17% of 58)	74 (46.83% of 158)	24 (41.37% of 58)	6 (35.29% of 17)	
Good result........	30 (93.75% of 32)	72 (97.29% of 74)	23 (95.83% of 24)	6 (100% of 6)	
Poor result........	2 (6.25% of 32)	2 (2.70% of 74)	1 (4.16% of 24)		
Dead...............	26 (44.82% of 58)	84 (53.16% of 158)	34 (59.64% of 57)	11 (64.70% of 17)	
Good result........	2 (13.33% of 15)	12 (17.64% of 68)	24 (100% of 24)	2 (18.18% of 11)	
Poor result........	13 (86.66% of 15)	56 (82.35% of 68)		9 (81.81% of 11)	
Total good result...	32 (68.08% of 47)	84 (59.15% of 142)	23 (47.91% of 48)	8 (47.05% of 17)	147 (57.87% of 254)
Total poor result....	15 (31.91% of 47)	58 (40.84% of 142)	25 (52.08% of 48)	9 (52.94% of 17)	107 (42.12% of 254)

TABLE 24

NO LYMPH NODES REMOVED, GRADE OF MALIGNANCY, AND RESULTS (RANKIN AND BRODERS)

	Grade 1	Grade 2	Grade 3	Grade 4
No lymph nodes removed*....	23 (60.52% of 38)	9 (23.68% of 38)	4 (10.52% of 38)	2 (5.26% of 38)
Information................	23 (100% of 23)	8 (88.88% of 9)	4 (100% of 4)	2 (100% of 2)
Living...................	19 (82.69% of 23)	2 (25.00% of 8)	1 (25.00% of 4)	
Good result.............	18 (94.73% of 19)		1 (100% of 1)	
Poor result.............	1 (5.26% of 19)	2 (100% of 2)		
Dead....................	4 (17.40% of 23)	6 (75.00% of 8)	3 (75.00% of 4)	2 (100% of 2)
Good result.............	1 (33.33% of 3)			
Poor result.............	2 (66.66% of 3)	6 (100% of 6)	3 (100% of 3)	1 (100% of 1)
Total good result........	19 (86.36% of 22)		1 (25.00% of 4)	
Total poor result........	3 (13.63% of 22)	8 (100% of 8)	3 (75.00% of 4)	1 (100% of 1)

* A one-stage operation was performed such as the Quénu-Tuttle or Harrison-Cripps.

duration of life since operation. It can be seen that the grade of malignancy plays practically no part in the average duration of life of those who are living, and it plays practically no part in the duration of life of those who died after a good result, but it does play a part in the average duration of life of those who died from carcinoma, since the average duration decreases as the grade of malignancy increases. By good results is meant that the patient has been free from carcinoma, as far as can be ascertained, for a number of years, the average of which is recorded in the table. If the patient is dead and the result is recorded as good it signifies that death occurred some years after operation from a cause unrelated to carcinoma. Poor results refer to cases in which there was reason to believe that death was due to carcinoma, even though in some instances death did not occur until more than seven years after operation.

Table 22 shows the relationship of metastasis and grade of malignancy to ultimate results. It is obvious that the grade of malignancy is the dominant factor since the total of good results decreases in inverse proportion to the grade, and the total of poor results increases in proportion to the grade.

Table 23 shows the relationship of absence of metastasis and grade of malignancy to ultimate results. The percentage of total good results decreases in inverse proportion to the grade of malignancy, and the percentage of total bad results increases in direct proportion to it. Although the grade of malignancy has its influence on the good and bad results in the absence of metastasis, this influence is not so marked as when metastasis is present. It can be noted also that in cases of carcinoma graded 3 or 4 without demonstrable metastasis the result is not much better than when metastasis accompanies carcinoma graded 1.

In Table 24 the grade of malignancy and the results are compared in a series of cases in which the nature of the operation precluded the removal of lymph nodes.

Dukes, in 1940, reported the results of a study of 985 cases of carcinoma of the rectum in which the carcinoma was removed surgically at St. Mark's Hospital, London. The specimens were graded by Broders' method, using the same sections as served for the grouping into "A," "B," and "C" cases (referred to under the heading immediately above) but, in order to avoid bias, without knowing how the cases had been classified. The results are reported in Table 25 which shows the number of the four grades of adenocarcinoma and colloid carcinoma in the cases previously classified as "A," "B," and "C."

Dukes' conclusions were as follows: "It will be seen that the majority of adenocarcinomas in all groups belong to grade 2, while

TABLE 25

RELATION OF SPREAD TO HISTOLOGICAL GRADE

(985 CASES—DUKES)

	Grade I		Grade II		Grade III		Grade IV		Colloid	
	No.	Per Cent	No.	Per Cent	No.	Per Cent	No.	Per Cent	No.	Per Cent
144 A Cases....	28	19.4	97	67.4	8	5.5	0	0	11	7.7
342 B Cases....	20	5.8	233	68.1	57	16.7	1	0.3	31	9.1
499 C Cases....	16	3.3	232	46.4	159	31.8	13	2.7	79	15.8

nearly all the grade 1 were A cases, and most grades 3 and 4, C cases. There appears therefore to be a definite relationship between the degree of differentiation of the malignant cells as estimated histologically and the extent of spread as measured by the A, B, and C classification."

TABLE 26

INCIDENCE OF GLANDULAR INVOLVEMENT

Grade 1 .... 27 per cent
Grade 2 .... 35 per cent
Grade 3 .... 50 per cent
Grade 4 .... 56 per cent

The results, he stated, "confirm the work of Rankin and Broders in that they show that the prospects of survival are best in grade 1 cases and progressively less good in grades 2, 3, and 4. All cases graded 1 are still alive and most of those graded 3 are dead, grade 2 proving an intermediate group."

Colon and rectum.—The preceding studies were confined either to the rectum or the colon. Recently one of us (Rankin) has made a comparative study of the various segments of the large intestine.

TABLE 27

FIVE-YEAR CURES IN RELATION TO GLANDULAR INVOLVEMENT

	With Nodal Involvement	Without Nodal Involvement
Right Colon		
Incidence..................................	34%	....
Five-year cures...........................	39%	.... 66%
Left Colon		
Incidence..................................	31%	....
Five-year cures...........................	20%	.... 56%
Rectum		
Incidence..................................	46%	....
Five-year cures...........................	20%	.... 48%

The material for this study consisted of 753 cases which were closed at the end of operation with a hopeful prognosis and which have resulted either in survival over a period of five years without recurrence or in death from recurrence. In every case the pathologic specimens were available for study. The distribution of the tumors is interesting and of significance prognostically. There were 187 cases of carcinoma of the right colon, 266 cases of the left colon, and 300 cases of carcinoma of the rectosigmoid and rectum. In this study, as in the previous studies, the incidence of glandular involvement was in direct ratio to the grade of the malignancy as shown in Table 26.

TABLE 28

GRADING OF MALIGNANCY IN RELATION TO POSTOPERATIVE LENGTH OF LIFE

	Grade 1	Grade 2	Grade 3	Grade 4
Right Colon				
Incidence	16%	53%	21%	10%
Five-year cures	68%	60%	48%	37%
Left Colon				
Incidence	13%	67%	16%	4%
Five-year cures	63%	51%	30%	18%
Rectum				
Incidence	13%	53%	24%	10%
Five-year cures	57%	44%	22%	19%

Table 27 shows very strikingly the influence of glandular involvement on five-year cures. The incidence of glandular involvement in the two halves was about the same, there being a slight advantage to the left side, namely, 31 per cent as against 34 per cent, which is an unusual observation, since the ultimate prognosis for the right colon is slightly better than that for the left. Glandular involvement in the rectum, however, was encountered considerably more frequently than in either half of the large bowel, 46 per cent of the cases being recorded as showing malignant lymph nodes resected with the specimen. It is apparent from Table 28 that there is definite correlation between the grade of malignancy and the prognosis as concerns not only ultimate cure but likewise the rapidity with which recurrence takes place. There is great pathologic similarity between carcinoma of the colon and the rectum so far as grading is concerned and one observes that little more than half of the growths in both locations fall into grade 2.

As one reviews these tables, considering the relationship of glandular involvement to recurrence and postoperative life, and compares as in Table 29 the five-year cures in the different grades, one can scarcely escape the conclusion that the intensity of malignant invasion is the most important factor in estimating prognosis, since

TABLE 29

RELATIVE PERCENTAGE OF CURES IN RELATION
TO SITUATION OF LESION

	Total	Dead	Cures	Percentage Cured
Right colon	187	81	106	57.6
Left colon	266	139	127	47.7
Rectum	300	186	114	38.0
	753	406	347	45.8

	Total Cases	Grade 1	Grade 2	Grade 3	Grade 4
Number	753	101	434	157	61
Incidence		13%	58%	21%	8%
Five-year cures		63%	51%	31%	24%

TABLE 30

GRADE OF MALIGNANCY AND MUCUS COMPARED WITH
LYMPHATIC INVOLVEMENT, RECURRENCE AND MORTALITY
(RANKIN AND CHUMLEY)

Mucus		Lymphatic Involvement		Recurrence		Living		Dead	
Grade	Cases	Cases	Per Cent	Cases	Per Cent	Cases	Per Cent	Cases	Per Cent
Malignancy Grade 1									
1	2	—	—	1	50.0	1	50.0	1	50.0
2	4	1	25.0	—	—	4	100.0	—	—
3	9	1	11.1	6	66.6	3	33.3	6	66.6
4	12	8	66.6	7	58.3	5	41.7	7	58.3
Malignancy Grade 2									
1	3	1	33.3	1	33.3	2	66.6	1	33.3
2	10	6	60.0	5	50.0	5	50.0	5	50.0
3	10	5	50.0	4	40.0	6	60.0	4	40.0
4	13	6	46.1	10	76.9	3	23.1	10	76.9
Malignancy Grade 3									
1	2	2	100.0	2	100.0	—	—	2	100.0
2	—	—	—	—	—	—	—	—	—
3	9	6	66.6	7	77.7	2	22.3	7	77.7
4	8	8	100.0	7	87.5	1	12.5	7	87.5
Malignancy Grade 4									
1	3	—	—	3	100.0	—	—	3	100.0
2	—	—	—	—	—	—	—	—	—
3	1	1	100.0	1	100.0	—	—	1	100.0
4	6	6	100.0	6	100.0	—	—	6	100.0

the incidence of local glandular metastasis and distant implants as well depend directly on it. It is significant, moreover, that the figures presented in these tables are the averages of a large group, while the study of the individual cases show considerable scattering from the median. What is prognostic for the average of a series is the dominant tendency of the individual case.

Colloid (mucoid) carcinoma.—In perusing the literature, considerable difference of opinion is noted as to the malignancy of mucoid carcinoma. Many regard the excess of mucinous substance as a degenerative phenomenon. Parham referred to it as an "uncontrolled function of secretion" and expressed the belief that "mucous formation is a sign of functional differentiation of the carcinoma cells." Opposed to that view, however, are the observations of Rankin and Chumley in their study of 158 cases of colloid carcinoma of the colon and rectum. They found that a high percentage of these carcinoma were of a low grade of malignancy, but of a high grade of mucous formation (see Ochsenhirt's method of grading mucous-forming cells under "Pathology"). In the lower grades of malignancy there was a tendency for the amount of mucus which was present to be inversely proportional to the grade of malignancy. The grading of the amount of mucus in colloid carcinoma proved to be of value as a prognostic factor. The influence of the grades of malignancy and mucus on lymphatic involvement, recurrence, and mortality in this series is shown in Table 30.

Dukes, in 1940, reported that nearly all patients with colloid cancer of the rectum who survived resection of the rectum for five years or longer were originally grouped as A and B cases, which shows "the important prognostic feature in colloid cancer is the extent of the growth, and not the presence of colloid degeneration."

REFERENCES

1. BRODERS, A. C.: The grading of carcinoma. *Minnesota Med.*, **8**: 726–730 (Dec.), 1925.
2. COLLER, F. A., KAY, E. B., MACINTYRE, R. S.: Regional lymphatic metastasis of carcinoma of the rectum. *Surgery*, **8**: 294–311 (Aug.), 1940.
3. CUTTING, R. A.: Carcinoma of anus and rectum. *Am. Jour. Surg.*, **10**: 547–556 (Dec.), 1930.
4. DALAND, E. M., WELCH, C. E., and NATHANSON, I.: One hundred untreated cancers of rectum. *New England Med. Jour.*, **214**: 451–458 (March), 1936.
5. DIXON, C. F., and OLSON, P. F.: Twenty-year cures of carcinoma of colon. *Surg., Gynec., and Obstet.*, **62**: 874–878 (May), 1936.
6. DUKES, C. E.: Classification of cancer of the rectum. *Jour. Path. and Bact.*, **35**: 323–332 (May), 1932.
7. DUKES, C. E.: Cancer of the rectum: analysis of 1000 cases. *Jour. Path. and Bact.*, **50**: 527–539 (May), 1940.
8. FITZGIBBON, G., and RANKIN, F. W.: Polyps of the large intestine. *Surg., Gynec., and Obstet.*, **52**: 1136–1150 (June), 1931.

9. GABRIEL, W. B., DUKES, C. E., BUSSEY, H. J. R.: Lymphatic spread in cancer of the rectum. *Brit. Jour. Surg.*, **23**: 395–413 (Oct.), 1935.
10. GILCHRIST, R. K., and DAVID, V. C.: Lymphatic spread of carcinoma of the rectum. *Ann. Surg.*, **108**: 621–642 (Oct.), 1938.
11. GILCHRIST, R. K., and DAVID, V. C.: A consideration of pathologic factors influencing five-year survival in radical resection of the large bowel and rectum for carcinoma. *Ann. Surg.*, **126**: 421–438 (Oct.), 1947.
12. GORDON-WATSON, C.: Treatment of cancer of rectum with radium by open operation. *Proc., Roy. Soc. Med.*, **21**: 9 (Dec.), 1927.
13. GLOVER, ROBERT P., and WAUGH, JOHN M.: The retrograde lymphatic spread of carcinoma of the "rectosigmoid region." *Surg., Gynec., and Obstet.*, **79**: 434–448 (Oct.), 1944.
14. GRAHAM, A. STEPHENS: Unpublished data.
15. GRINNELL, R. S.: The lymphatic and venous spread of carcinoma of the rectum. *Ann. Surg.*, **116**: 200–215 (Aug.), 1942.
16. LOCKHART-MUMMERY, J. P.: Two hundred cases of cancer of the rectum treated by perineal excision. *Brit. Jour. Surg.*, **14**: 110–124 (July), 1926.
17. LOCKHART-MUMMERY, J. P.: Prognosis in rectal cancer. *Lancet*, **2**: 1307–1309 (Dec.), 1926.
18. MILES, W. E.: Pathology of spread of cancer of rectum and its bearing upon surgery of cancerous rectum. *Surg., Gynec., and Obstet.*, **52**: 350 (Feb.), 1931.
19. MILES, W. E.: The present position of the radical abdominoperineal operation for cancer of the rectum in regard to mortality and post-operative recurrence. *Proc. Roy. Soc. Med., Sect. Surg., Subsect. Proct.*, **24**: 989–991 (May), 1931.
20. McVAY, J. R.: Involvement of lymph-nodes in carcinoma of rectum. *Ann. Surg.*, **76**: 755–760 (Dec.), 1922.
21. NEWMAN, GEORGE: Great Britain Ministry of Health Report on Public Health and Med. Subjects. London, Bulletin, 46, 1927.
22. OETTLE: Quoted by Shore, B. R.: Abstract in: *Am. Jour. Cancer*, **27**: 179 (May), 1936.
23. OTTENHEIMER, EDWARD J.: Cancer of the rectum: An analysis of cases occurring in Connecticut during 1935–1945. *The New England Jour. Med.*, **237**: 1–7 (July), 1947.
24. POSTLETHWAIT, R. W.: Personal communication to authors.
25. RANKIN, F. W.: The curability of cancer of the colon, rectosigmoid, and rectum. *Jour. Am. Med. Assn.*, **101**: 491–495 (Aug. 12), 1933.
26. RANKIN, F. W., and BRODERS, A. C.: Factors influencing prognosis in carcinoma of the rectum. *Surg., Gynec., and Obstet.*, **46**: 660–667 (May), 1928.
27. RANKIN, F. W., and CHUMLEY, C. L.: Colloid carcinoma of the colon and rectum. *Arch. Surg.*, **18**: 129–139 (Jan.), 1929.
28. RANKIN, F. W., and OLSON, P. F.: The hopeful prognosis in cases of carcinoma of the colon. *Surg., Gynec., and Obstet.*, **56**: 366–374 (Feb.), 1933.
29. SEEFELD, PHILIP H., and BARGEN, J. ARNOLD: The spread of carcinoma of the rectum: invasion of lymphatics, veins, and nerves. *Ann. Surg.*, **118**: 76–90 (July), 1943.
30. STEWARD, J. A., and RANKIN, F. W.: Blood supply of the large intestine; its surgical consideration. *Arch. Surg.*, **26**: 843–891 (May), 1933.
31. WOOD, W. Q., and WILKIE, D. P. D.: Carcinoma of the rectum: an anatomico-pathological study. *Edinburgh Med. Jour.*, **40**: 321–343, 1933.

CHAPTER VII

CHOICE OF OPERATION

Most of those who are interested in the treatment of patients with carcinoma of the colon and rectum, including surgeons, internists, and radiologists, consider surgery the treatment of election in practically all cases that are operable. This uniformity of opinion, however, does not extend to the multitude of problems that confront the surgeon dealing with such cases. Considerable differences of opinion are found among surgeons of wide experience in this field concerning the merits of the various operative procedures; the advantages of the one stage over multistage operations primary resection and anastomosis, with or without antecedent or concomitant complementary drainage, versus exteriorization measures; open anastomosis versus a closed, so-called aseptic technic; the relative value of chemotherapeutic agents; and, operations based on the principles of Miles versus procedures in which the anal sphincteric mechanism is preserved. It is as MacFee has recently said, "undoubtedly, these divergences of view have created uncertainty in the minds of the general surgeon who operates upon the occasional case. His experience with the disease has not been sufficient to permit him to have definite ideas based upon personal observation, and a review of the literature does not enable him to see clearly the course he should pursue."

Choice of operative procedure in cancer of the distal colon and rectum continues to hinge upon the acceptance or non-acceptance of colostomy, either temporary or permanent, as an integral part of the operation. For a period of somewhat more than a hundred years from 1839 when Amussat wrote in the defense of colostomy —this has been a debatable subject; yet, by 1938—the year in which we last made a complete survey of opinion in this field— most English speaking surgeons had accepted the proposition that abdominal colostomy is an essential adjunct to a proper extirpation of the rectum and rectosigmoid. Moreover, they undertook, in most instances, a multiple-stage resection of the distal colon, such as the Rankin obstructive resection. This near unanimity of opinion developed only after many years of painstaking groundwork by such pioneers as Miles and Lockhart-Mummery, and subsequent demonstration by an overwhelming array of statistical data of the soundness of their principles by Grey Turner, Gordon-Watson, Abel, and Gabriel in England; Wilkie and Fraser in Scotland; Graham of Toronto; and in this country, Daniel Fiske Jones, Mayo, Cheever, Rankin, Stone, T. E. Jones, Pemberton, David, Pfeiffer, Lahey, Brindley, Coller, and a few others. Almost alone among general surgeons of wide experience in surgery of the large bowel at this time was Babcock, who since 1932 had consistently condemned any procedure which required abdominal anus.

The tide of opinion, however, began to turn late in the 1930's. Several factors were influential. Those surgeons who are unable to become reconciled to a colostomy life for their patients were prodded to unusual activity by the stimulus of the pathologic researches of Gabriel, Dukes and Bussey (1935), Gilchrist and David (1938), and Coller and his coworkers (1940), in which it was determined that the inferior zone of spread of malignancy through the lymphatic channels in cancer of the rectosigmoid and rectum was relatively meager. Commenting on the findings of Dukes, Lynch in 1938 expressed an opinion in which many surgeons were soon to concur. "It permits," stated Lynch, "one to discard entirely such radical and unnecessary operations as that popularized by Miles."

Another factor has been the tremendous gain in popularity of surgery of the large bowel as compared with a decade ago—1938—when relatively few undertook most of the surgery in this field. Now almost every young general surgeon and an increasingly larger number of proctologists, on completion of their residencies, consider themselves fully qualified to undertake this type of surgery. Not only has this new generation felt the necessity of re-exploration of the question of colostomy, but also a considerable number of the older general surgeons and proctologists whose interest in resections of the colon and rectum for cancer was late developing.

Many of us who served in the Armed Forces returned to civilian status completely confused by the differences of opinion in this field. It was difficult to determine the true status of treatment for carcinoma of the colon and rectum. A few surgeons had published articles unequivocally accepting sphincter-saving operations as the procedure of choice, and others, notably Wangensteen, were less positive as to the ultimate merits but were nevertheless favorable to these measures, primarily it would seem because of a decided personal aversion to colostomy. Few who were pre-eminent in this field had recently published their opinions.

Allen, in 1947, reflected the concern we and many others felt when he said, "We have been disturbed by the trend of the times, indicating a great revival of interest in operations upon the rectum that include preservation of the anal sphincter. This tendency is growing. . . . "

In order to clarify this situation, questionnaires were sent in 1947 to surgeons in this country, Canada, and Great Britain. In addition to questions dealing with the choice of operation for cancer of the distal colon, rectosigmoid and rectum, inquiries were made concerning the employment of complementary proximal drainage and chemotherapy. One of us (Graham) has recently (1948) reported the detailed findings of this inquiry, a summary of which follows:

"1. A survey by questionnaire was undertaken to determine current trends in the surgical treatment of cancer of the distal colon and rectum as practiced by 50 surgeons with relatively large experience in this field. The opinions of 10 of these whose preeminence few would question have been contrasted with those of the remainder of the group. Identical opinions of approximately 20 qualified colleagues of these 50 were not included in this survey. The departments of surgery of 31 medical schools and seven clinics are represented.

"2. There was noted a decided trend away from extraperitoneal multi-stage operations for lesions of the distal colon. Sixty-two per cent of the combined groups estimate employment of primary anastomosis in 75 to 100 per cent of cases. In the smaller group 60 per cent believe they use this method in fewer than 25 per cent of instances; the remaining four estimate a performance of over 90 per cent (Table 31).

"3. Sixty per cent of the combined groups use a closed method of anastomosis; in the smaller group there is an even division between this and the open technic (Table 31).

"4. Fifteen, or 30 per cent, routinely establish complementary proximal drainage by means of appendicostomy, cecostomy, or transverse colostomy: seven preliminary to resection and anastomosis and the remainder at the time of operation. Three expressed preference for the Devine type of colostomy. Seventeen find decompression by means of an indwelling duodenal tube adequate in most instances. Five regularly utilize decompression by the Miller-Abbott tube before, during and after resections of lesions in the distal colon (Table 31).

"5. Forty-two, or 84 per cent, indicated regular use of chemotherapeutic agents. The small minority is equally divided between the two groups, constituting 10 per cent of the larger group and 40 per cent of the smaller one. Twenty-seven limited the use of sulfonamides to the preoperative administration of sulfasuxidine or sulfathalidine. Fifteen, or 36 per cent, of the 42 who regularly utilize chemotherapy also instill into the peritoneal cavity at the time of operation either sulfanilamide or sulfathiazole. All but one of these are of the larger group. Five regularly administer oral streptomycin preoperatively. Twenty-two use penicillin postoperatively (Table 31).

TABLE 31

RESECTION AND IMMEDIATE ANASTOMOSIS OF THE COLON

(50 Surgeons: Group I, 40; Group II, 10)

	Incidence of Employment			Method		Complementary Drainage			Chemotherapy		
	0–24%	25–74%	75–100%	Closed	Open	Routine	Pre-Resection	Pre- & at Resection	Routine	Pre-Op. Only	Pre-Op. & at Op.
Group I......	2 (5%)	11 (27%)	27 (67%)	25 (62%)	11 (27%)	11 (27%)	5	6	36 (90%)	22 (61%)	14 (39%)
Group II......	6 (60%)	0	4 (40%)	5 (50%)	5 (50%)	4 (40%)	2	2	6 (60%)	5 (83%)	1 (17%)
Both groups...	8 (16%)	11 (22%)	31 (62%)	30 (60%)	16 (32%)	15 (30% of 50)	7 (47% of 15)	8 (53% of 15)	42 (84%)	27 (64% of 42)	15 (36% of 42)

TABLE 32

Choice of Procedure in Cancer of Rectosigmoid and Rectum

	Anterior Resection of Rectosigmoid			Choice of Procedure in Cancer of Rectosigmoid and Rectum		
	Incident of Employment			Miles Operation	Anterior Resect. Rectum	Babcock-Bacon Operation
	Routine	Rare	None			
Group I........	7 (17.5%)	25 (62.5%)	8 (20.0%)	33 (82%)	6 (15%)	0
Group II........	2 (20.0%)	4 (40.0%)	4 (40.0%)	8 (80%)	1 (10%)	0
Both groups....	9 (18.0% of 50)	29 (58.0% of 50)	12 (24.0% of 50)	41 (82% of 50)	7 (14% of 50)	0

"6. Only nine, or 18 per cent, regularly perform anterior resection of the rectosigmoid for operable lesions. Seven of these are in the larger group. Twelve, or 24 per cent, never undertake this procedure, whereas 14 of the remaining 29 consider it justifiable only as a palliative measure when liver metastasis exists. Of the residual 15 who indicated use of the method in highly selected cases, half further emphasized infrequency of employment by appending such terms as, "rarely ever" or "very seldom." Eight commented on their former routine use of anterior resection which they no longer consider a proper procedure (Table 32).

"7. Forty-one, or 82 per cent, indicated the Miles operation as the procedure of choice both for lesions of the rectum and rectosigmoid. Two of the remaining surgeons elect the Miles operation for all lesions except those involving the rectosigmoid, for which they prefer anterior resection. Seven regularly practice anterior resection for all rectosigmoidal growths and for rectal growths located as follows: three for all which are at least 10 cm. above the ano-rectal line (one occasionally uses a pull-through operation for small, early growths); two for those 6 cm. above this line; and one each for lesions situated respectively 5 and 3 cm. above the anus. Nine who had in recent years performed operations of the Babcock-Bacon type expressed dissatisfaction with the procedure and a disinclination to employ it in the future. No one indicated proctosigmoidectomy as the operation of choice (Table 32).

"8. From the foregoing expressions of opinion by those in this country who probably undertake most of the surgery of the large bowel for cancer, it would seem that one may properly conclude that there no longer exists cause for the concern felt by many of us, and expressed before this Association last year by Dr. Allen, over what had appeared to be a widespread revival of interest in operations upon the rectum and rectosigmoid that include preservation of the anal sphincter. It would now appear that a transient trend in that direction has, as Jones recently predicted, the probability of being short-lived. One trend, however, will in all likelihood end in universal acceptance in suitable cases. Reference is made to the steadily growing tendency to perform single-stage rather than multistage operations for lesions in every segment of the large intestine. This is accomplished for the cecum, ascending, transverse, descending and sigmoid portions of the colon by immediate anastomosis after resection and for the rectosigmoid and rectum by a one-stage, combined abdominoperitoneal resection."

In regard to standardization of technical procedures employed in the treatment of carcinoma of the large intestine we can do no better than to quote Cheever who said: "Even were it desirable, it certainly is not possible completely to standardize the treatment of any disease. Such a multiplicity of variable factors are involved, in the patient himself, in the disease, in therapeutic measures, and in the physician who applies them, that any attempt at actual standardization is fallacious and unlikely to prepare the physician to meet an unusual and unforeseen situation when it arises. Nevertheless a classification of the types of a disease and a knowledge based on experience of what measures have proved best to meet each typical condition are absolutely essential to prompt and efficient action. Of no disease are these statements more true than of carcinoma of the colon, and yet, in the selection of operative measures in this condition very great divergence of opinion exists among surgeons of experience as to what methods are best." Although standardization is not wholly practical we feel with Daniel Fiske Jones that at least some agreement as to the fundamental principles of the treatment of patients with carcinoma of the colon and rectum can be reached. In a valuable contribution to the subject he quoted Grey Turner as having said: "The history of surgery of malignant disease is neither so discouraging nor so discreditable as many would have us believe, for it shows that when efforts of the surgeon have been *sufficiently thorough*, the results have often been commensurate with the sacrifice which the patient has had to make." It is our opinion that resection definitely is justifiable in all cases up to and frequently including those of borderline operability. Certainly, one loses little and perhaps gains much if a questionable growth is extirpated. Such extirpations, especially for lesions of the rectum, are often formidable and require not only skill but considerable courage. A case which is considered operable by one surgeon may be considered inoperable by another. The surgeon who is satisfied with an operability of 50 per cent may do posterior resection or even local excision with low mortality and a high percentage of patients who survive for three to five years, but by so doing he abandons another 25 per cent or more of those patients whose lesion might be resectable in the hands of a surgeon who is bolder and does more radical resection. The second surgeon who has 75 per cent or greater resectability may have higher mortality and a lower percentage of patients who survive for three to five years; yet he will have a much larger number of five-year "cures" in a given number of patients originally examined and on whom a diagnosis of carcinoma was made.

The controversy as to what is a "sufficiently thorough" operation for carcinoma of the rectum is continued to a considerable extent by those who object to permanent colostomy. No one, we believe, has more effectively answered these objectors than Pfeiffer when in 1937 he said: "It has been the dream of every surgeon interested in the surgery of malignant disease of the rectum and rectosigmoid to devise a plan which fulfills the requirements of adequate cancer surgery and at the same time permits restoration of continuity of the bowel. No artificial anus is equal to the natural mechanism. I am, however, impelled to interpolate right here that a well-made and properly located colostomy in a well patient is easily managed. The chief and most vociferous objectors to colostomy are those who do not have them and do not need them to remain alive.

"It is to be hoped that no one will advocate or condone deliberate sacrifice of sound cancer surgery for any lesser consideration. Good surgery cannot be founded upon the occasional lucky case or the unusual condition. The rock upon which most attempts at restoration of continuity have foundered has been the necessity of making adequate removal of tissue and at the same time preserving the blood supply of the bowel necessary for viability and healing. To this is added the technical difficulty of making a clean and satisfactory anastomosis between the sigmoid and rectum. That it is possible to do so is attested by many successful cases from Kraske down through Hochcncgg and other great masters of the surgery of this region. That it is dangerous and difficult is likewise evident from the trend in recent years toward increasing restriction of efforts in this direction. The lowest mortalities, the highest operability rates, the greatest percentages of cures are unquestionably in the hands of those whose practice it is to perform the widest removal of tissues.

"In my earlier experiences with carcinoma of the rectum and rectosigmoid, I tried a number of expedients to restore continuity, but my results were such that I felt that the occasional successes did not counterbalance the increased morbidity and mortality, as contrasted with frank adoption of permanent colostomy in all but highly selected cases. Of course, the uncontrolled perineal colostomy is indefinitely inferior to the abdominal anus in all respects except sentimental nonsense."

With the exception of the small group of patients who present themselves with acute intestinal obstruction, carcinoma of the large bowel may be relegated, in so far as its surgical treatment is concerned, into the category of chronic ailments. This is of not inconsiderable significance in that it allows time in which to institute preliminary measures aimed at increasing factors of safety in the extirpation of these lesions. (See "Preoperative and Postoperative Treatment.")

PROCEDURES FOR THE COLON

It is important to recognize the different surgical requirements of the two natural divisions of the large bowel, namely, the right half which extends from the ileocecal valve to the middle of the transverse colon, and the left half from the middle of the transverse colon to the rectosigmoid juncture. Developmentally, anatomically, and physiologically, the right and left halves of the bowel differ so much that the colon is virtually a dual organ (see Chapter I). The two halves are not only different anatomically so far as the structure of the wall is concerned, but they derive their blood supply from different sources, the superior mesenteric artery supplying the digestive or absorptive part of the gastro-intestinal tract, and the inferior mesenteric artery supplying the distal half. Moreover, the two arms of the colon harbor different types of pathologic lesions. In the right half of the colon large, bulky, ulcerating growths occur usually on the lateral wall and do not tend to obstruct because of (1) the liquid nature of the fecal current in this segment and (2) the lack of tendency to encircle the bowel, the lumen of which is greater here than elsewhere in its course. On the other hand, in the distal segment of the large bowel, carcinoma usually originates close to the mesenteric border and spreads laterally, diminishing the size of the lumen and consequently producing chronic, subacute, and even acute obstruction.

Right half of the colon.—Carcinoma of the right colon anywhere between the ileocecal juncture and a point just beyond the hepatic flexure is considered almost unanimously to be treated best by removal of the entire right segment of colon, followed by anastomosis between the terminal ileum and the transverse colon (ileocolostomy). The reasons for this have been well expressed by Cheever as follows: "(1) Removal of a lesser part hardly gives a wide enough margin of safety [see 'Lymphatics of the Colon']; (2) the proximal colon being incompletely covered by peritoneum and having a good deal of attached fat or membranous veils is less amenable to anastomosis; (3) the ileum has a rich blood supply which minimizes the liability to suture line necrosis; and (4) the operation is relatively easy." Opinion does differ, however, as to how the anastomosis should be made—whether end-to-end, end-to-side, or side-to-side, by open suture or one of the closed methods, with or without a special clamp, and whether it should be accompanied by a proximal safety valve ileostomy of some type—and, as to whether resection should be accomplished in one or two stages. "The one fundamental prerequisite, however," as T. E. Jones recently stated, "is to do as extensive and as radical an operation as possible. Whether this is done by the closed or open method, by the one-stage or two-stage method, or by any other technique makes little difference provided the surgeon can show that his results from the standpoint of mortality and morbidity are equal to those of the other techniques."

As the safety of primary resection and anastomosis has increased, there has developed a growing tendency toward performance of a single-stage instead of a multistage operation for uncomplicated carcinoma of the colon irrespective of the location. Ravdin and Abbott, Whipple, and Newton and Blodgett, have reported strikingly favorable results from the use of the Miller-Abbott tube before, during and after resection as a means of decompression in cases of carcinoma of the right colon, including those that produce obstruction. Ravdin et al., reported in 1947 that their experience with long tube decompression had been so satisfactory that a two-stage resection of the right colon had not been done by them since 1938. This experience, however, has not been shared by many other surgeons. Jones probably reflects the opinion of a majority of those who undertake most of the surgery of the large intestine when he said: "Because of the frequent difficulty in passing the tube, the intolerance of certain patients to it, and irritation from it which may produce pulmonary complications, when necessary for many days, the ileostomy tube may be more satisfactory." Coller and Vaughan have recently reaffirmed their continued adherence to a two-stage operation in most instances. While admitting certain drawbacks for the multistage procedures, they nevertheless believe that early mobilization of the patient has reduced hospitalization time with the two-stage operation until the time element is no longer an argument against it. At the Lahey Clinic where obstructive resection has long been considered the operation of choice for carcinoma of the large bowel, including the right colon, there appears to be some deviation from this rule with respect to the right half. In 1946, Cattell and Colcock reported on 77 resections of the right colon performed at the Lahey Clinic in 1945, of which 13 were accomplished by primary resection and anastomosis.

Our own choice in the absence of obstruction, subacute perforation or fixation is a one-stage procedure, accomplished by the closed, Rankin clamp method without complementary ileostomy proximal to the anastomosis. On the rare occasion in which advanced obstruction is present, a preliminary side-to-side ileotransverse colostomy is done and in two or three weeks is followed by resection. When subacute perforation or fixation is present without obstruction, a preliminary end-to-side ileotransverse colostomy is performed. We have not performed a two-stage resection of the right half of the colon in the past two years.

End-to-side anastomosis between the terminal ileum and the transverse colon in instances in which resection of the right half of the colon is desired either immediately or subsequently is, in our opinion, decidedly the most satisfactory method. The greatest advantage of end-to-side anastomosis is the ability thereby to sidetrack the fecal current completely from passing over an ulcerating surface. We believe that the necessity of graded operation is largely dependent upon the amount of infection around the primary growth, which not only renders immediate resection hazardous but gravely undermines the individual's powers of resistance. Reduction of this infection and rehabilitation are two steps which are not to be gainsaid in successful attack on right colonic lesions. Moreover, we have found it convenient in any case, first, to establish the end-to-side anastomosis between the terminal ileum and the transverse colon, and then to determine from the immediate condition of the patient if resection of the right segment of colon is justifiable at the initial operation. Occasionally a patient who appeared in satisfactory condition for a single-stage maneuver at the commencement of the operation was found to be in a less favorable state at the completion of the anastomosis of the ileum to the colon. Careful questioning of many patients who have borne end-to-side anastomosis over a period of more than a year has failed to elicit a history of abdominal discomfort or of sensations of pressure at the site of anastomosis, although this is a frequent complaint of patients in whom lateral union has been made.

Cannon and Murphy and others have demonstrated by animal experimentation that lateral anastomosis is an unphysiologic procedure. Severing the circular muscle fibres in lateral anastomosis abolishes peristalsis in the region of the anastomosis, and the blind pouches at the ends fail to empty completely. The stasis that tends to develop at the new juncture and the concomitant attempt on the part of the normal segment of bowel proximal to this point to overcome the obstacle probably accounts for the upper abdominal discomfort frequently mentioned by patients in whom lateral anastomosis has been established. Lockhart-Mummery lists these additional disadvantages of lateral anastomosis as applied to the colon in general: (1) It requires a much greater length of bowel; (2) it requires either more extensive freeing of the colon or less extensive removal of the diseased part as compared with axial union; (3) the operation takes much longer to perform as, in addition to the actual anastomosis, two ends of colon have to be closed; (4) the subsequent anatomic condition is not perfect and the blind end of the proximal portion is apt to give trouble. The observer reports several cases in which there has been abscess in this portion of the large bowel.

In contemplating any method of anastomosis between two segments of bowel one must take into consideration certain important technical factors, such as ability to approximate the edges of the bowel accurately, adequacy of blood supply, liability to obstruction from formation of stricture or excessive diaphragm, probability of hemorrhage, and danger from contamination or subsequent leakage at the line of suture. In well over 200 patients operated on by us with a special clamp (Rankin) not a single postoperative hemorrhage has occurred. In our cases there was no obstruction at the site of anastomosis, yet in not a single instance during graded procedures was enterostomy established proximal to anastomosis. The good clinical results of our clamp method, we believe, bear out the experimental advantages which were demonstrated by one of us (Graham) in Mann's laboratory. These animal experiments, which have been reported previously (1929), elicited the following results: Absence of postoperative hemorrhage, of leakage at the site of anastomosis, of circular constriction, almost complete absence of a diaphragm within the lumen, and absence of diminution in the diameter of the lumen (Figs. 86 to 88).

Controversy concerning the relative merits of the closed and open methods of intestinal anastomosis continues. Despite strenuous theoretical objections to the aseptic technics, particularly those that employ special clamps, by Whipple, Meyers et al., and a few others, their popularity has grown steadily since 1937, when a survey made by us revealed almost universal preference for open anastomosis. In a survey of 50 surgeons made in 1947, 60 per cent indicated preference for a closed type of anastomosis. Stone, Wangensteen, Waugh, White, Pemberton, Dixon, MacFee and ourselves are among those who believe mortality is favorably influenced by the closed technic. As advocates of aseptic anastomosis, we believe it is more desirable because it diminishes if it does not abolish the element of infection, and experience has shown that it may be accomplished with ease and satisfaction in the hands of most surgeons. At the same time it would be extremely dogmatic to urge that any single operative method to accomplish an objective so far outbalanced the disadvantages of all others as to make it indispensable. Elements of personality and circumstance must inevitably influence the choice of technic, and in consequence, the range of maneuvers continues wide and at the same time acceptable so long as fundamental principles are observed.

The danger of postoperative distention causing rupture of the suture line following ileocolostomy provided adequate blood supply to the two ends of bowel is insured, is not very great if routinely before the patient leaves the operating room the anal sphincters are thoroughly stretched or else an inlying rectal tube (or rectal spool) is employed from the time the patient leaves the operating room until firm healing has occurred at the site of anastomosis, that is, about six or seven days.

Left half of the colon.—Obstruction is the most alarming symptom in the left colon, by which is meant the major portion of the transverse colon, the descending colon and sigmoid. If the obstruction is acute, which has been quite infrequent in our experience, or of the chronic type which has failed to respond adequately to the usual medical measures of decompression, drainage by cecostomy or colostomy proximal to the growth is urgently indicated as a preliminary step to subsequent resection. While this is now a well-recognized surgical principle and is more or less the general practice, many surgeons continue to explore the abdomen at this time; relief of the immediate obstruction is the paramount consideration and manipulation of the colon under such circumstances is highly dangerous because of the likelihood of perforation or of spread of organisms which may have penetrated the distended, attenuated wall of the colon.

Routine establishment of proximal surgical drainage, prior to or at the time of resection of the distal colon or rectum, is less popular than formerly. In a recent (1947) survey by questionnaire undertaken by us (considered in detail in the foregoing general discussion), 15, or 30 per cent, indicated regular employment of appendicostomy, cecostomy, or colostomy; seven preliminary to resection and anastomosis and the remainder at the time of operation. These included Dixon, R. Graham, White, Whipple and Fallis. Tube cecostomy is favored over other methods. Only three expressed preference for the Devine type of colostomy. A number commented that this procedure is unnecessarily complicated and are in agreement with Dennis, Fallis, and Wangensteen who believe satisfactory defunctionalization as well as decompression can be attained by a simple loop colostomy. Stone, Waugh, Meyer et al., and Wangensteen have recently taken positive stands to the effect that proximal drainage is not essential to a low mortality in primary suture of the left colon. Ravdin considers decompression with the Miller-Abbott tube before, during and after resection to be an important contributory factor in the reduction of mortality in primary resection of the distal segment of the bowel. Only four other surgeons indicated that they made regular use of long tube decompression. Seventeen found decompression by means of an indwelling duodenal tube adequate in most instances.

Although we recognize the occasional advantage of preliminary cecostomy or colostomy as an adjunct to surgery of the distal colon, we do not consider such a step essential to safe surgery of the large intestine when obstruction is absent or has been relieved. The proof of this to us has been the practical experience with hundreds of cases in which incomplete obstruction, often to a marked degree, was relieved by a regime consisting of initial purgation, repeated colonic irrigations, and an essentially non-residue diet. Strict avoidance of oral administration of barium in conjunction with roentgenoscopic examination of the intestinal tract when an obstructive lesion of the colon is suspected has, we believe, reduced materially the necessity of preliminary procedures for drainage in our cases, for unquestionably such practice is responsible for many instances of acute obstruction superimposed upon chronic obstruction of long standing. Adequate care in preparing these patients for operation, taking five to seven days or more, is, in our opinion, secondary in importance only to early recognition of the malignancy. Emergency surgery rarely is necessary or justifiable in such cases since obstruction, when it develops, usually is slowly progressive and well tolerated even for a week or more after it becomes complete. The blood chemistry under the circumstances, in striking contrast to the findings in acute obstruction of the small intestine, may and usually does remain unaltered.

On a number of occasions, in consultation with other surgeons or on visits to their hospitals both in this country and abroad, we have observed the tendency to consider as acute obstruction cases which in our experience have, in scores of instances, responded to a medical regime aimed at decompressing the chronically obstructed bowel. Even if the response has not been wholly adequate there can be no doubt that the patient becomes a better operative risk for cecostomy or colostomy after a period of hospitalization in which measures to overcome dehydration have been instituted.

If complete diversion of the fecal stream is desired we agree with Cheever, Devine, Wangensteen, Fallis, Dennis, Gurd and Heyd that colostomy in the proximal transverse colon is the measure of choice. This will avoid the serious disturbance of fluid balance which is likely to occur if the cecum is mobilized and brought out on the abdomen as advocated by Gordon-Taylor and Horsley. In the latter circumstance the same problem would obtain as with the loss of fluid following establishment of ileostomy. Moreover, in our experience closure of transverse colostomy has been less difficult than closure of cecostomy that completely diverts the feces. The somewhat involved method of defunctionalization proposed by Devine and championed by Gurd and Heyd seems less satisfactory than a simple loop colostomy which can readily be performed under local anesthesia and in the experience of ourselves and many others satisfactorily diverts the fecal stream.

Choice of operation in lesions of the distal colon is between (1) an extraperitoneal excision such as obstructive resection, and (2) primary resection followed by immediate anastomosis, with or without antecedent or concomitant cecostomy or transverse colostomy. An analysis of findings in our recent survey by questionnaire (see page 175) revealed a decided trend away from extraperitoneal, multistage operations. One of the 50 surgeons in this survey stated that he never performed primary suture of the distal colon; three that they undertook it only on rare occasion, and four others claimed 100 per cent performance. Between these extremes are recorded in Table 31 a varied incidence of performance. Thirty-two or 62 per cent, estimate employment of primary anastomosis in 75 to 100 per cent of cases.

Although a difference of opinion prevails as to which single factor chiefly is responsible for reasonably safe accomplishment of resection and immediate anastomosis, most of the surgeons who made special comment on the subject considered the following to be contributory: (1) The advent of chemotherapeutic agents for oral use during the preoperative period; (2) a better understanding and utilization of preoperative preparation, especially as regards anemia and serum protein deficiency; and (3) improvement in anesthetic methods. In addition to these influences, a number of surgeons, especially Stone, believe that a closed type of anastomosis contributes materially to the success of this undertaking. Somewhat more controversial are values placed on antecedent or concomitant use of decompressive measures.

In 1942 considerable impetus was given to the developing trend toward resection and immediate anastomosis of the colon through Stone's influential advocacy of the method in a valuable contribution to the subject in which McLanahan collaborated. More recently technical methods and reasons for preference of primary anastomosis over extraperitoneal resection have been reported by White and Amendola, Whipple, Waugh and Custer, Clute and Kenny, Meyer et al., Hoxworth, Wangensteen, McFee, and Ravdin, et al.

T. E. Jones, Rankin, Lahey and Cattell, and David have repeatedly urged that the old-type Mikulicz operation not be confused with the newer concept of extraperitoneal resection, exemplified by obstructive resection of Rankin. They believe that in many, if not in most instances, an exteriorization measure, rather than primary suture of the bowel, is the proper choice; that ample statistical data on resectability, mortality and five-year survivals attest the adequacy of this mode of resection, by which as great an extent of colon and gland bearing mesentery can be removed as in resection and primary anastomosis. We are in full accord with Lahey's statement that, "it is important to state, because of the confusion which exists in many minds about the old and original type of Mikulicz operation and the modern modification, that the procedure [obstructive resection] in no way differs in the extent of its radicalness, either in amount of colon removed or in the area of adjacent mesentery and mesenteric glands included in the removal of the colon. It differs from primary removal and primary anastomosis only in the method of restoring the fecal stream and not in the radicalness of extent." Until recently we have considered primary anastomosis in the left half of the colon to be seldom desirable. We now find ourselves in the same category as McFee, who said that he was unable to accomplish such an anastomosis in more than 25 per cent of cases; yet, since 1938 he has been a strong advocate of primary resection and primary anastomosis. In 1947 he aptly expressed the concern with which a number of us have viewed the all-or-none attitude adopted by many surgeons in regard to primary suture of the distal colon when he said: "When primary resection is intended and an unforseen complication is encountered, there is always the inclination to proceed with the definitive operation as planned, bearing in mind, but at the same time disregarding, the fact that conditions for the operation are not ideal. The results may be chastening to the surgeon, and irreparably bad for the patient."

PROCEDURES FOR THE RECTOSIGMOID, RECTUM, AND ANUS

The ideal operation for removal of carcinoma of the rectum and rectosigmoid has not been devised because a radical extirpative measure cannot be accomplished satisfactorily with preservation of the sphincteric apparatus. The acceptance, however, of colostomy as routine was one of the great steps forward in surgical treatment of patients with such lesions. (This has already been considered in detail in the foregoing general discussion.) While there is small difference of opinion that radical surgery is the method of choice in its treatment, the rediscovery of the "pull-through operation" has in recent years created a certain amount of controversy as to the type of procedure most acceptable in the majority of cases. Since Miles's epic publication there have been innumerable surgeons both great and small who have tried to develop many procedures for the preservation of the anal sphincter in the treatment of cancer of the rectum. In the light of the recent studies of the lymphatics of the perirectal and pelvic tissues carried out by David and Gilchrist and again by Coller et al., there seems little justification for this effort. The bitter cry against colostomy as pointed out by Pfeiffer is raised by "those who do not have them and do not need them to remain alive." Again he observed that "Of course, the uncontrollable perineal colostomy is infinitely inferior to the abdominal anus in all respects except sentimental nonsense." With this thesis most surgeons who have had wide experience in this field are in accord, as has been revealed in our survey in 1947 of current literature and by questionnaire of 50 surgeons (Table 32).

It is interesting to observe that the proponents of the two conflicting schools of thought in the treatment of cancer of the rectum both find inspiration and guidance in the several pathologic studies of the lymphatic spread in rectal cancer. The most enthusiastic champions of preservation of the anal sphincteric mechanism, Babcock, Lynch, Bacon, Waugh, and Wangensteen, have all pointed to the common finding of these investigations namely, infrequent retrograde spread of rectal cancer as justification for operative methods which eliminate colostomy. On the other hand, the staunchest supporters of the principles of Miles include four surgeons—Gabriel, Coller, Gilchrist and David—who have played important roles in demonstrating the pattern of lymphatic metastasis in cancer of the rectum. The latter two, as a result of their most recent (1947) study, concluded that "Lesions which are partially or completely below the peritoneal reflection have a high incidence of local and liver recurrences and pull-through or sleeve resections are not much better than a local resection." Rankin, Jones, Lahey, Stone and many others have referred to these pathologic studies as additional proof of the necessity for the radical rather than the conservative resection of the rectum. Jones found that the relatively high incidence of local recurrence in the cases recently reported by Gilchrist and David "prove further that radicalism is necessary and that revival of the pull-through operations and low anastomosis will be short-lived."

Combined abdominoperineal and perineo-abdominal resection in one stage.—In our judgment a radical combined operation in a single stage by which the local growth and the gland-bearing tissue in immediate juxtaposition to it are extirpated in toto after the manner of Miles, or some modification which suits the individual surgeon's fancy such as the perineo-abdominal excision of Turner or of Gabriel, is the most desirable one. More familiarity with technical details and more meticulous preoperative preparation and postoperative care have allowed us in recent years to utilize the single-stage procedure in a higher percentage of cases than hitherto. That this may not be carried out in some cases where the rectal tumor is removable, yet hazardously so because of complicating co-existing debilitating diseases and the patient's inability to stand formidable operative procedures, is quite evident. These occasions, however, are now exceedingly rare.

Abel lists three fundamental principles of surgery involved in operating on a patient with carcinoma of the rectum and states that the only operation which fulfills these principles is the radical abdominoperineal excision introduced in 1907 by Miles: (1) Not only the growth but also all removable fields of lymphatic spread must be extirpated as widely as possible. In this instance the upward spread demands the most careful attention and should be

removed just up to the point at which the left colonic artery arises
from the inferior mesenteric artery. (2) When an operation involves
two different fields of maneuver of which one is sterile and the other
relatively infected, the aseptic field should be dealt with first and
closed off, and the infected area should be dealt with last, in order
that the former may not be infected from it. (3) Before a primary
growth is tampered with or manipulated in any way, the blood and
lymph vessels, which are liable to transmit metastatic cells into the
venous and lymphatic circulations, should be ligated. Primary dissection should be carried out as far as possible from the original
growth. Posterior excision following colostomy will not fulfill any
of these requirements and perineo-abdominal excision will fulfill
only the first principle, since the initial approach is through the
relatively infected perineal region and the segment containing the
growth is manipulated prior to ligation of blood and lymph vessels.

Gabriel, who is the principal advocate of the one-stage perineo-
abdominal operation, takes a somewhat different view from that of
Miles and Abel. Admitting the merits of the abdominoperineal
excision by the Miles technic, he states that the considerable number of two-stage modifications which have been described indicate
the desire and the attempts of surgeons to minimize the risks of the
original operation. He enumerates the following advantages which
the one-stage perineo-abdominal excision possesses over the operation of Miles: (1) it is an easier operation to perform provided the
operator has the experience which enables him to do neat perineal
dissection; (2) it overcomes the serious difficulties of a narrow male
pelvis, especially in those cases with a large tumor at the rectosigmoid juncture; (3) the dangers of sepsis and shock are largely
eliminated—the former by avoiding intraperitoneal division of the
colon, and shock by doing the perineal part of the operation first
so that no turning of the patient is required after completion of the
abdominal operations; and (4) it fulfills all the requirements of a
radical operation in regard to high sections of the vascular and
lymphatic pedicle and, in regard to the length of bowel which is
removed, is slightly more radical than the Miles technic.

Formerly Gabriel performed the operation as a "blind" one-
stage procedure in carefully selected cases in which a freely mobile
growth was situated low in the rectum. In 1945, however, in the
third edition of his book, he stated that in all cases a preliminary
exploration is done. In 1935 one of us (Rankin) reported a series of
cases in which exploration was carried out through a McBurney
incision and cecostomy established; subsequent perineo-abdominal
resection was consummated. We believed that this maneuver would
be applicable in many instances in which the Miles operation would
be contraindicated. Our present belief, however, is that the com-

bined operation of Miles is applicable in almost every instance and as a consequence have not employed perineo-abdominal resection in recent years.

To the question in our recent survey, "Do you consider combined abdominoperineal resection the operation of choice for carcinoma of the rectosigmoid and rectum?" 41, or 82 per cent of those queried answered in the affirmative. Two of the remaining nine employ the Miles operation for all but rectosigmoidal lesions; the residual seven perform anterior resection not only for lesions of the rectosigmoid but also for carcinomas situated at varying levels of the rectal ampulla as well (Table 32).

Combined abdominoperineal and perineo-abdominal resections in two stages.—Although we advocated a two-stage operation for the less sturdy risks in our earlier publications, we have more recently utilized the one-stage procedure almost exclusively. With the steady improvement in preoperative preparation, in anesthesia and postoperative care, more and more patients including the elderly, the feeble, and the depleted are being submitted to radical resection in one-stage with lower mortality and higher curability rate. The only remaining indications for a two-stage operation, as we see it, are firm fixation of the growth to adjacent viscera or structures, or definite evidence of infection about the growth. Obstruction unrelieved by preoperative medical measures will, of course, require preliminary drainage by cecostomy or transverse colostomy. We are not certain but that the same type of preliminary drainage measure is indicated when fixation or infection exists, rather than a two-stage type of combined operation such as that described by one of us (Rankin) or by Lahey. Upon relief of obstruction or fixation, if there is no other contraindication, a one-stage combined type of maneuver may then be undertaken.

The two-stage combined operations now in vogue vary somewhat in technical details and in scope, but the fundamental principle of all of them may be traced to the classical one-stage procedure of Miles. The type advocated for many years by Daniel Fiske Jones had much to recommend it. An advantage which it possessed was that a radical procedure was carried out at the first stage without the need for opening the bowel; a disadvantage was that loop colostomy was required. The results, both immediate and remote as reported by Jones, were good. The operation now, however, is obsolete owing to the advantages which the Miles operation possesses over it. One of us (Rankin), in 1929, described a procedure in which at the first stage a single-barreled or end colostomy is made and the divided distal end is inverted and dropped back; at the second stage a perineo-abdominal excision is consummated. One year later Lahey modified this operation by bringing the lower end of divided sigmoid out of the exploratory incision for purposes of irrigation between stages.

Because of the many disadvantages of the Coffey operation we see little justification for its employment under any circumstances. The mortality attending this procedure, judging from most reports, is prohibitively high. From the technical standpoint it may be impossible to telescope the distal end of the bowel through the constricted lumen of the bowel at the site of the growth, and failure of collateral circulation may and not infrequently does give rise to necrosis of the inverted distal end of bowel and pelvic cellulitis.

Colostomy and posterior resection (perineal excision).—For growths beneath the peritoneal reflection, particularly if low in the rectum, this procedure is satisfactory from the standpoint of operative mortality and the comparative ease with which it can be accomplished. On the other hand, this operation does not permit excision of the node-bearing tissue in the vicinity of the rectosigmoid and in the mesentery of the sigmoid as thoroughly as by the combined abdominoperineal maneuver. The high rate of recurrence following perineal excision led Miles to design the combined operation. In his series of 58 survivals of perineal excision, 55 were known to have died from recurrence, a rate of recurrence of 94.8 per cent. While it is still true that recurrence is more frequent after posterior excision than when the radical combined maneuver is employed, nevertheless, there is ample statistical proof that the former can be carried out in a group of cases which are such grave operative risks that the latter is not to be considered, and with five-year "cures" of 38 per cent in 300 cases (Rankin) and 50 per cent in 209 cases (Lockhart-Mummery). This type of operation is a useful procedure in certain desiccated, devitalized and depleted patients upon whom one hesitates to do a Miles operation. Its utility is steadily decreasing and in the past few years only an occasional case has been submitted to this type of procedure by us.

Contrary to an apparently widespread belief, Lockhart-Mummery neither advocates nor employs perineal excision to the exclusion of all other procedures. He states that his operative procedure is suitable in any case in which the growth is at the anus or anywhere in the rectum proper, provided it is not fixed to important structures; it cannot be performed if the growth is at or above the rectosigmoid junction unless the growth is small and the sigmoid fairly lengthy. A high growth, he states, ordinarily "should be removed by an abdominoperineal operation, or if the surgeon finds himself in difficulties owing to the fact that the growth is too high to be removed safely from the perineum, he may reverse the procedure, and, after freeing the rectum below, close the posterior wound, turn the patient on his back, and complete the operation from the abdomen—in short, do a perineo-abdominal resection."

Anterior resection of the lower sigmoid, rectosigmoid and rectum.— Neoplasm situated low in the sigmoid occasionally constitutes a separate problem. It cannot be exteriorized without extensive mobilization of the rectosigmoid, hence the patient is subjected, as a rule, to abdominoperineal operation of some type. From the standpoint of curing the disease such a course is entirely satisfactory, but unquestionably there are instances, admittedly rare, in which a more conservative procedure without sacrifice of the rectum is justifiable. If the growth is situated well within the peritoneal cavity, at least 5 cm. from the reflection of the peritoneum on the bowel, we will consider an anterior resection with immediate restoration of the continuity of the bowel provided that: (1) the growth is small and of a low grade of malignancy (grades 1 and 2), as determined by biopsy through the sigmoidoscope; (2) the growth is a polypoid one of doubtful benignancy; or (3) the patient refuses permanent colostomy. However, not infrequently factors are present which make such procedure inadvisable, chief among which is marked inflammatory reaction or formation of abscess in the vicinity, marked adiposity, and instances of a short sigmoid flexure. In 1936 we described for the low sigmoidal lesion modified obstructive resection, employing the Rankin clamp. David previously had described a similar procedure which differed somewhat in the details of technic. Although convinced that these procedures may be employed advantageously in certain carefully selected cases, we do not lose sight of the fact that even in instances of low sigmoidal growth the ideal procedure, in the absence of contraindications, is combined abdominoperineal operation, either in one or two stages. With Pfeiffer we feel that the occasional success which attends anterior resection of the rectosigmoid does "not counterbalance the increased morbidity and mortality, as contrasted with frank adoption of permanent colostomy in all but highly selected cases." We have not employed obstructive resection for low sigmoidal lesions in many years and very few anterior resections with immediate anastomosis. For growths which are situated in the rectosigmoid at or below the reflection of the peritoneum onto the bowel we believe a combined operation is the maneuver of election.

Only nine, or 18 per cent, of the 50 surgeons to whom we sent questionnaires indicated that they regularly undertake anterior resection of the rectosigmoid for operable malignant growths. Twelve, or 24 per cent, signified that they never perform this operation, whereas 14 of the remaining 29 especially commented that they consider it justifiable only as a palliative measure when liver metastasis exists. As evidence of a trend away from anterior resection are statements volunteered by eight to the effect that formerly they favored this measure as the operation of choice in all cases, but now use it only as an expedient or not at all. White and several others in this group give credit for their decision to the recent (1947) report of David on their pathologic studies of lymphatic spread in cancer of the rectum. The objection to anterior resection most frequently expressed is the high incidence of local recurrence. Others were influenced by a high morbidity incident to leakage at the suture line, with subsequent pelvic infection, fistula formation or occurrence of stricture at the site of anastomosis.

The principal advocates of anterior resection are Dixon, Wangensteen and Mahorner. Their thesis is simply this: (1) carcinoma of the rectosigmoid does not ordinarily metastasize downward; (2) contrary to longstanding belief, the superior hemorrhoidal vessels may be sacrificed without impairment of the circulation of the divided ends of sigmoid and rectum; and, (3) avoidance of colostomy is a pre-eminent humanitarian consideration. To date, the number of cases undertaken by this method have been too few in any one series, and the length of time which has elapsed since they were undertaken has been too short, to permit its proper evaluation. From the foregoing it would appear, nevertheless, that a decided majority of those who probably undertake most of the surgery of the large bowel in this country question the wisdom of restoring intestinal continuity after resection of the rectosigmoid when cure is the objective.

Waugh, Wangensteen, Mahorner and four others, or 14 per cent of those whose questionnaires comprised our recent study of trends in surgery of the large intestine, have extended the scope of anterior resection to include lesions at varying levels of the rectal ampulla as follows: three for all lesions more than 10 cm. above the pectinate line (one employs a pull-through operation for small, early growths); two for all lesions more than 5 cm. above this line; one for selected, small growths 6 cm. above the anus; and for one all lesions at least 3 cm. above the ano-rectal line (Table 32). All employ the Miles operation when cancers are situated below the levels which have been indicated.

Of those who utilize anterior resection or the pull-through operation for rectal growths, only a few, notably Babcock, Bacon, and Garlock, include lesions situated as low as 3 cm. from the ano-rectal line. Wangensteen is convinced, despite the failure of Coller and his associates to find evidence of lateral lymphatic spread in lesions lying more than 3 cm. above the anus, that in low-lying lesions, failure to excise the levator muscles in juxtaposition to the bowel invites local recurrence. "I have learned," he states, "the bitter lesson that it is unwise to attempt to salvage sphincters in such low lesions. If one does so, he compromises on the cure."

Another factor to be considered in the evaluation of anterior resection of the rectosigmoid and rectal ampulla for cancer is the malignant potential of the entire rectum when a single area of malignancy has been observed. It has recently been suggested by one of us (Graham) and by Baker that perhaps the high incidence of so-called local recurrence which accompanies anterior resection of the rectum and rectosigmiod might in part be due to the development of new cancers on the basis of satellite polyps which are frequently noted in excised specimens of the rectum. Baker emphasized the importance of repeated sigmoidoscopic examinations following resection and prinary anastomosis of the upper rectum. He pointed out that such sessile polyps are not always visualized through the proctoscope and might not be demonstrated until the removed colon or rectum has been evaginated.

Proctosigmoidectomy (Abdominoperineal resection in one stage without abdominal colostomy).—Recent renewed interest in procedures designed to eliminate the establishment of an abdominal anus would seem to have been inspired by pathologic studies of lymphatic spread of rectal cancer reported by Gabriel, Dukes and Bussey, Gilchrist and David and by Coller and his associates. Lynch, for instance, in referring to the investigations of Gabriel, Dukes and Bussey, remarked, "It permits one to discard entirely such radical and unnecessary operations as that popularized by Miles." Yet, Gabriel, Gilchrist, David, and Coller are themselves staunch supporters of the principles of Miles and therefore consider abdominal colostomy essential to an adequately radical resection of the rectum. In 1947, Gilchrist and David as a result of their most recent study of lymphatic spread in rectal cancer concluded that "Lesions which are partially or completely below the peritoneal reflection have a high incidence of local and liver recurrences and pull-through or sleeve resections are not much better than a local resection. The Miles operation seems to give the best chance of cure here."

In our recent survey of opinion in regard to trends in surgery of the large bowel not one of the 50 surgeons to whom questionnaires were sent indicated proctosigmoidectomy as the procedure of choice. (This survey has been considered in detail in the foregoing general discussion.) Nine who had in recent years performed an occasional operation of the Babcock-Bacon type expressed dissatisfaction with the procedure and a disinclination to employ it in the future. Waugh supplemented his answers to these questions with the observation that he had used the pull-through operation of the Babcock type in over 100 patients whose lesions were between 5 and 10 cm. from the pectinate line. Although he believes that if used advisedly, this procedure is as curative as the Miles operation, he nevertheless found anal function to be less satisfactory than it is after anterior resection and anastomosis. For this reason he has extended downward the scope of end-to-end anastomosis to include growths 5 cm. from the anus. Wangensteen said in his additional remarks that he reserved the abdominoperineal procedure for large, fixed ampullary growths and for all growths lying within 6 cm.* of the anus. He further commented that the Babcock-Bacon type of operation, which he had performed on a number of occasions in recent years "fails to preserve the internal sphincter and in consequence fails to preserve continence." Also recently, in remarking on Babcock and Bacon's assertion that the sphincterless perineal colostomy is to be preferred to abdominal colostomy, he said: "Whereas for sentimental reasons, the perineum may appear to be a more desirable location for an artificial anus, it would seem better to have such an opening where it may come more directly under the watchful eye of its owner."

Daniel, who indicated that he considers the Miles operation the method of choice for all rectal lesions, provided us with unpublished statistics of his recent personal experiences with 20 anterior resections of the rectal ampulla in which primary anastomosis was done, 24 resections of the Babcock-Bacon type, and 34 abdominoperineal resections, all performed between December 1, 1945 and February 1, 1947. The incidence of secondary metastasis, or reappearance at the operative site, were: (1) for anterior resection, 15 per cent; (2) for the Babcock-Bacon procedure, 30.38 per cent; and, (3) for the Miles operation, 1 wound metastasis, or 3.4 per cent. In a previous study there were 22 wound metastases in 257 cases of abdominoperineal resection and colostomy and perineal resection, or an incidence of 7.7 per cent. Recurrences in the anterior resections were in the bowel itself. Of the seven secondary metastases in the pull-through operations, in three instances perirectal nodes and fat were involved and in four there was no discernible involvement outside the bowel wall.

The secret of proper adjustment to an abdominal colostomy, we believe, is the realization that this is the safest and best method of securing longevity. The surgeon who is a staunch advocate of the combined operation as the best possible means for saving the life of his patient, will not belie the confidence of his patient in a faltering dissertation of the pros and cons of an abdominal anus versus perineal colostomy or the doubtful possibility of retaining the use of the anal sphincter.

---

* In 1948 he reported a change of the limit to 8 cm. owing to the relatively high incidence of local recurrence when lesions nearer than 8 cm. to the anus were resected anteriorly.

The average patient's abhorrence of colostomy can be overcome readily by anyone who is, himself, convinced that it is a tolerable state, compatible with a normal, comfortable, contented, useful and profitable existence. Infinite tact and patience will be rewarded by almost invariable acceptance of artificial abdominal anus.

PROCEDURES FOR PALLIATION

The ultimate aim of all types of operation for cancer is cure, but it must be recognized that there is a definite group of cases in which cure being impossible, the ingenuity and resourcefulness of the surgeon may still be available in the application of palliative procedures. Such a decision, often difficult in the extreme, is a function which no surgeon may escape, for trying as it is, it demands a not inconsiderable amount of courage as well as keen surgical judgment One must often decide whether resection as a palliative measure is justifiable or whether because obstruction is not present the abdomen is closed and the individual permitted to languish agonizingly as a result of local extension of the lesion. It is a not uncommon experience to explore a patient with a cancer of the colon or rectum which is freely movable, and resectable with a reasonable mortality risk, and to find by palpation of the liver surfaces multiple umbilicated, irregular, malignant nodules. Removal of the local growth, precluding obstruction, fixation to neurogenic elements, and other painful complications, is often warranted under such circumstances, even though the mortality figures may be higher than in more hopeful cases. Death from cancer of the liver is a not too painful experience and in such circumstances, removal of the primary growth and consequent comfortable prolongation of life, is entirely praiseworthy.

It is now more the rule than the exception, when hepatic metastasis is encountered, to proceed with the resection as planned, regardless of the segment of bowel involved, provided local conditions permit. There are surgeons who, under these circumstances, will regularly undertake an abdominoperineal resection in one-stage for lesions of the rectosigmoid and rectum. Others who regularly employ the Miles operation for such lesions when operable will, however, resort to anterior abdominal resection of the rectosigmoid and upper ampulla, with immediate anastomosis, when secondary deposits in the liver are noted. The current trend toward more radical palliative resections is due to a better understanding and utilization of preoperative measures, the advent of chemotherapeutic agents and improved anesthetic methods—the same conditions which in the operable cases have been chiefly responsible for the steady rise in the resectability rate.

There will always be a few patients who are not sufficiently strong to withstand the more formidable resections, even the relatively safe obstructive resection of mobile segments of colon, or colostomy and posterior excision. Moreover, when obstruction supervenes with fixation, abscess formation or other local complications, resection of any type is out of the question. For this group of patients the following measures are available: (1) Simple exteriorization measures as those of Mikulicz or of Paul, for lesions of the colon; (2) local excisions without colostomy as those devised by Cripps, Quénu, Tuttle, and others for lesions of the rectum; and, (3) operations for overcoming obstruction as cecostomy, colostomy or by-passing measures as colo-colostomy. Before making the decision to establish a colostomy in a patient with an inoperable growth, but which is not producing obstruction, the surgeon should consider the fact that the average span of life of these patients is not prolonged by colostomy (Table 8). On the whole, our experience with palliative colostomies in elderly, markedly debilitated individuals has been most unsatisfactory. We are in agreement with Jones who recently stated that colostomy is often indiscriminately done and that obstruction is the only indication.

REFERENCES

1. ALLEN, A. W., WELCH, C. E., and DONALDSON, G. A.: Carcinoma of the colon, *Ann. Surg.*, **126:** 19–30 (July), 1947.
2. BABCOCK, W. W.: The operative treatment of carcinoma of the rectosigmoid with methods for elimination of colostomy. *Surg., Gynec., and Obstet.*, **55:** 627–632 (Nov.), 1932.
3. BACON, H. E.: Evolution of sphincter muscle preservation and reestablishment of continuity in operative treatment of rectal and sigmoidal cancer. *Surg., Gynec., and Obstet.*, **81:** 113–127 (Aug.), 1945.
4. BAKER, JOEL W.: Controversial trends in cancer of the lower sigmoid and rectum. *Bulletin of the Mason Clinic*, **1:** 83–92 (Sept.), 1947.
5. CANNON, W. B., and MURPHY, F. T.: The movements of the stomach and intestines in some surgical conditions. *Ann. Surg.*, **63:** 519–520, 1906.
6. CHEEVER, DAVID: The choice of operation in carcinoma of the colon. *Ann. Surg.*, **94:** 705–716 (Oct.), 1931.
7. COLLER, F. A., KAY, E. B., McINTYRE, R. S.: Regional lymphatic metastasis of carcinoma of the rectum. *Surgery*, **8:** 294–311, 1940.
8. COLLER, F.A., and VAUGHAN, H. H.: The treatment of carcinoma of the colon. *Ann. Surg.*, **121:** 395–411 (April), 1945.
9. CLUTE, H. M., and KENNEY, F. R.: Primary anastomosis in carconoma of the colon. *New England J. Med.*, **233:** 799 (Dec. 27), 1945.
10. DANIEL, W. H.: Personal communication to authors.
11. DANIEL, W. H.: Primary and secondary metastases from cancer of the colon and rectum. *South. Med. Jour.*, **39:** 480–482 (June), 1946.
12. DAVID, V. C.: Treatment of carcinoma at rectosigmoid junction by obstructive resection. *Surg., Gynec., and Obstet.*, **59:** 491–495 (Sept.), 1934.
13. DENNIS, C.: Treatment of the large bowel obstruction; transverse colostomy—incidence of incompetence of ileocecal valve; experience at university hospitals. *Surgery*, **15:** 713–734, 1944.

14. DIXON, C. F.: Anterior resection for carcinoma low in the sigmoid and recto-sigmoid. *Surgery*, **13**: 367–377 (March), 1944.

15. FALLIS, L. S.: Transverse colostomy. *Surgery*, **20**: 249–256, (Aug.), 1946.

16. GABRIEL, W. B. Perineo-abdominal excision of the rectum in one stage. *Lancet*, **2**: 69–74 (July 14), 1934.

17. GABRIEL, W. B., DUKES, C. E. BUSSEY, H. J. R.: Lymphatic spread in cancer of the rectum. *Brit. J. Surg.*, **23**: 395–413 (Feb.), 1935.

18. GILCHRIST, R. K., and DAVID, V. C.: Lymphatic spread of cancer of the rectum. *Ann. Surg.*, **108**: 621–642 (April), 1938.

19. GILCHRIST, R. K., and DAVID, V. C.: A consideration of pathologic factors influencing five-year survival in radical resection of the large bowel and rectum for carcinoma. *Ann. Surg.*, **126**: 421–438 (Oct.), 1947.

20. GRAHAM, A. STEPHENS: Quoted by Rankin.[44]

21. GRAHAM, A. STEPHENS: Current trends in surgery of the distal colon and rectum. *Ann. Surg.*, **127**: 1022–1034 (May), 1948.

22. GRAHAM, A. STEPHENS: One stage resection and anastomosis of the colon (Editorial). *Surg., Gynec., and Obstet.*, **88**: 264–266 (Feb.), 1949.

23. HORSLEY, J. S.: Resection of the rectosigmoid and upper rectum for cancer, with end-to-end union. *Surg., Gynec., and Obstet.*, **64**: 313–333 (Feb.), 1937.

24. HOXWORTH, P. I.: Technic of anastomosis of the colon following resection. *Surg. Clinics of N. America*, 1197–1208 (Oct.), 1946.

25. JONES, D. F.: The diagnosis and principles of treatment of carcinoma of the colon and rectum. *Ann. Surg.*, **94**: 860–870 (Nov.), 1931.

26. JONES, D. F.: Carcinoma of the rectum and colon. *South. Med. Jour.*, **29**: 339–344 (April), 1936.

27. JONES, T. E.: Personal communication to the authors.

28. JONES, T. E.: Consideration of elective surgical procedures in various segments of the colon. *Surgery*, **14**: 342–349, 1943.

29. LAHEY, F. H.: Two-stage abdominoperineal removal of cancer of the rectum. *Surg., Gynec., and Obstet.*, **51**: 692–699 (Nov.), 1930.

30. LAHEY, F. H.: In discussion of Stone and McLanahan.[51]

31. LAHEY, F. H.: A discussion of the modified Mikulicz operation for carcinoma of the colon and its technic. *Surg. Clinics of N. America*, 610–622 (June), 1946.

32. LEE, W. E.: Discussion: Horsley.[23]

33. LOCKHART-MUMMERY, J. P.: Excision of the rectum for cancer. *Am. Jour. Cancer*, **18**: 1–14 (May), 1933.

34. LYNCH, J. M.: Quoted by Bacon.[3]

35. MACFEE, W. F.: The management of carcinoma in the several parts of the colon. *Ann. Surg.*, **126**: 125–139 (Aug.), 1947.

36. MACFEE, W. F.: Personal communication to the authors.

37. MAHORNER, HOWARD, and SABATIER, JOSEPH: Modern procedures for lesions of the colon and rectum. *The New Orleans Med. and Surg. Jour.*, **99**: 313–317 (Jan.), 1947.

38. MILES, W. E.: Pathology of spread of cancer of rectum and its bearing upon surgery of the cancerous rectum. *Surg., Gynec., and Obstet.*, **52**: 350–359 (Feb.), 1931.

39. MEYER, K. A., SHERIDAN, A., and KOZOLL, D. D.: One-stage open resection of lesions of the left colon without complementary colostomy. *Surg., Gynec., and Obstet.*, **81**: 507–514 (Nov.), 1945.

40. PEMBERTON, J. DE J.: In discussion of Coller and Vaughan.[8]

41. PFEIFFER, D. B.: Discussion.[23]

42. POTH, E. J.: Sulfasuxidine and sulfathaladine in surgery of the colon. *South. Med. Jour.*, **40**: 368–375 (May), 1947.
43. RANKIN, F. W.: Technic of combined abdominoperineal resection of rectum. *Surg., Gynec., and Obstet.*, **49**: 193–203 (Aug.), 1929.
44. RANKIN, F. W.: Resection and obstruction of the colon (obstructive resection). *Surg., Gynec., and Obstet.*, **50**: 594–598 (March), 1930.
45. RANKIN, F. W.: Graded perineo-abdominal resection of the rectum and rectosigmoid. *Am. Jour. Surg.*, **27**: 214–222 (Feb.), 1935.
46 RANKIN, F. W., and GRAHAM, A. STEPHENS: Aseptic end-to-side ileocolostomy: clamp method; technic and statistical data. *Ann. Surg.*, 676–681 (April), 1934.
47. RANKIN, F. W.: The principles of surgery of the colon. *Surg., Gynec., and Obstet.*, **72**: 332–340 (Feb.), 1941.
48. RANKIN, F. W., and JOHNSON, C. C.: Surgical treatment of cancer of rectum and rectosigmoid. *Jour. Am. Med. Assoc.*, **136**: 371–375 (Feb. 7), 1948.
49. RANKIN, F. W.: In discussion of Gilchrist and David.[19]
50. RAVDIN, I. S., ZINTEL, HAROLD A., and BENDER, DORIS H.: Adjuvants to surgical therapy in large bowel malignancy. *Ann. Surg.*, **126**: 439–447 (Oct.), 1947.
51. STONE, H. B., and McLANAHAN, S.: Resection and immediate anastomosis for carcinoma of the colon. *J.A.M.A.*, **120**: 1362–1366, (Dec.), 1942.
52. TURNER, GREY: Quoted by Jones.[25]
53. WANGENSTEEN, O. H.: Intestinal obstruction, ed. 2, Charles C Thomas, Springfield, 1942, p. 448.
54. WANGENSTEEN, O. H.: Primary resection (closed anastomosis) of the rectal ampulla for malignancy with preservation of sphincteric function. *Surg., Gynec., and Obstet.*, **81**: 1–24 (July), 1945.
55. WANGENSTEEN, O. H.: Personal communication to authors.
56. WANGENSTEEN, O. H.: In discussion of Gilchrist and David.[19]
57. WAUGH, J. M., and CUSTER, M. D.: Segmental resection of lesions occurring in the left half of the colon with primary end-to-end aseptic anastomosis. *Surg., Gynec., and Obstet.*, **81**: 593–598 (Dec.), 1945.
58. WAUGH, J. M.: Personal communication to authors.
59. WHIPPLE, A. O.: Advantages of cecostomy preliminary to resection of colon and rectum. *Tr. Sect Surg., Gen. and Abd.*, *Am. Med Assn.*. pp. 362–368, 1931.
60. WHIPPLE, A. O.: In discussion of White and Amendola.[61]
61. WHITE, W. C., and AMENDOLA, F. H.: The advantages and disadvantages of closed resection of the colon. *Ann. Surg.*, **120**: 572–581, 1944.
62. WHITE, W. C.: Personal communication to authors.

CHAPTER VIII

RADIOTHERAPY OF CARCINOMA OF THE RECTUM

FRED M. HODGES, M.D.

Carcinoma of the rectum is a surgical disease in operable cases except under unusual circumstances, as for instance, in extremely poor surgical risks.

Opinion in regard to the value of radiotherapy in carcinoma of the rectum has changed little during the past ten years. At first there were three very different and distinct schools of thought: One considered radiotherapy of little value in carcinoma of the rectum; another thought radiotherapy would supplant surgery; while a third group felt that radiotherapy was an important adjunct to surgery and would become progressively more important through technical improvement, through a greater knowledge of tumor sensitivity or resistance and normal tissue resistance and protection, and finally, as a result of a better understanding of the near and distance effects of radio-active energies. My experience agreed ten years ago and does now with the latter group. Papers written prior to ten years ago on this subject now are more or less obsolete owing to marked changes in dosage and other technical factors. Many who were some years ago extremely skeptical of the value of radium and the roentgen-ray are now convinced that these agents properly applied are of certain value in some cases of carcinoma of the rectum, especially papillary adenocarcinoma which is clinically the bulky, fungating type. It is my feeling, though, that when possible the opinion of a surgeon experienced in this field should be obtained before radiotherapy is employed.

Instead of quoting from the literature a large number of opinions, series of cases and technics, most of which are more or less obsolete, this discussion will be limited to the results which are being obtained by a few experienced investigators with proven cases of carcinoma of the rectum, treated by radiation alone or radiation in conjunction with colostomy.

Merritt, of Washington, in 1937, reported excellent results in advanced cases in which patients had survived for periods of several years, but there had been no five-year survivals. He employed heavy doses of external roentgen-rays, the total dose ranging between 4,500 and 6,000 r measured in air, 200 kv.p. at 50 cm. distance, thoraeus 2 filters, administered through three ports, namely, anterior, posterior, and perineal. With this he also uses radium locally, the dosage being dependent on the size, shape, and location of the growth. The following case report of a patient who refused operation is illustrative of his technic:

A woman, aged 46 years, the wife of a physician, was observed first in August 1934, at which time she gave a history of having bled from the rectum during the preceding three months. Digital examination revealed a hard nodular tumor on the anterior wall of the rectum, at the tip of the examining finger. Proctoscopic examination demonstrated an ulcerating growth three by four centimeters in diameter; examination by Lindsay and Bloodgood of tissue removed showed adenocarcinoma, graded 2. Treatment consisted of (1) deep roentgen-ray therapy, 1,400 r through each of three ports, anterior, posterior, and perineal, extended over a period of twenty-four days; and (2) 2,520 milligram hours of radium, applied directly to the lesion with a heavy filter of 1 mm. of gold and through the posterior vaginal wall. The patient gained twenty-five pounds in weight and was still free of symptoms when last observed in May 1937, at which time there was no evidence of a rectal lesion and her general health was excellent. The sole reason for treating this case by radiotherapy was the fact that the patient's husband, a physician, refused to consider an operation of any kind.

In one of Merritt's very advanced cases of adenocarcinoma, graded 2, the patient was administered external irradiation alone, receiving a total of 6,000 r, measured in air, and now more than three years after the treatment there is demonstrable no evidence of the local growth or distant metastasis. In his opinion all of these cases should receive both types of treatment, but in this instance, because of the marked sensitivity of the growth, it had disappeared completely before radium could be applied.

In 1948, Dr. Caulk, an associate of the late Dr. Merritt, stated that there had been no change in their attitude toward the treatment of carcinoma of the rectum during the past decade. The physician's wife treated by Dr. Merritt in 1934 was, he stated, still living in 1947. There was at the time of the last examination no evidence of local or abdominal recurrence but there had developed a destructive lesion in the cervical vertebrae. It could not be determined whether or not this was a metastatic lesion.

Burnham and Neill have noted very promising results in certain cases of carcinoma of the rectum following radiation. In a personal communication Neill, in 1937, stated:

"In our experience, it has been almost impossible to standardize the technique for treating rectal carcinomas. The variations in sensitiveness, in size, extent, and location, make absolutely indispensable a thorough individualization of each case. Cures can be obtained in some of the very early cases where conservative operation has not been very satisfactory, and where there is a real disinclination to do radical surgery, either because of the general condition of the patient or because of the dislike of interfering with the normal bowel movements and normal sphincteric control. The extensive, inoperable cases often can be very greatly improved symptomatically. It is possible, also, by preoperative radiation to reduce the bulk of borderline and early inoperable cases and to render radical operation a possibility. In extensive, inoperable cases our best results have been obtained by the use of heavy cross-firing from the outside either with roentgen-ray or teleradium. This is also generally the method of choice in borderline cases where a preliminary course of radiation precedes operation. In some of these, however, direct treatment with radium through the proctoscope, or by implantation, has been helpful. In early cases readily accessible by proctoscopic examination, chief reliance has been put on the use of radium. Depending upon the amount of infiltration and the size of the growth, either implantation or repeated daily applications are carried out. In those situated in the region of the anal sphincter extra-rectal implantation has been of great value. As a rule, in addition to the radium, cross-firing with roentgen-ray is employed as an adjunct procedure."

Schreiner, in 1935, reported eight cases of inoperable, proven cases of carcinoma of the rectum which were successfully treated by irradiation alone. These eight cases averaged a little more than ten years following treatment with no local recurrence. Six of the eight patients were living and apparently well at the time of the report. One of the eight died of pneumonia eleven years and nine months after treatment; no carcinoma was found. Another died of metastasis to the liver seven and one-half years after treatment; there was no evidence of carcinoma in the rectum.

Schreiner later commented: "Since this report there have been quite a number more which have regressed completely but are not yet free from the disease for five years. My impression is that the tumors which are papillary and not annular, are the ones that do the best by irradiation. The technique used for treatment of these cases is varied all the way from daily x-ray treatment with one anterior and one posterior field, administering 280 r daily, alternating front and back, and supplemented with seeds or tubes in the rectum; to other cases which are treated over four fields drawn out with 200 r daily until each field has from 2,000 to 2,500 r, then using rectal tubes against the lumen of the stricture. In several cases there has been complete regression with the use of 4.5 gm. radium pack treatment, giving 100 to 200 r per field, 3 fields each day front and back, and supplemented with intracavitary and interstitial irradiation."

Bowing also reports encouraging results. He believes, however, that few cases are cured by radiation alone but that marked palliation is obtained in many instances.

The Chaoul method, in which the lesion of the rectum is exposed directly to the roentgen-rays by operative procedures and special roentgen tubes which can be brought almost in contact with the growth, enables the administration of very heavy doses of radiation directly into the diseased tissues. From 10,000 to 15,000 r per field can thus be used without damage to surrounding structures. Regional lymph nodes are usually favorably influenced by this dosage. Of 9 patients treated in this manner during the two-year period in which the method has been tried, 6 were free of any evidence of cancer for periods of several months to two years. Of course, more time must elapse before a proper evaluation of this form of therapy is possible, but it certainly seems to promise something in carefully selected cases.

It should be borne in mind that, although a few cases of carcinoma of the rectum apparently have been cured by radiation alone, this method of treatment has not been so perfected that operable cases should receive it instead of surgery. This point cannot be stressed too strongly. That surgery still remains the method of choice in operable cases is owing largely to the fact that the majority of rectal lesions are radio resistant, are frequently inaccessible, and the surrounding tissues are more or less radio sensitive.

In a number of cases which I have treated, the temporary results have been excellent, but in not a single instance has a patient survived a period of five years without local recurrence or distant metastasis. Recent patients who have received not only roentgenotherapy but adequate radium therapy as well, should do better. Contrary to most statements in the literature, some metastatic lesions have in my experience regressed for periods of several months up to three years. All of these have finally died of cancer, but they were almost free of symptoms for a period of time. One such case was that of a white male, approximately 60 years of age, who had radium applied interstitially to the growth in the rectum in January, 1933. The local lesion disappeared, but in February, 1934, he showed evidences of a very markedly enlarged, nodular liver with ascites and had lost a great deal of weight. He received during February and March a total dose of about 6,000 r measured in air, through four ports, two over the abdomen and two over the back. The following factors were used: 200 kv.p. and filters of 2 mm. of copper and 2 mm. of aluminum at 50 cm. distance. The mass in the abdomen together with the ascites disappeared and he was able to continue his work for more than a year. He finally died of carcinoma about eighteen months after treatment.

In a number of instances of large secondary growths in the abdominal wall, around the colostomy opening, with almost complete closure of the stoma, the masses have more or less completely regressed following external radiation alone.

My technic is as follows: Each case must be individualized and a definite method of attack outlined. As a rule my total dose of external irradiation ranges from 4,500 to 6,000 r measured in air and administered through three or more ports. We employ 200 or more kv.p. filtered through at least the equivalent of 2 mm. of copper at a distance of 50 cm. or more by the Coutard or semi-Coutard method. After three or more weeks, radium is applied locally. By this time, if the growth is more or less radio sensitive, infection is less, the growth is smaller, and radium can be more effectively applied. Radium in gold or platinum seeds seems to give the best results, though some prefer contact applications of radium heavily filtered with 1 mm. gold, or more fractionally administered. The dosage here usually averages from 2,500 to 5,000 mg. hours. When seeds are used doses ranging between 3,500 and 10,000 mg. hours are necessary, depending upon the size, shape, and position of the growth. In order to obtain the best results it is essential that such care be exercised in placing the seeds that the entire growth receives a more or less homogeneous radiation.

A few doctors have had sufficient training in surgery, proctology, and radiology to treat carcinoma of the rectum without assistance from others, but in a large majority of instances radium, whether applied interstitially or in tubes, should be applied by one thoroughly familiar with such procedures. External radiation should be under the charge of an experienced radiologist.

When large quantities of radium are available, several grams can be used with a heavy filter at a distance of from 10 to 15 cm. from the skin. Some feel that this possesses an advantage over the roentgen-ray. For over two years we have used 360 to 400 kv.p. constant potential at a distance of 90 cm. with a filter of 2.25 mm. copper and .8 of tin. Different cases vary so much in their ratio of sensitivity, regardless of the pathologist's grading, that it has been very difficult to say definitely a better result has been obtained than was the case with 200 kv.p. filtered with 2 mm. of copper.

SUMMARY

1. Carcinoma of the rectum is primarily a surgical disease.
2. This is a highly specialized field of surgery and many cases which are inoperable in the hands of the average surgeon are oper-

able in the hands of the surgeon thoroughly experienced and skilled in this field.

3. Even when the best surgery is obtainable, between 20 and 40 per cent of cases are seen after the lesion becomes inoperable.

4. Great advances have been made in radiation therapy of rectal carcinoma and it is becoming an increasingly important adjunct to surgery.

5. This method of treatment alone or in conjunction with colostomy has resulted in a very small percentage of cases surviving a period of five years.

6. Constant improvements in technic and a wholehearted co-operation between the surgeon and radiotherapist should very definitely increase the percentage of cures or instances of marked palliation.

REFERENCES

1. Bowing, H. H., and Fricke, R. E.: Primary rectal carcinoma under radiation treatment; statistical review of 500 cases. *Am. Jour. of Roentgenol.,* **32**: 635–645 (Nov.), 1934.
2. Burnam, Curtis F., and Neill, William, Jr.: Personal communication.
3. Caulk, R. M.: Personal communication.
4. Merritt, Edwin A.: Personal communication.
5. Schreiner, B. F.: Successful irradiation treatment of 8 cases of inoperable rectal carcinoma. *Am. Jour. Cancer,* **24**: 326–333 (June), 1935.
6. Schreiner, B. F.: Personal communication.

CHAPTER IX

OPERATIVE MORTALITY AND END-RESULTS

Mortality following radical operations on the colon and rectum, contrary to an apparent widespread opinion, is not prohibitive, nor are fatalities from recurrence so discouragingly numerous as was the case a quarter of a century ago. At about that time barely 25 per cent of the diagnosed cases were operable, 20 to 50 per cent of those who were operated on died in the hospital, and well over 75 per cent of the survivors eventually succumbed to recurrence. In striking contrast to these results, surgeons during the past decade have reported operability rates as high as 90 per cent for large series of cases, while a comparative study of the mortality rate for individual surgeons and institutions by five-year and ten-year periods has revealed a progressive decline until now the general rate for all types of operations, in the hands of experienced surgeons, approaches 5 per cent. Moreover, the incidence of recurrence as determined for numerous large groups of cases varies from 25 to 50 per cent, which is an improvement of 40 to 60 per cent over the best available figures several decades ago. In other words, until relatively recent years fewer than ten out of one hundred patients in whom a diagnosis of malignancy of the large bowel was established, were alive five years after operation, whereas now we can reasonably expect between thirty and fifty to be living at the end of such a period. As a matter of fact, a study of any statistical data which are available indicates that more patients with carcinoma of the large bowel and rectum are found to survive over a given period of years than those with carcinoma of any other portion of the gastro-intestinal tract.

Mortality statistics are always comparative, and although it is highly desirable to have a small number of immediate deaths in hospital from any type of operation, we believe that in the main one must regard resectability as the main key to successfully combating malignancy. That is, one should rather consider how many persons out of a hundred will be benefited either by operative measures or curative interference over a term of years than how many brilliant technical procedures may be accomplished with a low hospital death rate.

Among the various factors that have in our experience been influential in the reduction of mortality, there are several that deserve special consideration, such as the preoperative preparation of the patient, the choice of anesthesia and operative procedure, and the postoperative care. Adequate care in preparing these patients for operation is, in our opinion, secondary in importance only to the early recognition of the malignancy. Emergency surgery rarely is necessary or justifiable in such cases since obstruction, when it develops, is slowly progressive and well tolerated, even after it becomes complete. The blood chemistry under such circumstances, in striking contrast to the findings in acute obstruction of the small intestine, may remain unaltered. It is always advisable to hospitalize the patient for a period of time sufficient to enable decompression of the obstructed colon and restoration of the hypertrophied and often edematous bowel to a healthier state, to combat dehydration, and the effects of malnutrition, and to permit an investigation of the function of the other organs of the body. Our regime, during this preoperative interval has been described in detail under "Preoperative Treatment."

Too much emphasis cannot be placed on the importance of carefully regulating the postoperative regime as a factor in reducing mortality. Complications are of frequent occurrence and considerable variety but many of these may be prevented, or by early recognition their progress be stayed. Sepsis, shock, and collapse, pulmonary complications, and urinary disorders are the chief causes of immediate death. Shock and collapse are more readily prevented than relieved and, since many of the patients under consideration are debilitated or must undergo drastic and time-consuming procedures, it is well to institute preventable measures while the patient is still on the operating table. In some cases this will entail merely the subcutaneous administration of normal saline solution, or intravenous injection of glucose solution, but in many instances a transfusion will be indicated. Immediately following any resections of the colon, and all resections of the rectum, it has been our custom for many years to give a blood transfusion of 500 cc. of citrated blood. Our regime during the postoperative period is described in detail under "Postoperative Treatment."

Individual statistics on operative mortality for carcinoma of the colon and rectum are of value only after a careful consideration of certain modifying influences such as (1) the experience and general surgical ability of the operator; (2) the type of operation performed, particularly if originated by the surgeon in question, for he should be able to do his special procedure better than one less familiar with its principles and technic; (3) the number of cases on which the report is based; (4) the sex of the patient; (5) the exact location of the growth; (6) the operability; and (7) whether the cases reported are private cases or charity hospital cases, for experience has demonstrated that the mortality varies considerably in these two groups. D. F. Jones reported a mortality for the combined operation in private cases (136) of 12.5 per cent, in charity hospital cases (132) of 33 per cent; Lockhart-Mummery for the perineal excision in private cases (100) of 3 per cent and hospital cases 14 per cent. Lockhart-Mummery feels that this marked difference is due to several factors. The private cases are better nursed, while in the charity hospital the staff is more or less chronically overworked and the same individual attention cannot be given, and probably a more important factor is that the ordinary charity patient is not in such good general condition; they seek treatment in a more advanced state of the disease and are relatively older at the same age as a result of hard work. By prolonging his preoperative period Lockhart-Mummery believes he has considerably improved the mortality risk in this group of cases.

In addition to the foregoing factors one must study the mortality experience of the individual surgeon over a period of years in order to appreciate the real worth of his statistics. Unfortunately these figures are somewhat confusing because such essential facts as the number of cases and the operability rate are not reported, or because the total series has been subdivided into many small groups. Surgeons sometimes fail to state which of the deaths they regard as directly attributable to the operation. The general trend was to consider a death "operative" if it occurs within one month of operation, but most surgeons now include deaths beyond this period if the patient dies in the hospital.

In view of the appreciable percentage who develop recurrence in the fourth and fifth year after operation, it seems unwise to consider anything less than a five-year survival as a "cure." It would seem to us that the more satisfactory appellation is that employed by Newman in his report to the British Ministry of Health, namely, three-year and five-year survivals. In compiling end-results, it is the practice of some authors to eliminate the cases which cannot be traced and assume the result would correspond to the ones which have been traced. That this can lead to serious errors when large numbers of cases are concerned has been demonstrated by Newman, who overcame the difficulty to a great extent by employing Survivorship Tables. In a study of 2,543 persons submitted to radical operations, of which number 759 were known to have died within the first year, 373 could not be traced. In regard to these cases Newman said:

"If we say that the probability of dying within one year is 759/2,543 we tacitly assume that none of those lost sight of die within the first year and that those operated upon less than a year ago will certainly live to the end of the year. This is too optimistic an assumption.

"If, alternatively, we assume that all those lost sight of are actually dead, and that all those operated upon within the year will die before its end, our numerator becomes $759+373=1,132$ and the fraction measuring the probability of dying $1,132/2,543$. This is too pessimistic a use of the material. The 'real' death rate must in fact be between.

"A middle course is to assume that the floating 373 persons not really under observation a whole year (or until death) were under observation half of the year and so to modify not the numerator but the denominator by subtracting from the latter half of 373, viz., 186.5 and stating the probability of dying as $759/2,543-186.5$ $=759/2,356.5$. This really amounts to saying that the floating population did have a chance of contributing to the recorded deaths for the first six months of the year after operation, and has an analogy with the method adopted by actuaries in treating lapses of policies when contructing real life tables. At the end of the first year the balance retained is to be substracted and the floating population of the second year similarly dealt with." On computing a Survivorship Table on the basis of Newman's figures it can be estimated that the approximate number of five-year survivors, as determined for the alternative methods given above, will be 329, 114, and 297 respectively, the latter figure representing the "middle course." Until such a method as this one becomes a general practice in computing end-results there will continue to exist much confusion in the realm of postoperative statistical data.

TABLE 33

SUMMARY OF RESULTS IN CASES OF CARCINOMA OF THE RIGHT SIDE OF THE LARGE INTESTINE

Patients operated on (1910 to 1920)	150
Complete postoperative data on	133
Patients living	57 (42.8 per cent)
Deaths	76 (57.2 per cent)
Patients living more than three years after operation	62 (47 per cent)

POSTOPERATIVE PERIOD OF LIFE

	Patients Living
From 10 to 15 years	13
From 5 to 10 years	30
4 years	6
3 years	7
From 1 to 2 years	11
	57

RANKIN'S STATISTICS

Colon.—In 1922, Rankin reported on 150 resections of the right half of the colon performed at the Mayo Clinic during the year 1910 to 1920. The operative mortality was approximately 12 per cent. A summary of the results is given in Table 33.

In 1925, he reported on 183 Mikulicz procedures in which the immediate mortality was 9.6 per cent and in 14 instances, or 7 per cent, recurrence was noted in the abdominal wall, and two years later reported on a series of 493 cases of carcinoma of the left half of the colon. In this series a radical resection was accomplished in 333 cases, or 67 per cent of all cases diagnosed carcinoma of the colon; 54 operative deaths are recorded, a mortality of 16.2 per cent. A summary of results is given in Table 34.

TABLE 34

SUMMARY OF RESULTS IN CASES OF CARCINOMA OF THE LEFT SIDE OF THE LARGE INTESTINE

	Operations	Hospital Mortality
Total	509	97 (19.6 per cent)
Resection	333	54 (16.21 per cent)
Palliative	100	31 (31 per cent)
Explorations	73	12 (16.44 per cent)

RESECTIONS

	Cases	Per Cent
Resections (all data)	208	74.50
Subsequent deaths	105	50.48
Living	103	49.51

The percentage of three-year cures was 46.11.

Rankin, in 1929, in reviewing the mortality statistics following colostomy for carcinoma of the large bowel writes as follows:

"In order to arrive at some conclusions relative to the causal factors and percentage of mortality in a large series of cases, I have reviewed the records of 919 cases in which colostomy has been performed in the Mayo Clinic from 1920 to 1926 inclusive. Colostomy was performed in 385 cases in which further procedures were deemed impossible because of metastasis, extensive local involvement, or other factors which made it impossible to eradicate the malignant growth; there were 26 deaths. In 584 cases, at exploration for colostomy, the growth was deemed resectable; however, in 16 cases death occurred before the operation could be completed. From these figures it will be seen that a mortality of 7.67 per cent attends the performance of colostomy as a palliative measure and

2.7 per cent is the mortality rate of the operation in the group in which further operation is considered advisable (Table 35).

In 1929, the operability rate for malignant lesions of the large intestine reached 58 per cent, whereas the average operability for the years 1916 to 1924, reported in 1927, has been only 34.9 per cent. Of 381 such lesions 221 were resected with mortality of 12.3 per cent.

In 1933, Rankin reported the results of a study on the curability of cancer of the large bowel, rectosigmoid, and rectum. The 753

TABLE 35

CONDITIONS PROHIBITING RESECTION FOLLOWING COLOSTOMY IN GROUP OF 355 CASES WITH NUMBER OF DEATHS IN HOSPITAL

	Cases	Hospital Mortality	Per Cent
Metastasis to liver.............................	100	2	2
Fixed and extensive growth (obstruction in thirty)..	140	17	12.05
Acute obstruction..............................	7	3	42.85
Attachment to bladder and peritoneum...........	21	2	9.52
Peritoneal and retroperitoneal involvement........	17		
Pelvic metastasis.............................	9	1	11.11
Involvement of bladder........................	8		
Involvement of prostate and bladder.............	6		
Attachment to prostate........................	3		
Metastasis to inguinal lymph nodes..............	7		
Metastasis to mesentery........................	4		
Multiple intestinal metastasis...................	6	1	16.66
Poor general condition (age, secondary anemia)....	6		
Epithelioma of larynx..........................	1		
Total......................................	335	26	7.76

cases studied were closed at the end of operation with a hopeful prognosis and either resulted in survival over a period of five years without recurrence or ended fatally of recurrence. There were 187 cases of cancer of the right colon, 266 cases of the left colon, and 300 cases of cancer of the rectosigmoid or rectum. Table 36 shows the relative percentage of cures in relation to the segment of colon involved.

TABLE 36

RELATIVE PERCENTAGE OF CURES IN RELATION TO SITUATION OF LESION

	Total	Dead	Five-year Cures	Per Cent Cured
Right half of colon including cecum......	187	81	106	57.6
Left half of colon including sigmoid......	266	139	127	47.7
Total...........................	453	220	233	51.3

It will be noted that the prognosis is definitely more favorable for lesions of the right half of the colon.

The effects on end-results of the size of the growth, lymphatic involvement, and of the relative degree of malignancy, as determined by Broders' classification, which were discussed in the foregoing report, have been considered in detail in the chapter on prognosis.

Rectum.—In 1927 Rankin made the following report:

"In this series which I am reporting the majority of the cases were treated by graded procedures of the following types: (1) Colostomy and posterior resection of the growth; (2) the Jones or the Miles procedure, especially applicable to carcinoma of the rectosigmoid and high rectal growths; (3) the Coffey operation, and (4) the Quénu-Tuttle or Harrison Cripps type of perineal excision.

TABLE 37

DURATION OF LIFE AFTER ANY TYPE OF RESECTION

Patients Heard From		Patients	Per Cent
420	Lived three years or more	201	47.85
366	Lived four years or more	142	38.80
305	Lived five years or more	103	33.77
243	Lived six years or more	70	28.80
204	Lived seven years or more	55	26.96
165	Lived eight years or more	41	24.84
108	Lived nine years or more	23	21.29
58	Lived ten years or more	14	24.13

"From January 1, 1916 to January 1, 1926, resection was performed for carcinoma of the rectum in 602 cases at the Mayo Clinic. All of these growths were true rectal carcinomas and the series does not include malignant tumors situated at the rectosigmoid juncture, which present a different clinical picture and frequently necessitate the choice of a different surgical procedure. Of those patients dismissed from the hospital, 511 (93 per cent) were traced; 308 (60 per cent) had died and 203 (40 per cent) were living (Table 37). In this series the males predominated over the females in the proportion of 378 to 224. The hospital mortality of the whole group was 8.9 per cent (54 cases). Of the total number of cases (1,727) of malignant disease of the rectum, resection or excision was performed in 602 (34.9 per cent) and palliative procedures were carried out in 343 (19.8 per cent). Thus, in 54.7 per cent of the cases some type of operative treatment was given, although only about one-third were resectable while 782 (45.3 per cent) were found to be inoperable."

In computing the survivals at five years in the foregoing report the untraced cases were subtracted from the operative survivals. If instead these cases are treated as having died in less than five years the percentage becomes 37 rather than 40. These figures then can be compared on the same basis with those of Jones, Abel, and Gabriel (also revised). Of the 602 cases subjected to operation, 382 underwent colostomy and posterior resection. The operative mortality of this group was 9.4 per cent (36 cases) and there were 33.1 per cent five-year survivals. It was this low percentage of five-year survivals that convinced us that the perineal excision was not a sufficiently thorough operation and consequently led to the development of a modification of Miles's abdominoperineal excision in two stages. Although the operability of this series is admittedly low (34.9 per cent), it reached 58 per cent (221 out of 381 cases) for the year 1929 and since then has ranged from 50 to 68 per cent for yearly series of a similar number of cases. In a personal series of 578 cases of carcinoma of the rectum operated on by Rankin and reported by him in 1937 there was an operability of 71.4 per cent of the cases.

In a report which already has been discussed under "Prognosis," Rankin, in 1933, reviewed the results of a study of 300 cases of cancer of the rectum for which resections were performed. There were 114, or 38 per cent, five-year survivals. Of the total series, 46 per cent of the cases were recorded as showing malignant lymph nodes resected with the specimen. Only 20 per cent of these survived the five-year period, while of the cases without nodal involvement 48 per cent survived such a period. It was also shown in this study that there is a definite correlation between the grade of malignancy and the period of survival. The percentage of five-year survivals, according to the grade of malignancy were as follows: Grade I, 57 per cent, Grade II, 44 per cent, Grade III, 22 per cent, and Grade IV, 19 per cent.

At the American Medical Association meeting in 1937, one of us (Rankin) reported that "since January, 1927, I have operated on 578 patients for cancer of the rectum and sigmoid. This group upon which many different types of operations have been done—radical, exploratory, and palliative—serves as a background for some conclusions as to the merits of different surgical procedures and their accompanying mortality, morbidity, and applicability." The conclusions prompted by this experience are in accord with those of Daniel Fiske Jones who said: "I have gradually increased the number of one-stage operations and decreased the number of two-stage operations, and believe that this should be done as men find their ability to do the one-stage operation increasing. I still

TABLE 38
CANCER OF THE RECTUM AND RECTOSIGMOID

576 Cases 412 Resected	}Operability	71.4 per cent
576 Cases 75 Deaths	}Mortality	13　per cent
412 Resected 49 Deaths	}Mortality	11.8 per cent
164 Explorations or colostomy 26 Deaths...	Mortality	15.8 per cent

feel that there are a few cases in which I want to do and which are not fit for a one-stage operation."

Table 38 indicates the mortality and operability of the series. It will be observed that the gross mortality was 13 per cent including all types of operation, both resections and palliative procedures, but this was done with an operability of 71.4 per cent.

Table 39 indicates the mortality in the different types of operation. In the series of 44 combined abdominoperineal resections done by Miles's technic there were two deaths. This is too low a figure to be hoped for in a large series but it does tend to demonstrate that familiarity with technic and attention to other details permit one to employ this type procedure with a very satisfactory mortality.

It will be seen that the mortality figure for the combined abdominoperineal operation in one and two stages—133 cases with 10 deaths—was 7.5 per cent, as compared with 162 cases with 12 deaths, or 7.4 per cent, in the group operated upon by colostomy and posterior excision. This latter figure is higher than is customary for private cases among surgeons using colostomy and posterior excision routinely. This is explained, however, by the higher operability and a recognition of the fact that the worse risks which were submitted to resection of any type were done by this variety of operative procedure.

TABLE 39
CANCER OF THE RECTUM AND RECTOSIGMOID

Operations	Cases	Deaths	Per Cent
Combined abdominoperineal resection, 1-stage........	44	2 ...	4.5
Combined abdominoperineal resection, 2-stage........	89	8 ...	8.9
Total one- and two-stage operations.............	133	10	7.5
Colostomy and posterior excision....................	162	12 ...	7.4
Miscellaneous—anterior resection, tube resection Harrison-Cripps operations, etc...................	117	27 ...	23.0
Total...	412	49	11.8

In 1948, Rankin and Johnston reported that during a period of seven years, from 1934 to 1941, 336 patients suffering with cancer of the rectum and rectosigmoid were studied. Of this group 310 were subjected to operation, while for 26 it was felt that an operation was contraindicated. Of this entire group, in 167 patients the abdominoperineal resection of the rectum in one stage was performed with a mortality of 5.3 per cent. The two-stage combined operation was utilized in 9 cases, while in 56 colostomy and posterior resection were done. In 19 patients exploration revealed that no further procedure was indicated, whereas exploration and colostomy were done on 54 patients. In 1 patient a local excision was done, and in 4 cecostomy for obstruction (Table 40).

TABLE 40

MORTALITY FOLLOWING OPERATION FOR CANCER OF THE
RECTUM AND RECTOSIGMOID (RANKIN AND JOHNSTON—1948)

	Cases	Deaths	Mortality, %
One stage combined abdominoperineal resection..	167	9	5.3
Colostomy and posterior resection	56	9	16.0
Posterior resection without colostomy	1	0	0
Two stage resection (Rankin)	9	2	22.2
Exploration alone	19	3	26.3
Exploration with colostomy	54	17	31.5
Cecostomy (acute obstruction due to cancer)	4	4	100.0

310 cases, 233 resections............................ Resectability, 75.1%
233 resections, 167 one stage combined abdominoperineal
  resections.. Applicability, 71.7%

Of this series of patients 212 were males and 124 females. Fourteen of the men were found to have inoperable cancer in contrast to 16 of the women, while one hundred and ninety-eight and one hundred and eight operations, respectively, were done in the two groups (Table 41).

Of the 167 patients subjected to the Miles operation, only 9 patients succumbed, and the operative mortality was 5.3 per cent. There were also 9 deaths following the fifty-six operations of colostomy and posterior resection, a mortality of 31.5 per cent. The higher mortality is, of course, in keeping with what one would expect in making every effort to see what could be done for the depleted patient harboring the far advanced lesion.

Table 42 presents a review of the results of the Miles operation performed on 167 patients for carcinoma of the rectum and rectosigmoid with a yearly follow-up of the survival rate beyond the initial three year period. Here again it is evident that the majority

Table 41

SUMMARY OF RESULTS FOLLOWING ABDOMINOPERINEAL
RESECTION IN ONE STAGE FOR CANCER
(Rankin and Johnston—1948)

Number of Operative Cases	Number of Males	Number of Females	Number of Operative Deaths	Hospital Mortality, %	Number of Cases Traced
167	101	66	9	5.3	162

Postoperative Follow-Up	Patients	Percentage
3 to 4 years	102	63.0
4 to 5	91	56.1
5 to 6	58	36.0
6 to 7	45	28.0
7 to 8	36	22.2
8 to 9	23	14.1
9 to 10	18	11.1
10 to 11	6	4.0
11 to 12	2	1.2

of deaths, 44.5 per cent, occur within the first five years. Therefore, one can hardly view with assurance data accumulated over shorter periods. Of the 167 patients, in only 5 have we been unable to complete the follow-up to date. At this time 85 patients are alive and without evidence of recurrence. This represents a survival rate of 52.4 per cent.

In this group of 167 combined resections, 2 patients succumbed to vascular accident, 1 to a cerebral thrombosis and another to pulmonary embolism. Two patients died of peritonitis and in another the immediate cause of death was not determined at autopsy. The remaining 4 deaths were the result of intestinal obstruction which was a complication of peritonitis in 2 cases and due to adhesion to the pelvic floor in 2. In 1, an omental band adherent to a seam in the pelvic diaphragm constricted the terminal ileum, while in another the terminal ileum was obstructed by a second loop of small bowel which had become adherent at the same place.

Table 42

RESULTS OF ABDOMINOPERINEAL RESECTION IN ONE STAGE
AT FIVE YEARS (Rankin and Johnston—1948)

Grade	Pa-tients	With Glandular Involvement					Without Glandular Involvement					Living 1946
		Total	Living Over Five Years		Living Under Five Years		Total	Living Over Five Years		Living Under Five Years		
			Alive	Dead	Alive	Dead		Alive	Dead	Alive	Dead	
1	6	0	0	0	0	0	6	3	0	1	2	4
2	61	15	5	1	2	7	46	19	2	13	12	39
3	51	25	5	0	3	17	26	9	1	8	8	25
4	44	33	8	1	3	21	11	5	0	1	5	17
Totals	162	73	18	2	8	45	89	36	3	23	27	85
Percentage			24.6	2.7	10.9	61.6		40.4	3.3	25.8	30.3	52.4

Of the entire group of patients 233 were amenable to resection of the lesion, giving a resectability rate of 75.1 per cent. The one-stage combined abdominoperineal resection of the rectum was applicable to 167 patients, or 71.7 per cent of the group.

It should be noted that in 73 patients glandular metastasis was found to have already developed, whereas in 89 patients no glandular involvement was found. Of the 73 patients with glandular metastasis 27.3 per cent lived five years or longer while 10.9 per cent were alive and well under five years. In the group of 89 patients who were found to have no glandular involvement, 43.8 per cent survived the five year period while 24.7 per cent were liv-

TABLE 43*

CARCINOMAS OF THE ENTIRE COLON—RESULTS OF TREATMENT
(JOHNS HOPKINS)

Results	Dead Following Operation	Well 5 Years or More	Not Traced	Total Cases
Inoperable, no operation........	0	1	15	27
Inoperable, exploration..........	9	0	7	35
Inoperable, colostomy...........	11	0	6	25
Inoperable, entero-enterostomy...	2	0	1	8
Total inoperable cases.......	22–23.2%	1–1.5%	29–30.5%	95–49.5%
Resection, lateral anastomosis....	11	6	11	41
Resection, end-to-end...........	9	10	2	34
Mikulicz operation.............	3	0	0	7
Resection right colon...........	3	1	3	13
Total operated cases........	26–27.4%	17–32.1%	16–16.8%	95–49.5%
Grand total...........	48–25%	18–12.3%	46–23.9%	192†

* Condensation of table prepared by Raiford.

† Two cases added here were considered operable but refused operation.

ing under five years. Over 61.6 per cent of those patients with glandular involvement died within the first five years following operation, while only 30.3 per cent of those without metastasis to the regional nodes succumbed during this period. The five year survival rate is 52.4 per cent.

JOHNS HOPKINS HOSPITAL STATISTICS

Colon.—Miller, in 1923, published a detailed report of his review of all cancers of the colon, exclusive of the rectum, which had been admitted to the Johns Hopkins Hospital 1889–1919. One hundred and twenty-nine of these were operated on, 70 or (54 per cent) of which were resected with 24 deaths, a mortality of 35 per cent. There were 13 five-year survivals (10 per cent of admissions,

28 per cent of those who survived operation). Eight of the 13 cures were carcinomas of the cecum and ascending colon, 1 of the transverse colon, and 4 of the sigmoid.

In 1935, Raiford published a comprehensive report of the entire series of carcinomas of the colon and rectum observed at the Johns Hopkins Hospital, including the cases reported by Miller and all subsequent cases. During this period 192 carcinomas of the colon were observed. The distribution of the operable cases was as follows: cecum and ascending colon, 35; hepatic flexure, 6; transverse colon, 11; splenic flexure, 4; and descending colon and sigmoid, 34. The results of treatment are shown in Table 43.

The operative mortality according to the segments of bowel harboring the growth was as follows:

	Number of Resections	Operative Mortality
Cecum and ascending colon	35	8 (22.8%)
Hepatic flexure	6	1 (16.6%)
Transverse colon	11	3 (27.2%)
Splenic flexure	4	2 (50.0%)
Descending colon and sigmoid	34	11 (32.6%)

The fact is stressed by Raiford that although colostomy is a relatively simple procedure, the dangers of the operation have apparently been overlooked by many. Of 25 colostomies, both palliative and preliminary, 11, or 44 per cent, died from the effects of the operation. The major causes of death were as follows: peritonitis 31.9 per cent; pulmonary disorders (pneumonia, embolus, abscess) 19.1 per cent, and shock 14.9 per cent. Raiford presented comparative figures to show that there had been a gradual increase in the operability of large bowel cancer. During the five-year period 1900–1905, only 24.1 per cent were operable while for a similar period between 1925 and 1930 the rate had risen to 65.5 per cent. The results of treatment showed the same trend. In the abovementioned five-year periods, the percentage of five-year cures increased from 14.6 per cent to 28 per cent.

Rectum.—Three hundred and nineteen of the 511 cases reported by Raiford were located in the rectum. Table 44 summarizes the results following the various types of operation employed.

The operability, as determined by resection, was 36.7 per cent (117 out of 319); actually 33, or 10.3 per cent, additional cases were considered operable but refused surgery. The untraced cases were grouped with those who lived less than five years. In considering these figures it should be remembered that they apply to all cases treated during a period of forty-two years, a great many of which were admitted at a time when surgery of rectal cancer was undeveloped. From 1900 to 1905, 32.4 per cent of all cases were operable, whereas over a similar period from 1920 to 1925 the operability had risen to 63.5 per cent. The percentage of five-year arrests had risen during the same period from 25 per cent to 36 per cent.

TABLE 44*

JOHNS HOPKINS HOSPITAL STATISTICS (RAIFORD 1935)

Operation	Patients Operated On	Operative Mortality		5-Year Survivals		Not Traced
		Cases	Per Cent	Cases	Per Cent	
Abdominal resection..........	8	3	37.5	2	2.5	0
Abdominoperineal resection 1 stage...................	35	11	31.5	7	20	3
Abdominoperineal resection 2 stages..................	13	5	38.4	1	7.7	4
Sacral resection.............	39	6	15.4	5	12.8	9
Perineal resection............	22	1	4.5	1	4.5	6
Totals.................	117	26	22.2	16	23.2	22

* Condensation of table prepared by Raiford.

STONE'S AND MCLANAHAN'S STATISICS

In 1942, Stone and McLanahan reported on 191 carcinomas of the colon. Their operability rates, based on the ratio of the number of tumors removed to the number of patients actually explored, are shown in Table 45. Among the 44 patients with inoperable tumors 14 died, which is a mortality of 31.8 per cent.

TABLE 45

CARCINOMA OF THE COLON: OPERABILITY RATE
(STONE AND MCLANAHAN—1942)

	Cases	Resections	Operability
Right..........	37	33	89.1%
Transverse......	30	25	83.3%
Left...........	124	89	71.7%
Total........	191	147	77.0%

Their mortality rate for 104 resections with immediate anastomosis is shown in Table 46. In nine instances anastomosis was preceded by a preliminary proximal drainage operation; two elsewhere and seven were performed because of acute intestinal obstruction. There were a variety of procedures employed in this series in addition to aseptic anastomosis immediately following resections. Comparative mortality figures are given in Table 47. The authors con-

TABLE 46

CARCINOMA OF THE COLON: MORTALITY OF RESECTIONS
FOLLOWED BY ANASTOMOSES OF THE ASEPTIC TYPE
(STONE AND McLANAHAN—1942)

	Resections	Deaths	Mortality
Right...........	16	3	18.7%
Transverse......	16	1	6.3%
Left...........	72	7	9.7%
Total........	104	11	10.6%

TABLE 47

CARCINOMA OF THE COLON: COMPARISON OF MORTALITY
IN DIFFERENT TYPES OF OPERATION
(STONE AND McLANAHAN—1942)

	Cases	Deaths	Mortality
Exploratory or palliative...	44	14	31.8%
vs			
Resections...............	147	19	12.9%
Aseptic anastomoses.......	104	11	10.6%
vs.			
Open anastomoses........	34	7	20.6%

TABLE 48

CARCINOMA OF THE COLON: CAUSES OF DEATH
(STONE AND McLANAHAN—1942)

	Cases
All resections	
Directly related to operative procedure:	
Peritonitis....................................	13
Wound infection...............................	1
Indirectly related to operative procedure:	
Embolism......................................	3
Pneumonia....................................	1
Myocardial failure............................	1
Total..	19
Resection and immediate aseptic anastomosis	
Directly related to operative procedure:	
Peritonitis....................................	8
Indirectly related to operative procedure:	
Embolism......................................	2
Pneumonia.	1
Total..	11

tend that undue stress has been laid on anatomic and physiologic differences between the two sides of the colon. They believe that one may as safely undertake resection and immediate anastomosis on the left as well as on the right and point to their lower mortality rate for resections done on the left side. In emphasizing the importance of aseptic anastomosis they point to the mortality of 9.7 per cent for 72 cases in which such an astomosis was carried out for lesions of the left colon, whereas in 19 left sided lesions in which an open anastomosis was done following resection, there were five deaths, or a mortality of 26.3 per cent. The causes of death in this series of cases are recorded in Table 48.

In lieu of accurate recent statistics, Stone in 1947, submitted estimates which he considers close to the actual fact: (1) Of all cases seen, about 95 per cent are advised to undergo operation and most of these accept; (2) of those explored about 80 per cent have a resection done; (3) of the resections, about 25 per cent are palliative in nature; and (4) of the 75 per cent resected with hope of cure, about 45 or 50 per cent are living and well at the end of five years. Stone is of the impression that in recent years his mortality rate has become higher. This, he believes, is because he has intentionally accepted more cases of the very poor risk type which in 1946 included two patients aged 83 and 85 respectively who died following extensive resection for advanced disease which produced a great deal of pain.

MASSACHUSETTS GENERAL HOSPITAL STATISTICS

Colon.—Allen, in 1939, reported 107 consecutive cases of carcinoma of the colon in which the resectability rate was 93.6 per cent. In 1943, he reported 79 additional personally managed cases in which the resectability rate was 87.4 per cent. An analysis of resectability and mortality in these 186 cases is shown in Table

TABLE 49

CARCINOMA OF THE COLON

(MASSACHUSETTS GENERAL HOSPITAL, ALLEN, 1925–1942)

	1-Stage	Deaths	Mortality (%)	2-Stage	Deaths	Mortality (%)	Total	Deaths	Mortality (%)
Right colectomies........	13	7	53.8	44	7*	15.9	57	14	24.5
Left colectomies†	16	3	18.7	70	8	11.4	86	11	12.7
Total resectability of stage operations.............	29	10	34.4	114	15	13.1			
Other resections......						26	43	10	23.3
Not resectable.......						17			
Grand total (Resectability, 91 per cent)							186	35	18.8

* Includes 2 deaths after first stage when 2-stage procedure was planned. Complementary cecostomy was done in these 1-stage operations.

† Includes transverse colectomies not done with right or left colectomies, obstructive resections, turnout operations, and combined abdominoperineal resections (for sigmoidal lesions.)

49. Allen states that all patients failing to leave the hospital alive, regardless of the time elapsed following operation, are included in the failures of treatment. The over-all mortality rate was 18.8 per cent. This included those whose lesions were not resectable. The mortality for the 44 with resectable lesions of the left colon in the more recent group of 79 cases was 6.8 per cent. In the 25 patients with resectable lesions of the right and transverse colon suitable for right colectomy, there were 10 deaths, or a mortality of 40 per cent. It is always dangerous, he states, to report a run of successful cases unless it is of sufficient length. In his previous report he had called attention to 22 consecutive right colectomies in two stages without a death.

In his latest report (1947) Allen presented data on 105 additional patients observed and treated since January 1, 1943. The resectability and mortality rates of this group are compared in Tables 50 and 51 with those of the earlier group. During the period

TABLE 50

CARCINOMA OF THE COLON: RESECTABILITY AND MORTALITY
(MASSACHUSETTS GENERAL HOSPITAL—ALLEN, 1947)

Years	No. of Cases	Resectability (%)	Resection Mortality (%)
1925–1942.......	143	91	17.5
1943–1946.......	105	95	2.0

TABLE 51

CARCINOMA OF THE COLON: RESECTABILITY AND MORTALITY
(MASSACHUSETTS GENERAL HOSPITAL—ALLEN, 1947)

1943–1946	No. of Cases	Deaths
Resections		
For cure..........	87	0
Palliative.........	13	2
Nonresectable........	5	2
	105	4

in which the resectability rose from 91 to 95 per cent and the mortality descended from 17.5 to 2 per cent, Allen employed the Miller-Abbott tube more often than cecostomy, resorted less frequently to exteriorization procedures, and adopted routine employment of sulfathaladine in the preparation of patients for colon resection. He prefers long paramedian incisions, either right or left, except for lesions of the flexures and mid-colon, in which cases a transverse incision is preferred; delayed primary wound closure, as advocated by Coller and Valk, is practiced; and wounds are closed with No. 30 interrupted cotton and stay-sutures of heavy cotton for the skin and fat. Open anastomosis is preferred to closed, aseptic technics.

McKittrick's Statistics.—In 1948, McKittrick reported the immediate results following resection of the colon for cancer during the sixteen year period ending in 1947. The year 1942 has been used as the transition year from the earlier to the present methods (Table 52). More striking than the drop in mortality rate, he be-

TABLE 52

TYPES OF OPERATION AND MORTALITY RATES, 1932–1947
(McKittrick—1948)

Types of Operations	1932–1941			1942–1947			Total		
	Cases	Mortality		Cases	Mortality		Cases	Mortality	
		No.	%		No.	%		No.	%
Anastomosis with proximal decompression.....	40	6	15.0	12	2	16.6	52	8	15.3
Anatomosis without proximal decompression	2	0	0.0	67	4	5.9	69	4	5.8
Obstructive resection....	13	0	0.0	1	0	0.0	14	0	0.0
Right colectomy, 1-stage.	15	3	20.0	43	0	0.0	58	3	5.7
Right colectomy, 2-stages.	20	1	5.0	6	1	16.6	26	2	7.6
Total operations.....	90	10	11.0	129	7	5.4	219	17	7.7
Total resections with primary anastomosis.....	17	3	17.6	110	4	3.6	127	7	5.5

lieves, is the transition from staged operation to resection and primary anastomosis, proximal decompression being reserved for those who were admitted with advanced obstruction or where a difficult anastomosis had been performed low in the pelvis and there was some doubt as to the security of the suture line. McKittrick states that the mortality rate of 3.6 per cent for 110 operations in which a primary anastomosis was done seems to justify a continuance of the present method.

McKittrick favors a lateral anastomosis in resections of the right half of the colon. For lesions at or beyond the midtransverse colon his preference is a closed type, end-to-end anastomosis, using the Parker-Kerr basting switch technique. #1 plain catgut is used for the basting stitches, a continuous #000 chromic catgut suture for the inside, and interrupted #70 cotton for the outside layers.

Rectum.—Among the most detailed and accurate, and consequently the most valuable statistics published a decade ago were those of Daniel Fiske Jones, from his private practice and from the

TABLE 53

COMBINED ABDOMINOPERINEAL OPERATION—ONE AND TWO
STAGES (D. F. JONES 1929)

	No. Cases	Died in Hospital Per Cent	Cases Operated Three Years	Per Cent Living	Cases Operated Five Years	Per Cent Living
M.G.H.* and private	204	22.7	120	70	103	50
Private..........	102	11.7	67	71.6	56	53

COMBINED ABDOMINOPERINEAL OPERATION—ONE STAGE

Private..........	54	5.5	38	78.5	32	56

*Massachusetts General Hospital.

Massachusetts General Hospital. We quote directly from his report of 1929:

"In Table 53 are given the mortality and the percentage of cases living three and five years after the combined abdominoperineal operation in one stage done under the best conditions, that

TABLE 54

TOTALS OF PATIENTS SEEN, OPERATED UPON, AND
TOTAL MORTALITY (D. F. JONES 1936)

Total number of patients seen........................ 672 ..... Per cent
Total number of radical operations.................... 427
Percentage of operability............................. 63.5

Type of Operation

Combined abdominoperineal, 1 stage.................. 167 ......:. 39
Combined abdominoperineal, 2 stage .... 110 .... 25.7
Combined abdominoperineal, sphincter removal.......... 21 .... 4.9
Colostomy and posterior excision..................... 114 .... 26.7
Abdominal excision and colostomy.................... 15 .... 3.5
Mortality of all groups.............................. 81 .... 18.96

is, in private practice. It will be seen that in properly selected cases the mortality in the one-stage operation is not high, and the percentage of three-year and five-year cases is considerably higher than by any other operation. This is most gratifying and is conclusive proof, we believe, that the more extensive operation will give better results in those patients who can stand it than in those obtained from more limited operations. These are the statistics which should be compared with those of any other single operation, such as resection and suture, colostomy and posterior excision or any other single operation suggested for removal of cancer of the rectum."

TABLE 55

TOTAL NUMBER OF ONE AND TWO STAGE COMBINED ABDOMINO-
PERINEAL OPERATIONS (D. F. Jones 1936)

	Total No. Cases	Mortality Per Cent	Operated 3 Years +	Lived 3 Years + Per Cent*	Operated 5 Yrs.	Lived 5 Yrs. + Per Cent*
Hospital and Private						
Abdominoperineal, 1 stage	167	13	143	72.2	111	52.6
Abdominoperineal, 2 stages	110	27	107	61	106	51.3
Private						
Abdominoperineal, 1 stage	135	11	111	76.8	80	56.5
Abdominoperineal, 2 stages	51	17.6	48	67.5	47	61.5

* Operative mortality excluded.

It will be noted that Jones placed his 7 untraced cases in the
group of those living less than three years; many surgeons simply
eliminate such cases. Jones' most recent (1936) reports afford an
interesting and instructive comparison with the foregoing statistics (Tables 54 and 55). Despite an increase of 10 per cent in the
operability rate of his entire series including the 265 cases reported
above, the operative mortality has decreased and the percentage
of five-year survivals has remained at the same high level.

ST. MARK'S HOSPITAL STATISTICS

The statistics from St. Mark's Hospital (London), prepared for
the most part by Gabriel and Dukes, are important and highly
significant because they represent the total experience of that institution with perineal excision and perineo-abdominal resection
over a period of thirty-five years. Moreover, the detailed manner
in which the data are presented and analyzed provides an ideal
study from the standpoint of operability, mortality, and end-results. These are considered from the standpoint of the following
modifying factors: (1) In relation to increasing experience with the
operation; (2) in relation to age and sex; (3) in relation to site of
growth; (4) in relation to the stage of the disease; and (5) in relation to Broder's grade of malignancy.

Operability.—Goligher, in 1941, compiled operability figures for
St. Mark's Hospital, based on a total of 1,186 patients diagnosed
cancer of the rectum during the period 1930 to 1939, inclusive.

The manner in which operability is determined at St. Mark's
Hospital differs from the prevailing method of most authors. Nevertheless, all the data necessary for determining operability or re-

TABLE 56

ANALYSIS OF RECTAL CARCINOMA MATERIAL AT ST. MARK'S
HOSPITAL IN 1,186 CASES (1930–1939, INCLUSIVE—GOLIGHER)

Operable		Inoperable	
Expectant (refused operation).....	23	Expectant...............	42
Radium.....................	5	Curettage and diathermy..	4
Local excision................	38	Radium.................	17
Colostomy or caecostomy alone*.	23	Laparotomy alone........	10
Hartmann's operation..........	14	Colostomy...............	387
Perineal excision..............	291	Palliative excision........	11
Combined excision............	321		
Total.....................	715	Total.................	471
	(60.3%)		

* Died before the second stage of a radical excision or refused further treatment.

sectability by the methods currently popular have been presented
in Table 56. The over-all operability as determined by Goligher is
60.3 per cent. As computed for the other series of cases in this
chapter (based on ratio of the number of tumors removed to the
number of patients actually explored) the operability, or resectability rate, of St. Mark's Hospital is 57.9 per cent if only the cases
operated on with the view to cure are considered, or 59 per cent if
as is customary, the 11 palliative resections are also included. For
practical purposes, then, the statistical data of this hospital are
comparable to those of other institutions which are recorded in this
chapter. The importance of aiming at a high operability rate in the
upper age-groups is shown by the fact that more than half the patients were over 60 years of age (Table 57). The operability rate
was shown to be higher in women (64.5 per cent) than in men
(58.5 per cent). Goligher suggests that the difference is due to the
feasibility, in women, of dealing radically with advanced growths

TABLE 57

EFFECT OF AGE ON OPERABILITY IN CANCER OF RECTUM
(ST. MARK'S HOSPITAL—GOLIGHER)

Age Group	Cases in Each Group	Accepted as Operable	Operability Rate
20–29.......	25	15	60.0%
30 39.......	63	42	66.7%
40–49.......	145	106	73.1%
50 59.......	351	224	63.8%
60–69.......	443	260	58.2%
70–79.......	139	65	47.0%
80–89.......	5	3	—
All ages	1 171	715	61.1%

TABLE 58

INFLUENCE OF SITE OF GROWTH ON OPERABILITY
(St. Mark's Hospital—Goligher)

Site of Growth		Growths in Each Site	Accepted as Operable	Operability Rate
Completely annular	Male	225	110	48.9%
	Female	112	60	53.6%
	Total	337	170	50.4%
Centred on anterior quadrant	Male	165	66	40.0%
	Female	71	42	59.2%
	Total	236	108	45.8%
Centred on one or other lateral quadrant	Male	165	130	78.8%
	Female	60	47	78.3%
	Total	225	177	78.7%
Centred on posterior quadrant	Male	190	157	82.6%
	Female	75	65	86.6%
	Total	265	222	83.8%

centered on the anterior wall of the rectum. This is brought out clearly in Table 58 (in men when the growth was centered on the anterior quadrant operability was 40 per cent; in women it was 59.2 per cent). Growths situated in the posterior quadrant had the highest operability rate (83.8 per cent). In the decade reviewed by Goligher (1930–1939), the operability rate was 62 per cent. He found that the lowest operability occurred in connection with growths in the upper third of the rectum (Table 59).

Operative mortality after perineo-abdominal excision.—Gabriel found the operative risk to be least in females in fairly early cases,

TABLE 59

OPERABILITY OF GROWTHS IN VARIOUS SEGMENTS OF THE RECTUM (St. Mark's Hospital—Goligher)

	Growths in Each Segment	Accepted as Operable	Type of Treatment Employed			Operability Rate
			Combined Excision	Perineal Excision	Other Methods	
Upper third...	395	224	161	31	32	56.7%
Middle third..	314	183	95	74	14	58.3%
Lower third...	387	273	59	181	33	70.5%
Totals.....	1,096	680	315	286	79	62.0%

TABLE 60

OPERATIVE MORTALITY AFTER ONE-STAGE PERINEO-ABDOMINAL
EXCISION FOR CARCINOMA OF THE RECTUM, 1932–1947
(GABRIEL)

Total number: 660. Operative deaths: 83 = 12.6 per cent

Age-Group	Male			Females		
	No. of Cases	Operation Deaths	Percentage Mortality	No. of Case	Operation Deaths	Percentage Mortality
20–29.....	3	0	0	7	2	28.5
30–39.....	15	1	6.6	17	2	11.7
40–49.....	51	5	10	45	1	2.2
50–59.....	118	14	12	66	5	7.6
60–69.....	157	29	18.4	61	5	8.2
70–79.....	81	16	19.8	35	3	8.6
0–89.....	3	0	0	1	0	0
Total...	428	65	15.2	232	18	7.7

and in young or middle-aged subjects; it was greatest in advanced
or border-line cases, and in aged men over 65 or 70. Table 60 shows
the mortality in his entire personal series of cases. The advantages
of increasing experience and of collecting these cases in a special
clinic are shown in Table 61. Where these cases are grouped ac-

TABLE 61

MORTALITY AFTER PERINEO-ABDOMINAL EXCISION IN ONE-STAGE
(GABRIEL'S CASES IN ST. MARK S HOSPITAL)

Date	Number	Operation Deaths
1932 38........	First 100	17
1939–43.........	Second 100	5
1943–45.........	Third 100	9
1945–47.........	Fourth 100	6
Total.	400	37 or 9.25%

cording to Dukes' classification, some interesting facts emerge, particularly the insignificant mortality in the early A cases (Table
62). He believes that the high death rate (16 per cent) which took
place in the male C cases is probably an expression of the difficulty
of radical removal of massive and locally advanced growths when
occurring in the narrow male pelvis. The high incidence of lymphatic metastasis (C cases) among females in this series (62 per
cent) agrees with known earlier onset of carcinoma of the rectum.

Operative mortality after perineal excision.—Gabriel, in 1944,
stated: "In the years when perineal excision was used as one of the
main methods of eradicating a rectal carcinoma, the mortality was
progressively reduced to 5 per cent. Since, however, it became evi-

TABLE 62

OPERATIVE MORTALITY AFTER ONE-STAGE PERINEO-ABDOMINAL
EXCISION OF THE RECTUM (GABRIEL's CASES IN
ST. MARK's HOSPITAL, 1932–1944)

660 cases classified according to depth of spread

Group	Males			Female		
	No. of Cases	Operation Deaths	Operation Mortality Per Cent	No. of Cases	Operation Deaths	Operation Mortality, Per Cent
A........	50	6	12	32	2	6
B........	163	23	14	56	4	7
C1.......	161	22	14	99	9	9
C2.......	54	14	27	45	3	7
Total..	428	65	15.2	232	18	7.7

dent that this operation was relatively ineffective in dealing with
the zone of upward lymphatic spread, and also when the frequency
of double carcinomas was realized, perineal excision has, at St.
Mark's Hospital, been done much less frequently. The tendency
has been in recent years to perform this operation in the very bad
risk cases, sometimes after a preliminary colostomy under local
anaesthesia, and also in locally advanced cases, perhaps associated
with fistulae or a fungating growth, when the operation was clearly
more in the nature of a palliative one than a radical procedure.
Hence it is not surprising that the operative mortality of this operation now shows a marked increase from the low level of 5 per cent
to above 10 per cent." Table 63, covering the St. Mark's Hospital
cases, over a period of more than thirty years, shows the gradual
decline and then the recent rise in the mortality rate.

Survival rate.—After analysis of 905 cases of rectal carcinoma

TABLE 63

OPERATIVE MORTALITY AFTER PERINEAL EXCISION
(ST. MARK's HOSPITAL STATISTICS)

Mean Operative Mortality, 10.7%. Males, 10.7%; Females, 10.7%

	Males	Females	Date	Operative Mortality	Males	Females
First 100 cases.	68	32	1910–22	16	11	5
Second 100 cases.	66	34	1922–27	13	11	2
Third 100 cases.	68	32	1927–29	10	8	2
Fourth 100 cases.	69	31	1930–33	8	5	3
Fifth 100 cases.	69	31	1933–36	5	3	2
Sixth 100 cases.	65	35	1936–39	11	4	7
Next 70 cases.	42	28	1939–47	9	6	3
Total 670 cases.	447	223	1910–47	72	48	24

treated by radical excision at St. Mark's Hospital (514 by combined and 391 by perineal excision), Dukes has shown that, including operative deaths, approximately 40 per cent of the total entry were alive at five years after operation. After recovery from operation the majority of subsequent deaths took place during the first three years after operation. The influence of early diagnosis on the ultimate results is shown when cases are classified according to the depth of spread by Dukes' classification (Table 64). This table

TABLE 64

FIVE-YEAR SURVIVAL RATE AFTER EXCISION OF THE RECTUM
(St. Mark's Hospital Statistics—Dukes)*

(Operation deaths excluded)

Group	Perineal Excision, Per Cent	Combined Excision, Per Cent
A.............	82.2	83.9
B.............	61.7	62.3
C.............	17.9	31.0
Total.	44.9	47.1

* 905 cases: 514 by perineo-abdominal and 391 by perineal excision.

shows that in A and B groups the results of the two operations, in their respective spheres, are closely similar, but in C cases the superiority of the combined excision is evident by an improvement of the 13 per cent over the results given by perineal excision.

Gabriel states that "When we consider that C cases, that is cases with lymphatic metastases, constitute at least 50 per cent of the cases treated, it can readily be seen that they form a very important group in regard to prognosis. The figures at present available show that when the upward lymphatic spread has reached the upper limit of the vascular pedicle removed surgically (C2 cases), the expectation of cure is very poor whether the operation has been a perineal or a combined one. When, however, a clear margin of uninfected glands has been obtained (C1 cases), the prognosis is distinctly better; here the advantage of the combined operation is undoubted and to be expected by all the knowledge now available on the spread of rectal cancer.

"Table 64 shows that in C1 case combined excision has given results almost twice as good as the perineal. Indeed, the superiority of combined excision in C cases is much greater than mere figures can indicate, because many late cases, if treated by perineal excision, would be classified as C2 with a survival rate of 9.7 per cent, whereas as if a combined excision were to be done the longer lymphatic pedicle obtained might enable a sufficient clearance to be

achieved to raise the category to the C1 group with a survival rate
of 42.5 per cent, a *difference of more than 30 per cent*. This is indicated by the fact that in my series of 400 perineo-abdominl excisions, out of 208 C cases there were only 61 C2 cases, that is less
than one-third of the C cases; whereas out of 102 C cases treated
by perineal excision at St. Mark's Hospital in the last ten years,
there were no less than 58 C2 cases, that is more than half of the
C cases. The difference in the prognosis between a C2 perineal and
a C1 perineo-abdominal is marked by the figures in heavy type in
Table 65."

TABLE 65

FIVE-YEAR SURVIVAL RATE AFTER EXCISION OF THE RECTUM IN
CASES WITH PROVED LYMPHATIC METASTASES (C CASES)*
(ST. MARK'S HOSPITAL STATISTICS—DUKES)

Group	Perineal Excision, Per Cent	Combined Excision, Per Cent
C1.............	24.8	**42.5**
C2.............	**9.7**	11.9
Total.	17.9	31.0

* 905 cases: 514 by perineo-abdominal and 391 by perineal excision.

Gabriel states that histological grading by Broders' method
provides valuable information as to the malignancy and the rate of
growth. The method has been in routine use at St. Mark's Hospital
for many years.

MILES'S STATISTICS

For forty years Miles utilized his procedure, finally perfecting it to the point where the mortality was entirely reasonable
and the end-results more satisfactory than for any other type of
operation.

It is true that Czerny under stress of circumstances did the first
combined abdominoperineal operation in 1883, demonstrating his
great versatility and courage as a surgeon; but it remained for
Miles, beginning in January, 1907, to establish the principles of
this operation, to work out the anatomical and technical details
and to demonstrate that radical dissection of the gland-bearing
tissue of the pelvis along with removal of the offending growth was
applicable to malignancy in this location. Basically the operation
of Miles fills the same niche in surgery for cancer of the rectum as
the Halsted operation occupies in surgery of the breast.

Too much credit cannot be given this pioneer surgeon for his
sturdy courage in forwarding surgery of the rectum during a period
when it was attended by high mortality and unquestionably poor

end-results, because of both the inaptitude of general surgeons in applying operative maneuvers as well as their lassitude and lack of interest in extirpative procedures in this portion of the gastro-intestinal tract.

In 1923 Miles reported on a series of 116 cases with an operability of 29.3 per cent in which the mortality was 25 per cent (23.4 per cent for 64 men and 26.9 per cent for 52 women). Of forty-four traced patients (many were lost sight of during the war) 70.5 per cent survived five years. In 1931 he reported a series of cases from 1920 to 1925 for the purpose of showing the percentage of cures. He does not state the number of deaths from operation, but gives the number of survivals for five years as 94. Of these, 8 are untraced. Known to be alive and well, there are 69, or 73 per cent, five-year survivals (Table 66). Although Miles failed to give the mor-

TABLE 66

RESULTS OF RADICAL ABDOMINOPERINEAL OPERATIONS AT
FIVE YEARS (MILES 1931)

Variety of Cancer	Sur- vivals	Un- traced	Died from Other Causes	Died Recur- rence	Alive and Well	Recur- rence Per- centage
(a) Papilliferous...	11	1	2	0	10	0
(b) Adenoid.......	73	7	6	9	58	14
(c) Colloid........	8	0	0	7	1	87.5
(d) Melanotic......	2	0	0	2	0	100
	94	8	8	18	69	27

tality rate for the entire series, he states that for different series (number of cases not given) the mortality is 32 per cent, 15 per cent, 9.8 per cent, and finally 7.6 per cent. He attributes this to three main factors: (a) the employment of more suitable anesthesia (spinal or caudal block and gas-and-oxygen); (b) the estimation of cardiac energy (Moots-McKesson index) when assessing operability; and (c) the adoption of blood transfusion as a routine measure immediately after the completion of the operation.

CANCER HOSPITAL STATISTICS (ABEL)

In a report to the Clinical Congress of the American College of Surgeons in 1934, Abel presented data on the 164 survivals after the radical abdominoperineal operation, operated on by the staff of Cancer Hospital, London, during the ten-year period 1920–29 inclusive. He analyzed the cases under the following headings: (1) incipient cancer (localized) without glandular involvement; (2) cancer that has extended to the lymph nodes; and (3) extensive

TABLE 67

FIVE-YEAR CURES OF CANCER OF THE RECTUM BY THE RADICAL
ABDOMINOPERINEAL EXCISION (CANCER HOSPITAL—ABEL)

Group		Survivals	Died in Less than 5 Years	Alive and Well after 5 Years	Un-traced	Percentage of 5-Year Cures
Rectosigmoid	I	6	1	5		83
	II	3	2	1		33
	III	8	7	1		14
Ampulla	I	22	4	16	2	73
	II	19	2	15	2	79
	III	8	6	1	1	14
Anal canal	I	2	0	2		100
	II	2	2	0		0
	III					
Total.........		70	24	41	5	58.5

local invasion with metastases. In 70 of the total series the exact
pathological condition is known. These are analyzed in Table 67.

From Table 68 the following facts emerge: Early cases without
glandular involvement have, on the whole, a higher five-year survival rate than more extensive ones. In the central portion of the
rectum the radical combined operation is as efficacious in effecting
five-year survivals in those with lymph nodes involved as it is in

TABLE 68

COMPLETED SERIES (CANCER HOSPITAL—ABEL 1935)

Survivals...	164
Died in less than five years...........................	47
Alive and well after five years........................	104
Untraced...	14
Percentage of five-year cures........................	63.4

those in which lymphatic invasion cannot be demonstrated pathologically.

Of the total series of 164 survivals, 47 cases died within five
years of operation, 104 were alive and well five years and more
after, and 14 are untraced (Table 68).

Out of all survivals 63.4 per cent were known to be alive and
free from signs of disease five years after operation. Abel suggests
that if the untraced cases are ignored (i.e., subtracted from the
survivals as is done by Lockhart-Mummery and by Gabriel) 104
out of 150 cases traced represent a five-year cure of 69.3 per cent.

TABLE 69

CARCINOMA OF THE RIGHT COLON AND HEPATIC FLEXURE:
TYPES OF OPERATION AND MORTALITY
(COLLER AND VAUGHAN—1945)

	Number	Deaths	Mortality
1. Palliative (nonresectable lesions):			
Ileotransverse colostomies..........		3	23.0%
Open anastomosis.................	4		
Closed anastomosis...............	9		
Total.........................	13	3	23.0%
2. Resectable lesions:			
One-stage right colectomies........	6	0	0
Two-stage right colectomies:			
(1) Ileotransverse colostomy:			
Open anastomosis....... 22			
Closed anastomosis...... 18			
(2) Right colectomy..............	40	1	2.5%
Obstructive resection.............	1	0	0
Total resectable lesions, right colon.	47	1	2.15%
Total.........................	60	4	6.6%

TABLE 70

CARCINOMA OF THE SIGMOID COLON TYPES OF OPERATION
AND MORTALITY (COLLER AND VAUGHAN—1945)

	Number	Deaths	Mortality
1. Palliative (nonresectable lesions):			
Celiotomy—only..	1	0	0
Celiotomy with colostomy..........	11	1	9.9%
Cecostomy—peritonitis............	1	1	100%
Total..	13	2	15.4%
2. Resectable lesions:			
End-to-end anastomosis:...........	51		
Closed.. 30		0	0
Open....................... 21		1	4.7%
Obstructive resections.............	6	0	0
	57	1	1.8%
Total.........................	70	3	4.2%
Preliminary cecostomy........ 12			
Preliminary colostomy......... 8			
Complementary cecostomy..... 31			
No decompression............ 6			

UNIVERSITY HOSPITAL, ANN ARBOR

Colon.—In 1945, Coller and Vaughan reported on the treatment of 173 patients with carcinoma of the colon managed in the University Hospital by 14 different surgeons of the permanent and resident staff between January 1, 1940 and September 1, 1944. The disposition of 60 cases with involvement of the cecum, ascending colon and hepatic flexure is shown in Table 69; and to cases with involvement of the sigmoid colon in Table 70. Of the total group of 173 cases 145, or 83.8 per cent were resectable. Nineteen per cent of these, however, had gross metastases in the liver or peritoneum that were beyond removal; therefore the resections were palliative in nature. In 112 patients, or 64.7 per cent, resection was undertaken without evidence of gross metastasis. Death occurred in only one patient in this group in which there was a chance of operative cure. They deliberately refrained from using the sulfa drugs in this series of cases in order that there would be a control group for comparison with similar groups of cases in which sulfa drugs have been used.

In 1947, Coller prepared for us the statistics which are shown in Tables 71 and 72. The number of cases of carcinoma of the colon observed at University Hospital has increased since 1944 from 173 to 406. The gross resectability then was 83.8 per cent and now is

TABLE 71

SUMMARY OF THE MANAGEMENT OF 406 CARCINCMAS OF THE COLON (UNIVERSITY HOSPITAL, ANN ARBOR—COLLER, 1948)

		Number	Per Cent
(1) No operative procedure		32	7.8
1. In extremis upon admission or condition too poor to warrant any surgical procedure	18		
2. Surgery elsewhere with recurrence. Palliative x-ray or no treatment	9		
3. Diagnostic only. No surgery	3		
4. Incidental findings at autopsy	2		
Total	32		
(2) Patients operated upon		374	92.2
Lesions not resectable			
Palliative operation		48	12.8
Lesions resected		326	87.2
(a) Other gross carcinoma irremovable			
(1) Liver metastases	55		
(2) Peritoneal carcinomatosis	42		
Total	97		
(b) Gross carcinoma removed with cure possible		229	61.2

TABLE 72

MORTALITY GRADIENT IN OPERABLE, RESECTABLE AND GROSSLY
CURABLE LESIONS OF CANCER OF THE COLON
(ANN ARBOR UNIVERSITY HOSPITAL—COLLER, 1948)

		Deaths	Mortality Rate
Total cases operated upon........	374 (173)	31 (13)	8.3% (7.5%)*
Palliative operations............	48 (28)	14 (7)	29.2% (25%)
Resected lesions.................	326 (145)	17 (6)	5.2% (4.1%)
Resected lesions in which liver or peritoneal metastases were present.........................	97 (33)	13 (5)	13.4% (15.1%)
Gross cancer removed with cure possible....................	229 (112)	4 (1)	1.7% (0.89%)

* In parentheses are the figures reported by Coller and Vaughan in 1944.

87.2 per cent; on the other hand, resection with cure possible was
64.7 per cent and now is 61.2 per cent. Mortality rates in the two
series of cases is compared in Table 72.

Rectum.—A review of the statistical data of University Hospital, Ann Arbor for surgery of the rectum for cancer were reported
in 1936 by Coller and Ransom. From 1931 to 1936 they endeavored
to follow the teachings and methods of Miles in the treatment of
carcinoma of the rectum, and it is with this period that their report
is concerned. A total of 270 cases diagnosed carcinoma of the rectum were observed. Of these, 46 came for diagnosis only, refused
treatment, or were operated upon elsewhere. Two hundred and
twenty-four remained for treatment: 114, or 51 per cent, proved
inoperable. The fate of the inoperable cases was as follows: No
treatment, 16; colostomy, 85; radium, 2; electrocoagulation, 2;
cystostomy, 2. The mortality for the palliative colostomies was 22
per cent. The fate of the operable cases is shown in Table 73.

The authors stated that their mortality was only 8.3 for the first
48 combined abdominoperineal operations in one stage. With an
increase in the operability rate the mortality likewise rose. Their

TABLE 73

CASES UPON WHOM CURATIVE OPERATIONS WERE ATTEMPTED
(UNIVERSITY HOSPITAL ANN ARBOR—COLLER AND RANSOM)

	No.	Mortality Cases	Per-centage
Colostomy—did not return for second stage......	4	0	
Colostomy with perineal excision...............	7	1	14
Two-stage abdominoperineal operation..........	27	7	26
One-stage abdominoperineal operation...........	72	12	16.5
	110	20	18.8

first cases were selected with great care, subsequently they accepted for operation patients aged more than 60 years and of these 7 died, 6 as a result of pneumonia or heart disease. Their early experience strikingly emphasizes the fallacy of deductions based on a small series of selected cases; their later experience convinced them of the advisability of returning to a somewhat more conservative selection of patients for the radical operation.

In 1944, Coller and Ransom published the results of their observation and treatment of 571 patients with carcinoma of the rectum and rectosigmoid, during the period from January 1, 1936 to July 1, 1942. In the group there were 352 males (61.6 per cent) and 219 females (38.4 per cent). Sixty-three patients refused any form of treatment or went elsewhere. There remained 508 patients who were admitted to the hospital for detailed investigation. Thirty-seven of these, or 7.3 per cent, were regarded as hopelessly inoperable and in the absence of obstruction received no definitive treatment. The disposition of the remaining 471 patients and the operative mortality rates were as follows:

	Cases	Deaths	%
Exploratory laporatomy only	7	1	14.3
Cauterization or radiotherapy	25	1	4.0
Local excision of polyp	3	0	0.0
Cecostomy	7	5	71.4
Colostomy	144	25	17.4
Total exploratory and palliative operations	186	32	17.2
Abdominoperineal resection (1-stage)	269	24	8.9
Abdominoperineal resection (2-stage)	5	2	40.0
Colostomy and posterior resection	9	2	22.2
Perineal resection with anastomosis	2	0	0.0
Total radical operations	285	28	9.8
Over-all mortality	471	60	12.7

Resectability, as determined by Coller and Ransom, was 56.1 per cent (ratio of resections to number of patients admitted to the hospital for study); as determined by most surgeons it would be 60.5 per cent (ratio of resections to number of patients actually explored). An abdominoperineal operation was performed in 96 per cent of the resections.

In regard to palliative colostomy the authors stated that: "In general with the known short life expectancy and the high mortality of colostomy in the terminal stages of rectal cancer, and the questionable benefits afforded by the operation, the trend in our clinic has been to employ it much less frequently than formerly. After observing the subsequent course of many of these patients, one agrees with the philosophy of the late Daniel Fiske Jones who urged removal of the tumor whenever possible since 'the condition of the patient after removal of the growth and a colostony cannot be compared with the physical discomforts, displeasures, and mental effect which follows a simple colostomy.'" In 144 of their cases simple loop colostomy only was performed. In 140 it was a palliative operation performed for non-resectable lesions, whereas in the four remaining cases it constituted the first stage of a proposed two-stage resection. The incidence of palliative colostomy among patients hospitalized was 27.8 per cent. The mortality rate was 17.4 per cent.

LAHEY CLINIC STATISTICS

Colon.—In 1943, Cattell reported 503 patients treated at the Lahey Clinic for carcinoma of the colon and rectum during the period of 1938 to 1941, inclusive. Four hundred and twenty had some type of resection, making a resectability rate of 83.5 per cent. The resectability of the colon and rectum separately was not given. A two-stage exteriorization procedure (obstructive resection) was performed in all carcinomas of the colon during this four-year period. There were 133 resections with 15 deaths, a mortality of 11.3 per cent. The number of palliative resections is not given. Cattell stated that if the curable cases were separated from the incurable, the operative mortality is materially improved; however, he feels that the only fair way to present one's experience with resection is to include all cases in which resection was performed.

Colcock, in 1947, reviewed the case histories of 337 patients with carcinoma of the colon and rectum treated at the Lahey Clinic prior to 1936; 307 of these patients were followed for at least 10 year. There were 103 patients with carcinoma of the colon. Eighty-one of the 103 patients were submitted to some type of resection, including 14 palliative resections. This is a resectability rate of 78.6 per cent. The disposition of the 22 patients in whom resection was not considered feasible is shown in Table 74. An exteriorization procedure of the obstructive resection type was done in 76, or 94 per cent, of the patients submitted to resection. Primary resection and anastomosis was performed in only one case. The operative mortality was 16.0 per cent in the resected cases, all of which were performed prior to 1936. The mortality for a similar group of patients in 1945 was 2.3 per cent, while the operability rate had risen to 90.7 per cent. The number of patients was not specified.

Of the patients with favorable lesions, that is, those in whom the adjacent lymph nodes were not involved and there was no local invasion of the surrounding tissues, 64.3 per cent survived five years without recurrence and 57.1 per cent are living and well without recurrence 10 or more years following resection of their malig-

TABLE 74

RESULTS OF OPERATION FOR CARCINOMA OF COLON AT FIVE AND TEN YEARS (LAHEY CLINIC—COLCOCK, 1947)

Type of Operation	Hospital Deaths	Patients Dying of Carcinoma Following Operation							Living and Well 10 or More Years	Deaths from other Causes	Total
		1–6 Mos.	6–12 Mos.	12–18 Mos.	18–24 Mos.	24–36 Mos.	3–5 Years	5–10 Years			
Laparotomy only	1	2	1	0	0	0	0	0	0	0	4
Ileocolostomy or cecostomy	2	6	5	0	0	0	0	0	0	0	13
Resection; liver metastases present	0	0	0	2	1	0	0	1*	0	0	4
Resection; liver negative; metastases in lymph nodes	8	1	4	3	3	3	1	1	3	0	27
Resection; liver negative; lymph nodes negative	5	1	2	0	2	1	4	2	16	5	38
Sarcoma	0	0	0	1	0	0	0	0	0	0	1

* Nodules noted in liver at time of operation; biopsy not done and may not have been metastases.

nant tumor. Of the patients with unfavorable lesions, 15 per cent were living and well five years after operation. Eleven per cent are living and well 10 or more years following resection (Table 75)

Rectum.—In 1934, Cattell and Lahey reported a review of 124 cases of carcinoma of the rectum and rectosigmoid (1928–33 inclusive). Sixty-six or 53 per cent were considered operable. The 66 resections done in this series were divided as follows: Lahey abdominoperineal (two stages), 33; Miles abdominoperineal (one stage), 5; anterior resection of rectosigmoid, 11; posterior resection following colostomy, 16; and local excision, 1. There were 9 operative deats, or a mortality of 13.6 per cent for the entire series; five died after resection and four died after colostomy. A sufficient length of time had not elapsed in order to permit computation of five-year results. In 1936, Lahey stated that for a two-year period his operability had been 73 per cent.

In 1943, Cattell again reviewed the total experiences of the Lahey Clinic in the treatment of 503 patients with carcinoma of the colon and of the rectum, who were observed during the period 1938 to 1941, inclusive. The resectability was 83.5 per cent. The rate for the colon and rectum separately was not given. There were

TABLE 75

CARCINOMA OF COLON: RESULTS AT FIVE AND TEN YEARS IN RELATION TO GLANDULAR INVOLVEMENT (COLCOCK—1947)

Group	Percentage of Patients Living and Well for 5 Years	Percentage of Patients Living and Well for 10 Years
Unfavorable lymph nodes involved and local invasion)	15.0	11.0
Favorable (lymph nodes not involved)	64.3	57.1

42 resections, 287 of which were for carcinoma of the rectum or rectosigmoid. The number and percentage of the four different types of resection performed for the rectum and rectosigmoid during the four-year period and for the year 1941 only are shown in Table 76. They consider the one-stage abdominoperineal resection

TABLE 76

CARCINOMA OF RECTUM: TYPES OF OPERATION AND MORTALITY
(LAHEY CLINIC—1938 TO 1941, CATTELL)*

	1938–1941				1941			
	Case		Mortality		Cases		Mortality	
	No.	%	No.	%	No.	%	No.	%
One Stage								
Abdominoperineal (Miles)	168	58 5	11	6 5	79	76.7	3	3.8
Anterior resection..	17	5.9	4	23.5	5	4.8	1	20.0
Total.	185	64 4	15	8.1	84	81.5	4	4.7
Two Stage								
Abdominoperineal (Lahey)....	87	30.3	12	13.8	15	14.5	1	6.7
Colostomy & perineal excision..	15	5.3	3	20.0	4	3.9	1	25.0
Total.	102	35.6	15	14.7	19	18.5	2	10.5
Total resections	287	100.0	30	10.4	103	100.0	6	5.8

* Consolidation of tables prepared by Cattell.

(Miles) the operation of choice for all lesions of the rectum and rectosigmoid; it was performed in good-risk patients of any age. Two-stage abdominoperineal resection (Lahey) is employed for poor-risk patients, some with moderate obstruction, for all patients who have perforated lesions with abscess, and for doubtfully operable patients, particularly those with marked adherence, in whom it is impossible to tell whether the cause is inflammation or extension of malignancy.

The operative mortality following the different types of operation is shown in Table 76. The mortality following the two-stage resection of the Lahey type was double that of the one-stage abdominoperineal operation, owing to the more extensive and complicated lesions in these patients. Approximately 10 per cent of their patients had liver metastasis at the time of operation while 22 per cent, including those having liver metastasis, had invasion of other structures.

Colcock, in 1947, reported on 337 patients with carcinoma of the colon and rectum treated at the Lahey Clinic prior to 1936, 307 of these patients were followed for at least 10 years. There were 234 patients with carcinoma of the rectum and rectosigmoid. One hundred forty-six patients were submitted to some type of resection. This is a resectability rate of 62 per cent. A two-stage Lahey procedure was performed in 83, or 56.8 per cent of the 146 patients, a one-stage abdominoperineal resection in 24, or 16.4 per cent, posterior resection in 22 or 15.0 per cent, and an anterior resection (with permanent colostomy) in 17, or 11.6 per cent. A steady tendency toward the increasing use of the one-stage Miles abdominoperineal resection is shown by the fact that this procedure was used in 16.4 per cent of the above group, 76.7 per cent in the year 1941, and 97.5 per cent in 1945. Resection was not carried out in 88 cases, a colostomy having been done in 62, a first stage Lahey procedure in 10, and a laporotomy only in 11. No operation was performed in 5 cases. Of the 146 patients who were submitted to resection, including 18 palliative resections, there were 11 deaths, or a mortality for the resected cases of 7.5 per cent. Since 1936 the operative mortality has dropped to 3.8 per cent in 1941 (79 cases) and 6.2 per cent in 1945. At the same time the operability rate has increased from 62 per cent to 83 per cent.

Follow-up data is shown in Table 77. In the favorable group

TABLE 77

RESULTS OF OPERATION FOR CARCINOMA OF THE RECTUM
AND RECTOSIGMOID AT FIVE AND TEN YEARS
(LAHEY CLINIC—COLCOCK 1947)

Type of Operation	Hospital Deaths	Patients Dying of Carcinoma Following Operation							Living and Well 10 or More Years	Deaths from other Causes	Total
		1–6 Mos.	6–12 Mos.	12–18 Mos.	18–24 Mos.	24–36 Mos.	3–5 Years	5–10 Years			
Laparotomy only	1	7	1	0	0	0	0	0	0	0	9
Colostomy only	29	18	15	2	1	1	1	0	0	0	67
Resection; liver metastases present	0	1	5	3	0	0	1	0	0	0	10
Resection; liver negative; lymph nodes involved	5	1	6	2	9	5	7	3	10	4	52
Resection; liver negative; lymph nodes negative	6	1	3	1	10	8	1	5	31	7	73
Sarcoma	0	0	0	1	0	0	0	0	0	0	1

(adjacent lymph nodes negative for carcinoma, no local invasion) 60 per cent were found to be well without recurrence at the end of 5 years; at the end of 10 years this figure had dropped to 51.6 per cent. In the less favorable group (lymph nodes showing metastatic carcinoma or invasion of the surrounding tissues by carcinoma), 30.2 per cent survived 5 years without recurrence. Only 22.2 per cent are living and well ten or more years following their operation (Table 78). In both instances the figures were arrived at after the postoperative deaths and patients who had died from other causes than malignant disease were omitted.

TABLE 78

CARCINOMA OF RECTUM: RESULTS AT FIVE AND TEN YEARS
IN RELATION TO GLANDULAR INVOLVEMENT (Colcock—1947)

Group	Percentage of Patients Living and Well for 5 Years	Percentage of Patients Living and Well for 10 Years
Unfavorable (lymph nodes involved and local invasion)...................	30.2	23.2
Favorable (lymph nodes not involved) .	60.0	51.8

CLEVELAND CLINIC STATISTICS

Colon.—Jones, in 1943, discussed his methods of choice in the treatment of carcinoma in the various segments of the colon. He emphasized the importance of perfecting one technic rather than trying every new procedure that is introduced unless one has an abundance of material. There are, he stated, many ways of accomplishing resection in the various segments but the fundamental prerequisite is to do as extensive and as radical an operation as possible. Whether this is done by the closed or open method, by the one-stage or two-stage method, or by any other technic makes little difference, he believes, provided the surgeon can show that his results from the standpoint of mortality and morbidity are equal to those of other technics.

Right colon.—Jones' preference in this group of cases is a one-stage right colectomy in which continuity is restored by a closed end-to-side ileotransverse colostomy over a Rankin clamp. He no longer employs enterostomy proximal to the anastomosis. He now uses instead the Miller-Abbott tube prior to operation. If, however, the tube has not reached the ileum before operation, enterostony is established. A review of 45 unselected cases revealed an average hospitalization of 20 days. The mortality was 13 per cent. The resectability is not given. Jones believes morbidity and mortality can be lower in resections of the right colon and the splenic flexure, particularly in fat persons in whom peritonealization of the large denuded areas following resection is extremely difficult, if a Mikulicz pack, which he has described, is utilized.

Left colon.—Previous to 1938, Jones favored resection of the sigmoid in one-stage procedure with end-to-end anastomosis and frequently with complementary colostomy or cecostomy. The mortality in this group including descending colon and sigmoid in 128 cases was 14 per cent. He felt this mortality could be improved upon, consequently in January, 1938, started a series of the Rankin obstructive resection. He felt then that one could do as radical an operation with this method as with primary resection and immediate anastomosis and now, in 1948, after ten years' experience he is fully convinced of this and uses obstructive resection to the exclusion of all other methods in dealing with lesions of the left colon.

From January, 1938, to July, 1942, the series totalled 77 cases. The mortality was five cases, or 6.5 per cent. Preliminary cecostomy for the relief of acute obstruction was done in 10 cases, or 13 per cent. Cecostomy was done once at the time of operation. The colostomy was closed as a secondary procedure in 66 cases. Spontaneous closure occurred in 11 cases, or 14.3 per cent of the series. Jones states that the principal objection to exteriorization procedures has been that it is a stage operation which requires prolonged hospitalization, not only for the resection, but also for closure of the colostomy. This, however, he found need not be so. In his experience the total duration of disability is only slightly longer than that following resection with anastomosis. The total hospital stay in this entire group of cases averaged 28 days. This included preoperative treatment in all cases, in 10 of which a cecostomy had to be performed for obstruction, and the hospital stay for closure of the colostomy, the latter averaging eight days. It was not necessary to do a second operation for closure in a single case.

In 1946, Jones reported that from January, 1940, to July, 1944, his series of Rankin type obstructive resections totalled 117 cases, 61 being in the left colon, the remainder in the transverse colon and splenic flexure. The mortality was 6 cases, or 5 per cent.

In the treatment of the low sigmoidal growth Jones believes one must be committed to a higher mortality and morbidity if the rectum is to be saved. The choice in such an event lies between two procedures: (1) colostomy followed by resection and end-to-end anastomosis, and (2) the anterior resection, or Hartmann procedure. The former, in his opinion, will carry a higher mortality and a lower curability rate, particularly in obese patients or those with an unusually short sigmoid. He states that, "In the young I would do an anastomosis and preserve the continuity of the bowel. In people over 60 years of age I would do the anterior resection and eliminate the two other surgical procedures."

Rectum.—In a personal series of 151 abdominoperineal resections in one-stage, reported by Jones in 1936, there were 16 deaths, or a mortality of 10.5 per cent. Fifty-two per cent survived five years. In 1943, he reported a mortality of 7.2 per cent in a series of more than 600 resections of the rectum and rectosigmoid for carcinoma. His most recent 128 consecutive cases were done without a fatality, yet liver metastasis was present in eight instances, 25 had arteriosclerotic heart disease with hypertension, five had coronary heart disease, and four had diabetes. The total hospital stay for this entire group averaged twenty-two and a half days. Only ten had a hospital stay of over thirty days. The operability rate is not stated.

Jones, in a personal communication in 1947, stated that between January, 1940, and November 1, 1947, he had operated upon 802 patients diagnosed carcinoma of the rectum and rectosigmoid

TABLE 79

ABDOMINAL WOUND MORBIDITY IN ONE STAGE-COMBINED
ABDOMINOPERINEAL RESECTIONS*
(JONES, NEWELL AND BRUBAKER)

| Group | Type of Closure | Infections | | | | | Disruptions | |
		No. Cases	Slight	Mod- erate	Se- vere	Per Cent	No. Cases	Per Cent
I	Catgut in layers with stay sutures........	76	3	17	3	27.5	3	3.9
II	Catgut and alloy steel. No stay sutures....	64	0	7	2	14.0	0	0.0
III	Alloy steel figure-of-eight sutures. No stay sutures........	116	0	1	0	0.85	0	0.0

* Comparison of types of wound closure in 256 cases.

with the intention of performing a combined abdominoperineal resection. The operability for the entire group is not known, but for the first ten months of 1947, of 105 patients operated upon, 88 had abdominoperineal resections, or a resectability rate of 87 per cent. The mortality for the 802 cases was 24, or 3.1 per cent.

In 1941, Jones, Newell, and Brubaker reported a comparison of types of wound closure in 256 cases of carcinoma of the rectum and rectosigmoid in which a one-stage combined abdominoperineal resection was undertaken. Table 79 reveals the incidence of wound morbidity in 76 cases in which closure was done with catgut in layers and with silkworm stay sutures; 64 cases in which catgut and alloy steel was used but no stay sutures; and 116 cases in which alloy steel figure-of-eight sutures alone were employed. In the latter group the wound morbidity was reduced to an extremely low incidence: the incidence of infection was reduced from 27.5 per cent with the use of catgut and stay sutures to 0.85 per cent with the use of interrupted figure-of-eight alloy steel sutures. Chemotherapeutic agents were not administered in any of these cases.

SCOTT AND WHITE CLINIC

In 1942, Brindley reported findings in an analytical study of 190 case records of patients with cancer of the colon who were seen at the Scott and White Clinic over a period of twenty-two years

(Table 80). The surgical mortality of one-stage resections was four times as high as that of multiple-stage procedures. Seventy-two per cent of the patients who survived surgery lived more than three years and 58.4 per cent lived more than five years.

TABLE 80

SUMMARY OF RESULTS IN CASES OF CARCINOMA OF THE COLON
(SCOTT AND WHITE CLINIC-BRINDLEY—1942)

A—Total number of patients seen.................................... 190
    No operation advised... 30

B—Operation advised.. 160
    Patient refused operation...................................... 10

C—Operation undertaken.. 150
    Inoperable at operation....................................... 50

Resection completed... 100
Resectability in relation to "A" (52.6%); to "B" (62.5%); to "C" (66.6%)

Type of Operation	Cases	Hospital Mortality
Resection for cure............................	100	17 (17.0 per cent)
Right colon...............................	46	7 (15.2 per cent)
Left colon...............................	54	10 (18.5 per cent)
One-stage...............................	20	7 (35.0 per cent)
Multiple-stage...........................	70	6 (8.6 per cent)
Hartmann s resection.....................	10	0
Palliative operations.......................	50	6 (12.0 per cent)
Exploration only.........................	12	0
Cecostomy...............................	11	4
Entero-enterostomy.......................	13	2
Exploration & drainage of abscess...........	2	0

PRESBYTERIAN HOSPITAL—UNIVERSITY OF ILLINOIS STATISTICS

In 1947, Gilchrist and David reported a detailed study of 200 patients operated upon more than five years ago for carcinoma of the large bowel where there was a reasonable chance of cure. Palliative resections for removal of tumors where known metastases could not be removed are not included in this group. The operability rate was approximately 75 per cent. There were 19 operative deaths, or a mortality of 9.5 per cent. One hundred and twenty-five, or 62.5 per cent, had lymph node metastasis; 114, or 57 per cent, were alive from five to ten years; and there was a 96.5 per cent five-year follow-up. All operations were performed before the era of chemotherapy.

Owing to the manner in which this tremendously important study has been presented, lesions of the rectosigmoid and rectum will be discussed in this section along with lesions of the colon. Since the term "rectosigmoid junction" means different things to different surgeons, and as their study has demonstrated the very different prognosis, recurrence, and mortality rate in different regions of the large intestine, the authors decided that a new set of landmarks should be used. They have designated those carcinomas which are partially or completely below the peritoneal reflection as "extraperitoneal carcinoma of the rectum." There were 112 of these. Those lesions which are entirely covered by peritoneum, anteriorly, and which are below the promontory of the sacrum were designated as "intraperitoneal carcinoma of the rectum." There, were 41 of these. Fourteen were in the redundant loop of sigmoid above the promontory of the sacrum. These last two, which total 55, are grouped as one in this discussion as all findings were identical. Thirty-three were in the remaining portions of the colon.

Right half of the colon.—There were fifteen carcinomas of the right colon, which included the cecum, ascending, hepatic flexure and the first three inches of the transverse colon. All had ileotransverse colon anastomoses at the time of resection. There were three deaths, or a mortality of 20 per cent. Thirteen, or 86.6 per cent, of these had metastases to nodes and, in spite of three postoperative deaths and one lost to follow-up, nine were known to be alive after five years (61.5 per cent).

Left half of the colon.—There were eighteen carcinomas in the

TABLE 81

END-RESULTS IN 55 INTRAPERITONEAL RECTAL AND SIGMOID
CARCINOMAS (GILCHRIST AND DAVID—1947)

	Per Cent
36 alive 5 years	65.4
4 postoperative deaths	7.2
3 deaths not due to carcinoma	5.5
2 had no follow-ups	3.6
35 had no node metastases	63.3
18 with node metastases alive 5 years	51.4
20 had no node metastases	
18 without node metastases alive 5 years	90.0
1 no follow-up	
1 postoperative death	
27 obstruction resections	
18 alive 5 years	66.6
16 had node metastases	
9 with node metastases alive 5 years	56.2
2 postoperative deaths	
1 short follow-up	
11 without node metastases	
9 without metastases alive 5 years	81.9
1 postoperative death	
1 no follow-up	

transverse or descending colon or at the splenic flexure. All of these had obstructive resections. There were no operative deaths. Only eight had node metastasis (44.4 per cent). Five of these died of recurrence within five years. Eleven were alive after five years (61.1 per cent).

Intraperitoneal rectum and sigmoid.—There were 55 carcinomas situated between the lower end of the descending colon and the reflection of peritoneum onto the pelvic colon (Table 81). Twenty-seven of the patients had obstructive resections performed. In many, the extraperitonealization of the resected area was done as described by David in 1934. In the more unfavorable cases, abdominoperineal resections were performed. This, state the authors, probably accounts for the fact that the results with obstructive resections were about the same as with abdominoperineal resections. Eighteen, or one-tenth per cent, of the 55 died of recurrence within

TABLE 82

RECURRENCE IN 112 EXTRAPERITONEAL RECTAL
CARCINOMA (Gilchrist and David—1947)

Recurrence	69 with Node Metastases		43 without Node Metastases	
Local........................	16	23.2%	2	4.6%
Liver.......................	11	15.9%	2	4.6%
Lung, bone, general...........	3	4.3%	1	2.3%
	30	43.5%	5	11.6%

five years, the recurrence rates being similar in the two types of operations. The low incidence of recurrence here contrasts sharply with the 43.5 per cent in carcinomas which are extraperitoneal. There were four postoperative deaths in this group of cases, or a mortality of 7.2 per cent.

Extraperitoneal rectum.—One hundred and twelve carcinomas were partially or completely below the peritoneal reflection. There were 12 postoperative deaths, or a mortality of 10.7 per cent, and four had no follow-up. Only 26 of the 69 with node metastasis were alive after five years (37.5 per cent), whereas 32 of the 43 with node metastasis were alive five years (74.4 per cent). All told 58, or 51.8 per cent, survived five to ten years. The incidence of local and liver recurrences in these low lying growths is striking (Table 82).

End-results.—If one excludes those patients who had died of other causes without any sign of recurrent carcinoma and those who had follow-up and those who died postoperatively, the prognosis would be as shown in Table 83.

New carcinomas have developed in seven of the 200 patients.

In each of these cases there is strong evidence to suggest that these are new tumors and not metastasis.

The following conclusions were reached by the authors:

1. In each of the regions of the bowel studied, patients in whom no lymph node metastasis could be found in the surgical specimens had a five- to ten-year survival rate of 78.5 per cent. If those who were lost to follow-up and those who died postoperatively and of other causes after leaving the hospital were taken into account, this figure would be even more impressive (90.9 per cent).

TABLE 83

END-RESULTS IN 166 CASES OF CARCINOMA OF THE LARGE INTESTINE (GILCHRIST AND DAVID—1947)*

		Per Cent Alive 5 Years
114	alive 5 years	68.7
58/89	extraperitoneal rectal	65.2
36/48	intraperitoneal rectal	75.0
9/11	right colon	82.8
11/18	left colon	61.1
54/100	with involved nodes	54.0
60/66	without involved nodes	90.9
26/53	extraperitoneal with involved nodes	49.1
32/36	extraperitoneal without involved nodes	88.8
18/30	intraperitoneal with involved nodes	60.0
18/18	intraperitoneal without involved nodes	100.0
7/9	right colon with involved nodes	77.7
2/2	right colon without involved nodes	100.0
3/8	left colon with involved nodes	37.5
8/10	left colon without involved nodes	80.0

* Excluding patients who died from other causes, those who had no follow-up and those who died postoperatively.

2. The 37.5 per cent survival rate of those having carcinoma of the left side of the colon when node metastasis are present indicates, the authors believe, the need for wider resection of mesentery in this area.

3. Resections of fixed tumors and structures to which they are adherent give a better prognosis than might be expected, a 40 per cent five-year survival. Twenty per cent died postoperatively. This figure will be much improved when chemotherapy is used (see Table 13).

4. Retrograde metastasis to nodes one to five centimeters below the tumor occurred in seven of the 153 tumors below the promontory of the sacrum (4.6 per cent). This finding reemphasizes the necessity for extensive resection in those having enlarged nodes and large tumors.

5. Postmortem examination of those dying in the hospital after resection for carcinoma of the rectum showed that the ordinary post-mortem examination will usually fail to demonstrate small metastases to nodes in the retroperitoneal tissues. In three of these, complete removal of all node metastases would have been obtained if the field of resection had been 1.5 cm. wider.

6. The liver was the site of recurrences in 10 per cent of the tumors. These were probably due to blood-borne metastasis.

7. Two of three patients who developed carcinoma of the rectum while pregnant lived over five years. This suggests that the gloomy prognosis given pregnant women with neoplasms may not be justified in carcinoma of the rectum.

8. New carcinomas developed in seven patients who had had resections. This does not include carcinoma of the skin. Patients who have had one cancer of the colon should be reexamined carefully whenever any symptom suggesting cancer appears.

9. In evaluating the type of procedure used in treating carcinoma, the survival rate is important. Of those who died of recurrence in less than five years, two-thirds occurred within three years and one-third between three and five years. Six of those listed as five cures developed recurrences and were dead or dying in less than seven years. In view of the appreciable percentage who develop recurrence in the fourth and fifth year after operation, it sems foolish, the authors state, to consider anything less than a five-years survival as a cure. Moreover, they believe such short term survivals should not be included in discussions since they lead the general practioner to false conclusions.

10. Finally, the authors are of the opinion that their study indicates the need for the widest possible resection in carcinoma of the large intestine. Lesions which are partially or completely below the peritoneum, they emphasize, have a high incidence of local and liver recurrence and pull-through or sleeve resections are not much better than a local resection. The Miles operation seems to give the best chance of cure here.

UNIVERSITY OF PENNSYLVANIA HOSPITAL, SURGICAL SERVICE "B"

In 1947, Ravdin prepared for us the following unpublished statistics. Between the years 1923 and 1946, there were admitted to Surgical Service "B," Hospital of the University of Pennsylvania 359 cases of malignancy of the large intestine: 358 carcinomas and one lymphosarcoma. The resectability (with no gross, remote metastasis) was 64.5 per cent for the colon and 62.5 per cent for the rectosigmoid and rectum. The number of cases encountered in the various segments of the large bowel was not given. The hospital mortality (within 30 days following operation) for the years 1923 to 1938 was 18.4 per cent, whereas for the years 1938 to 1946, it was 4.2 per cent. Ravdin, Zintel and Bender, in 1947, in a discussion of adjuvants to surgical therapy in large bowel malignancy, gave an explanation for this marked reduction in their mortality rate. It is due, they believe, to the adoption of a program of preoperative and postoperative measures consisting of (1) correction of existing anemia and plasma protein deficiency (hypoproteinemia); (2) administration of adequate vitamins to make up for losses of certain vitamins incident to oral chemotherapy; (3) long tube (Miller-Abbott) decompression before, during and after operation; and (4) routine employment of chemotherapy and the antibiotics, particularly oral streptomycin. In 1938, a portion of this program was commenced namely, routine employment of decompression by the Miller-Abbott tube for lesions of the right colon and correction of hypoproteinemia. In recent years the use of long tube decompression has been extended to include the preparation of patients with lesions in the more distal segments of the colon and oral streptomycin is regularly employed for a number of days prior to resection.

During the year 1946, total resectability for the colon rose to 73.6 per cent, whereas the over-all mortality in 53 resections of the colon for malignant lesions was 3.8 per cent. Forty, or 74.1 per cent, were done in one stage. Eighteen of the latter were performed by the open method.

MAYO CLINIC STATISTICS

The most recent available general report on surgery of the large intestine at the Mayo Clinic is the Annual Report for 1943, published December 27, 1944. Of the 1,034 lesions for which operations were performed 781, or 75.6 per cent were malignant (777, or 99.5 per cent of these were carcinoma). Four hundred and twenty-six, or 54.5 per cent involved the colon. The resectability rate is not given. In commenting on the probable causes for the considerable reduction in the general operative mortality rate following surgery of the large intestine, it was stated that in 1933, the rate was 13.1 per cent; in 1935, 12.0 per cent; in 1939, 9.4 per cent and in 1941, it was 5.6 per cent. The improved results coincided with the intraperitoneal employment of vaccine and the introduction and gradual extension of the use of the sulfonamide group of drugs. Intraperitoneal vaccination was used as early as 1939, whereas it was not until 1943 that routine administration of adequate doses of succinylsulfathiazole was begun as a preoperative measure. The routine instillation of sulfathiazole powder at the time of operation is considered a valuable aid.

Pemberton, in 1947, wrote of the effect of chemotherapy on surgery of malignant lesions of the colon. He stated that other than the introduction of chemotherapy, there has been no major change in the management of colonic and rectal lesions during the past twelve years at the Mayo Clinic. In the fall of 1939, they began to use sulfonilamide crystals in the peritoneal cavity. It was some while, however, before the sulfa compounds were used routinely. In 1942, they began the routine use of sulfasuxidine. A comparison was made between the incidence of peritonitis and pneumonia as causes of death in those cases in which the patient had received little or no sulfonamide compound with those in which the patient had received adequate doses. During the period 1934 to 1940, inclusive, 6.1 per cent of the patients operated on died of peritonitis, whereas only 1.8 per cent of those subjected to operation in the period 1941 to 1943, inclusive, and 1.6 per cent of those operated on in the period 1944 to 1945, inclusive, died of peritonitis. Similarly 2.2 per cent of the patients of the first period died of bronchopneumonia, as compared to 0.7 per cent and 0.5, respectively who died of this complication in the later period.

Right half of colon.—In a review of 885 cases of malignant lesions of the cecum and ascending colon in which operation was performed at the Mayo Clinic in the years 1907 to 1938, inclusive, the resectability rate was found to be 590, or 67 per cent. In 247 of the 590 cases, the lesion was situated in the cecum and in 343 cases it was in the ascending colon. The over-all mortality was 23.5 per cent. These cases include those in which only palliative procedures were carried out. A one-stage operation was done in 315 cases with a mortality of 22.2 per cent, a two-stage procedure in 246 with a mortality of 28.9 per cent and in 29 cases more than a two-stage procedure was undertaken with a mortality of 34.6 per cent. The survival rates in cases in which operation was performed with a view to cure are shown in Table 84.

TABLE 84

SURVIVAL RATES IN CASES IN WHICH OPERATION WAS
PERFORMED WITH A VIEW TO CURE; RESECTIONS
OF RIGHT COLON FOR CANCER
(Mayo Clinic, 1907–1938)

Period After Leaving Hospital	Patients Who Survived Operation		Survived Beyond Indicated Period	
	Total	Traced	Number	Per Cent of Traced Patients
5 years..........	302	298	170	57.0
10 years..........	225	219	104	59.5
15 years..........	155	150	56	37.3
20 years..........	91	88	22	25.0

In another review of cases in which resection of the right half of the colon was performed at the Mayo Clinic from January 1, 1940 through December 31, 1947, the following changes from the preceding report (1909–1938) are evidenced: 1, The resectability rate has risen from 67 to 84 per cent; 2, primary resection and ileotransverse colostomy in one stage has superseded multi-stage operations (77 per cent were one-stage operations); 3, of the one-stage operations, in 40 per cent primary resection and end-to-end ileotransverse colostomy were performed; 4, during the year 1947, resection

TABLE 85

OPERATIONS FOR MALIGNANT LESIONS RIGHT COLON,
1940–1947, INCLUSIVE
(MAYO CLINIC—1948)

	All Cases		
		Hospital Deaths	
	Patients	Number	Per Cent
Resection right colon, one-stage...............	393	11	2.8
Resection right colon, two-stage...............	66	4	6.1
Extraperitoneal resection of lesion.............	44	5	11.4
Local excision of lesion.......................	12	0	
Subtotal colectomy..........................	1	0	
Total cases with resection of lesion..........	516	20	3.9
Ileocolostomy, 1st stage of two-stage resection...	18	8	
Palliative ileocolostomy......................	99	8	8.1
Ileostomy.................................	1	0	
Colocolostomy..............................	2	0	
Abdominal exploration.......................	28	1	3.6
Total cases without resection of lesion........	148	17	11.5
Total, all cases........................	664	37	5.6

of the right portion of the colon was performed for malignant lesions in seventy-four cases with 2 hospital deaths (all but six were performed in one-stage); 5, mortality for the one-stage operation has decreased from 22 per cent to 2.8 per cent for the one-stage operation and from 29 per cent to 6 per cent for the two-stage operation (Table 85).

Left half of colon.—In 1945, Waugh reported that during the preceding 15 months he had performed at the Mayo Clinic 50 consecutive primary aseptic anastomoses over the Rankin three-bladed clamp in restoring continuity of the bowel after resection of lesions located variously between the midtransverse colon and the upper part of the rectum. The distribution of the lesions were as follows: transverse colon, 8; splenic flexure, 2; descending colon, 5; upper and middle sigmoid, 19; low sigmoid, 1; rectosigmoid, 14; and upper rectum, 1. Two of the 50 patients died, giving a mortality rate for this series of 4.0 per cent. The mortality for the 34 resections of the colon was 2.9 per cent; the mortality for the remaining 16 resectons was 6.3 per cent. In six cases there was metastasis to the liver or nodal involvement beyond the limits of resectability. Preparation with succinylsulfathiazole and employment of aseptic anastomosis are considered important factors in reducing the mortality rate. Proximal colostomy is considered unnecessary for lesions of the middle part of the sigmoid or above but, for lesions below the middle of the sigmoid, either proximal colostomy or passage of rectal tube beyond the point of anastomosis is thought to be indicated.

TABLE 86

ANTERIOR RESECTION 1930–1947: HOSPITAL DEATHS BY PERIODS
MAYO CLINIC (DIXON—1948)

Date	Cases	Deaths	
		Number	Per Cent
1930–1935..............	47	4	8.5
1936–1940..............	109	14	12.8
1941–1947..............	270	7	2.6
All years.............	426	25	5.9

Rectum and rectosigmoid.—Dixon, in 1948, reported his results in a personal series of 426 cases of anterior resection of malignant lesions between 6 and 20 cm. from the dentate line, performed with a view to cure. For lesions more than 10 cm. from this line the resectability rate was 86 per cent. Involvement of the bladder, ureter or small intestine did not prevent resection. For lesions at 10 cm. from the dentate line the resectability was 80 per cent and for those at 8 cm. it was 44 per cent. This was considered to be the lowest level of general applicability of the operation. In his opinion anterior resection is rarely applicable when the lesion is situated as low as 6 cm.

The hospital mortality in this series of cases is shown in Table 86. There were 25 deaths (5.9 per cent). Dixon states that the rise in mortality rate to 12.8 per cent during the years 1936 to 1940 was owing to the fact that more tissue was excised at operation than previously. He attributes reduction in mortality to 2.6 per cent for the next seven years principally to the routine use of sulfonamides.

Prior to 1938 the majority of these operations were carried out in three stages, including transverse colostomy. Since 1938 colostomy has been performed at the time of resection unless there was severe obstruction. In recent years antecedent colostomy has been performed less frequently; yet the mortality rate has been found to be considerably higher when colostomy is omitted. This was shown by Mayo and Smith (1948) who reported on 200 cases of carcinoma of the rectum, rectosigmoid and lower sigmoid situated from 5 to 15 cm. from the anus and treated by anterior segmental resection. Concomitant colostomy was performed in 100 consecutive cases. With colostomy mortality rate was 3 per cent and with-

TABLE 87

ANTERIOR RESECTION (NON-PALLIATIVE OPERATION): FIVE-YEAR SURVIVAL RATES FOR DIFFERENT LEVELS
(DIXON—1948)

Distance from Dentate Line, Cm.	All Cases		No Nodal Involvement		Nodal Involvement	
	Number	5 Yr. Survival Rate, %	Cases	5 Yr. Survival Rate, %	Cases	5 Yr. Survival Rate, %
6–10.............	74	63.7	32	72.4	42	57.1
11–15.............	97	70.2	58	78.8	39	57.7
16–20.............	101	66.9	60	71.5	41	60.4
All Levels.........	272	67.7	150	74.0	122	58.5

out it 6 per cent. The greatest difference between the two groups was in morbidity. In the series without colostomy, 82 per cent of the patients were out of the hospital within one month, and 65 per cent were dismissed from care within that period. In those with colostomy, 4 per cent were out of the hospital but none were dismissed from care within one month. Only 7 of 97 surviving patients were dismissed from care at 2 months.

Table 87 gives the five-year survivals for each level in cases with and without nodal involvement. The best rest results were obtained from removal of lesions occurring 11 to 15 cm. from the dentate line. Figure 67 shows graphically the survival rate in these 272 cases which had been performed at least five years previously. After five years 67.7 per cent of the patients were alive; 49.8 per cent were alive after ten years.

When it was found at exploratory operation that the lesion was too low in the bowel to be removed by anterior resection, colostomy was performed and the lesion removed by posterior resection two or three weeks later. Dixon contends that when properly carried out, posterior resection is much more radical locally (for growths below the pelvic peritoneal fold) than combined abdom-

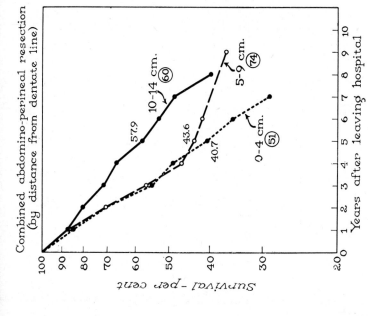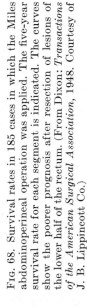

Fig. 68. Survival rates in 185 cases in which the Miles abdominoperineal operation was applied. The five-year survival rate for each segment is indicated. The curves show the poorer prognosis after resection of lesions of the lower half of the rectum. (From Dixon: *Transactions of the American Surgical Association*, 1948. Courtesy of J. B. Lippincott Co.)

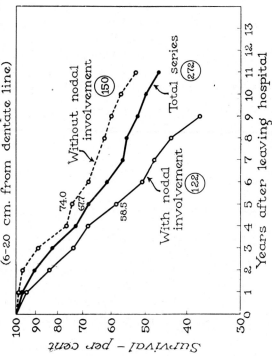

Fig. 67. Survival rates of 272 cases in which the operation of anterior resection was performed. Palliative operations are omitted. The five-year survival rates are indicated. (From Dixon: *Transactions of the American Surgical Association*, 1948. Courtesy of J. B. Lippincott Co.)

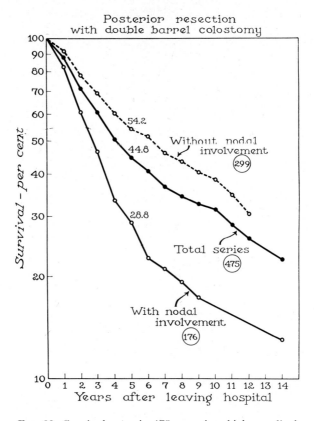

FIG. 69. Survival rates in 475 cases in which a radical posterior resection was performed. This figure is a complement to figure 67, for these are cases in which the lesion was too low for performance of the operation of anterior resection. This figure includes the lesions in the distal 6 cm. of rectum plus those occurring up to 10 cm. from the dentate line, in which the lesion was too extensive for anterior resection. The curves show that resection of lesions of the terminal portion of the rectum is attended by a poorer prognosis and that nodal involvement in this region is of graver significance than in cases in which anterior resection could be performed. (From Dixon: *Transactions of the American Surgical Association*, 1948. Courtesy of J. B. Lippincott Co.)

inoperineal resection and can be radical along the pelvic mesocolon. To evaluate his contention he selected a group of 185 cases in which a one-stage abdominoperineal resection was undertaken during the same time interval as the anterior resections were performed (Figure 68) and similarly has shown the survival rates in 475 cases of posterior resection performed during this period of time (Figure 69). In both instances the cases have been divided according to the distance between the lesion and the dentate line. The

TABLE 88

MALIGNANT LESIONS OF THE LARGE INTESTINE; ONE-STAGE
COMBINED ABDOMINOPERINEAL RESECTION
(MAYO CLINIC—1948)
Hospital Mortality

	Total			Males			Females		
		Hospital Deaths			Hospital Deaths			Hospital Deaths	
	Pa-tients	Num-ber	Per Cent	Pa-tients	Num-ber	Per Cent	Pa-tients	Num-ber	Per Cent
1908–1919..	21	6	28.6	13	4	30.8	8	2	25.0
1920–1929..	29	8	27.6	21	7	33.3	8	1	12.5
1930–1939..	169	28	16.6	111	20	18.0	58	8	13.8
1940–1946..	841	27	3.2	561	19	3.4	280	8	2.9
Total....	1060	69	6.5	706	50	7.1	354	19	5.4

TABLE 89

MALIGNANT LESIONS OF LARGE INTESTINE; ONE-STAGE
COMBINED ABDOMINOPERINEAL RESECTION
(MAYO CLINIC—1948)
Five-year survival rates by metastasis and grade of malignancy

	Patients*		Lived 5 or More Years after Leaving Hospital	
	Total	Traced	Number	Per Cent of Traced Patients
Without metastasis				
Grades 1 and 2.......	100	95	66	69.5
Grades 3 and 4.......	12	12	7	58.3
Grade not stated.......	7	7	6	85.7
Total............	119	114	79	69.3
With metastasis				
Grades 1 and 2.......	63	59	26	44.1
Grades 3 and 4.......	28	27	5	18.5
Grade not stated.......	6	6	2	33.3
Total............	97	92	33	35.9
Total series..........	216	206	112	54.4

* Inquiry as of January 1, 1946. Included are only those patients operated on
five or more years prior to the time of inquiry, i.e. 1940 or earlier. Hospital deaths
are omitted from the calculations.

five-year survival rate in the series of cases of posterior resection was 44.8 per cent; the corresponding five year survival rates for the combined operation were 40.7 per cent for lesions 0 to 4 cm. and 43.6 per cent for lesions 5 to 9 cm. from the dentate line.

Unpublished data from the Statistical Division of the Mayo Clinic (1948) on the total experience of that institution with the combined abdominoperineal resection in one-stage is shown in Table 88. Table 89 reveals the five-year survival rates of this series by metastasis and grade of malignancy. Included are only

TABLE 90

SURVIVAL RATES OF PATIENTS HAVING ADENOCARCINOMA
OF THE RECTUM AND SIGMOID COLON TREATED
BY ABDOMINOPERIEAL RESECTION
MAYO CLINIC—WAUGH AND KIRKLIN (1949)

Level of Lower Edge of Lesion Above Anal Margin	Nodal Metastasis	Patients	Traced Patients	Lived 5 or More Years After Operation*	
				Number	Per Cent of Traced Patients
0–5 cm.	All cases	100	93	43	46.2
	Without	56	50	33	66.0
	With	44	43	10	23.3
6–10 cm.	All cases	201	182	93	51.1
	Without	105	94	71	75.5
	With	96	88	22	25.0
11 cm. or more.	All cases	87	80	43	53.8
	Without	54	47	32	68.1
	With	33	33	11	33.3

* Inquiry was as of January 1, 1946. All operations were performed in 1940 or earlier.

those patients operated on five or more years prior to the time of inquiry i.e., 1940 or earlier.

Waugh and Kirklin, in 1949, further analyzed these cases in order to show the importance of the level of the lesion in the prognosis and treatment of carcinoma of the rectum and lower sigmoid colon (Table 90).

OCHSNER CLINIC STATISTICS

Colon.—In 1946, Ochsner and Hines reported the 113 cases of carcinoma of the large bowel observed at the Ochsner Clinic in the four years from its opening, January 1, 1942 to January 1, 1946. Their findings in regard to resectability and hospital mortality have been summarized in Table 91. The right colon was involved in 22 (19.5 per cent), the left colon in 42 (43.3 per cent). Sulfathalidine is employed routinely. Spinal anesthesia was used in 109 cases (96.4 per cent); in 34 cases the continuous technic was employed. In 42 of their cases an end-to-end anastomosis with colonic resection was done in 27 (64.4 per cent) and an obstructive resection in 15 (35.5 per cent). Of the resections with end-to-end anastomosis, an aseptic technic—their preference—was used in 17 and an open anastomosis in 10.

TABLE 91

ANALYSIS OF 113 CASES OF CARCINOMA OF THE LARGE INTESTINE (OCHSNER CLINIC, 1942–1945, INCLUSIVE)

Total number of patients observed		113
Right colon	22	
Left colon	40	
Rectosigmoid & rectum	51	
Resections performed		96 (84.8%)
For cure	87	
For palliation	9	
Right colon	18	
Left colon	26	
Rectosigmoid & rectum	43	
Palliative operations other than resections		17 (15.2%)
Colostomy	10	
Short-circuiting anastomosis	5	
Exploration only	2	
Total number of operations performed		113
Mortality rate (113 cases)		8 (7.1%)
Resection, right colon (18 cases)	0	
Resection, left colon (30 cases)	2 (6.6%)	
Resection, rectum (48 cases)	2 (4.1%)	
Palliative measures (17 cases)*	4 (23.5%)	

* Other than palliative resections.

These authors state that whereas they resect and reestablish continuity of the bowl in sigmoidal lesions with the exception of those at or near the rectosigmoidal junction, "we believe that this procedure is not justifiable in low-lying lesions, as has been advocated by Dixon, Wangensteen, Waugh and Custer, Babcock and Bacon, and we have used it in only one patient." It is interesting, they state, that although Gilchrist and David emphasize that Miles' operation is necessary to eradicate rectosigmoidal and rectal lesions, their investigations should be the basis for the procedures advocated by the above mentioned surgeons.

Rectum.—Resectability and mortality for lesions of the rectum are shown in Table 91. Of the 51 carcinomas of the rectosigmoid and rectum 43 were excised, which is a resectability of 84.3 per cent; an abdominoperineal resection was done in 41, or 95 per cent of the resectable cases. There were two deaths (4.1 per cent) in 48 resections of the rectosigmoid and rectum for carcinomas of these structures or of the lower sigmoid.

Ochsner and Hines emphasize the dangers of the current enthusiasm for procedures which permit preservation of the anal sphincters. They concur in the following dictum of Gilchrist and David: "Radical removal with resection of the superior hemorrhoidal artery as high as possible and wide resection of the levator ani muscles is necessary in order to give the best chance of permanent cure," and their conclusion, "A Miles type of operation seems the ideal one from the standpoint of wide removal of lymphatic node bearing area."

UNIVERSITY OF MINNESOTA STATISTICS

Colon.—In 1943, Wangensteen reported their experience with 61 operations on the colon and rectosigmoid during the two-year period from April 1, 1941 to April 1, 1943. Among the 61 patients, 46 had malignant lesions; 36 of these were situated in the colon and 10 in the rectosigmoid. In all but one of the 46 patients removal of the growth actually was accomplished, which is a resectability of 97.8 per cent. Five of these patients had hepatic metastasis. Simultaneous cholecystectomy or appendectomy was done on several occasions; coincidental hysterectomy was performed once; partial excision of the urinary bladder was undertaken twice; and the right kidney was removed twice for perforated lesions of the ascending colon. There was one death, or a mortality of 2.1 per cent, in the 36 resections of the colon.

The anastomosis in each instance was an end-to-end oblique, closed (aseptic) one, without antecedent complementary or supplemental cecostomy or colostomy except in several instances of acute obstruction. Sulfathiazole was implanted about the anastomosis. Sulfonamides were not administered prior to operation and none after operation until the elapse of forty-eight hours, when a total of 1 to 2 GM. of sulfadiazine is given subcutaneously in divided doses for two or three days if an indwelling urethral catheter still remains in place.

In 1945, Wangensteen reported an additional 78 patients who had undergone resection of the colon and rectosigmoid during the 19 month interval (April, 1943 to November 1, 1944) which had elapsed since their previous report. The resectability rate is not given nor is it specifically stated how many of the resections were for carcinoma. Moreover, the distribution of the lesions in the different segments of the colon and rectosigmoid is not presented. The over-all mortality was 7.6 per cent.

Rectum.—In 1945, Wangensteen reported for the period January 1, 1941 to November 1, 1944, 27 resections of the rectal ampulla and an undisclosed number of resections of the rectosigmoid (included with primary resections of the colon). Three of the resections were undertaken for chronic ulcerative colitis. There were two deaths among the 24 cases of carcinoma, or a mortality of 8.3 per cent. The types of operation performed were: Hochenegg "pull through" with Whitehead excision of the mucosa of the lower segment, eight cases; same type, leaving mucosa in distal segment, two cases; suture anastomosis through proctoscope, three cases; and primary closed anastomosis (suture from above), 14 cases. Of the 22 patients surviving ampullary resection for ampullary cancer, there was evidence of local recurrence in five. In four of these resection was undertaken as a palliative procedure. "Yet," stated Wangensteen, "even in these patients the abdominoperineal operation would have given better assurance against local recurrence. This matter of local recurrence in large fixed lesions has been the most disappointing experience in this effort directed at preserving sphincteric function in ampullary resection." He further stated that "ampullary resection in such instances can be indicted on the score of failing to remove the lateral zone of lymphatic spread as well as in its failure to deal adequately with the item of local invasion." And, "From the standpoint of cure of rectal cancer, obviously, the abdominoperineal operation is the best procedure."

In 1948, Wangensteen and Toon reported their experience with primary resection for carcinoma of the "true" rectum and low pelvic colon from January 1, 1945, to December 31, 1946. Their study of local recurrence in those instances in which the curative operative was undertaken (Table 92) has led Wangensteen to de-

TABLE 92

LOCAL RECURRENCE IN CURATIVE GROUP OF CARCINOMA
OF RECTUM AND LOW PELVIC COLON RESECTED
WITH PRESERVATION OF THE SPHINCTER
(WANGENSTEEN AND TOON—1948)

Distance in Cm. from Anus	No. Cases	No. Cases of Recurrence	Per Cent of Cases	Per Cent of Total Local Recurrence
0– 5 cm. incl.	7	2	30	30
6– 8 cm. incl.	12	3	25	40
9–13 cm. incl.	32	2	6.3	30
14–20 cm. incl.	12	0	0	0
Total	63	7	14	100

crease again the scope of the conservative operation for carcinoma of the rectum. A few years ago he resected lesions as low as 4 cm. from the anorectal line, last year the lower limit was 6 cm. and now (1948) he states that "For lesions in the lower rectal segment, at 8 cm. or less from the anus, the conservative operation is not a good operation for primary rectal cancer, primarily because it does not deal effectively with the invisible lateral spread of cancer as does the more radical abdominoperineal resection. Our own experience suggests quite definitely that for the upper group (14 to 20 cm. from the anus) the anastomostic operation holds out just as much promise of cure as does the abdominoperineal operation. The controversial group, it seems to me, is the intermediate group between 9 and 13 cm. from the anus. There is no debate about the superiority of the abdominoperineal operation for this group; that is granted. The question is: How much better is it from the standpoint of curability of cancer than anastomostic procedure? This is the group in which some case selection may have to be done."

During the two year period of their most recent survey, 100 consecutive cases of carcinoma of the lower sigmoid and rectum were observed. Seventy-eight per cent of these were resectable. In 56.4 per cent of instances the abdominoperineal operation was done and in 43.6 per cent the more conservative procedure of excision of the cancer with sphincter preservation was done. Mortality in 67 cases with carcinomas situated 0–13 cm. from the anus was: 51 cases of resection and primary anastomosis, 5.88 per cent; 15 cases of resection and Hochenegg pull-through, 6.65 per cent; and one case of Babcock-Bacon procedure which survived. There was one death among 20 patients who underwent resection for lesions situated 14 to 20 cm. from the anus. The over-all mortality was 3.76 per cent. The cases were treated between January, 1942 and June, 1947. Sixty-three (72.4 per cent) were operated on with a view to cure.

COLUMBIA-PRESBYTERIAN MEDICAL CENTER

Colon.—In 1943, Whipple reported the mortality for all operations performed on the colon during the years 1933 to 1942, inclusive. The operability rate and end-results are not given. Table 93

TABLE 93
MORTALITY FOLLOWING RESECTION OF THE COLON FOR CARCINOMA
(COLUMBIA-PRESBYTERIAN MEDICAL CENTER, 1933–1942, WHIPPLE)

	Ileocolectomies			Resections with Anastomosis						Rankin			Mikulicz		
				Left Colon			Transverse								
Cases	Year and P.O. No.	Deaths Per Cent		Cases	P.O. No.	Deaths Per Cent	Cases	P.O. No.	Deaths Per Cent	Cases	P.O. No.	Deaths Per Cent	Cases	P.O. No.	Deaths Per Cent
1933–1937:															
38	8	21.0		36	8	22.2	9	3	33.3	18	5	27.7	14	3	21.4
1938–1942:															
57	7	12.3		75	6	8.0	14	2	14.3	18	1	5.5	13	5	38.4
Total:															
95	15	15.8		111	14	12.6	23	5	21.7	36	6	16.6	27	8	29.6

summarized the results with ileocolostomies, resections with anastomosis, obstructive resections of the Rankin type, and Mikulicz resections. Strikingly favorable results in decompressing the small intestine in cases of inflammatory ileus and ileus due to bands and adhesions by the use of the Miller-Abbott tube led Whipple and his associates to use it in the preparation of patients with lesions of the right colon. The immediate improvement in the morbidity and mortality figures (Table 94) has convinced them that this

TABLE 94

MILLER-ABBOTT INTUBATION: ILEOCOLECTOMIES
(WHIPPLE, 1938 TO 1942)*

Ileocolo-stomies	No.	P.O. Deaths	Mor-tality %	With M.-A. Tube		Without M.-A. Tube	
				Cases	P.O. Deaths	Cases	P.O. Deaths
Cancer.......	57	7	12.3	41	4	16	3
Other diseases	29	4	13.8	18	1	11	3
Total......	86	11	12.8	59	5 (8.5%)	27	6 (22.2%)

* Of 86 ileocoloectomies, 59 or 68.6 per cent of the patients had the Miller-Abbott intubation prior to operation. In all but five of these the tube passed beyond the stomach.

method was far superior to an enterostomy done at the time of resection. Furthermore, it enabled them to discard the two-stage procedure, with the hazard of spillage and contamination eliminated, Whipple believes that anastomosis by the open method, with careful protection of the wound and remaining peritoneum and accurate suture technic, is as safe as the so-called aseptic methods, and more certain of giving an adequate lumen and avoiding subsequent leakage.

In 1947, Grinnell furnished us with unpublished statistics, the result of a comprehensive study of their total experiences with carcinoma of the colon and rectum for the year 1916 to 1942, inclusive and 1942 to 1946, inclusive. Table 95 shows in considerable detail all the factors having to do with resectability and mortality in 332 cases of carcinoma of the colon. The resectability rate based on the ratio of the number of lesions removed to the number of patients actually explored, as is the current trend, was 79.9 per cent. It is also possible from their data to determine operability in relation to total patients observed or as regards the number in which operation for cure was advised. Their figures are of particular value because of the minute detail in which they are presented. End-results are shown in Table 96.

TABLE 95

SUMMARY OF RESULTS IN CASES OF CARCINOMA
OF THE COLON
(COLUMBIA-PRESBYTERIAN HOSPITAL, GRINNELL—1947)

A—Total number of patients seen (1942–1946)...................... 332
    No operation advised............................... 15
    Palliative operation advised.......................... 10 25

B—Operation for cure advised............................... 307
    Patient refused operation....................................... 9

C—Operated on for cure.. 298
    Inoperable at operation...................................... 60

Resection completed... 238
Resectability rate in relation to "A" 71.9%); to "B" (77.5%), to "C" (79.9%)

Type of Operation	Cases	Hospital Mortality
Resections for cure......................	238......	16 (6.7 per cent)
Ileocolectomy.......................	88	3 (3.4 per cent)
Partial colectomy.....................	144	13 (9.0 per cent)
Local excision........................	6	0 (0 per cent)
Palliative operations....................	70	20 (28.5 per cent)
Total operations.......................	308*.....	36 (11.7 per cent)

    * For the period 1916–1941 there were 360 resections with 75 deaths, or a mortality of 20.8 per cent.

Rectum.—The summary of results in 248 cases of carcinoma of
the rectum and rectosigmoid observed at Columbia-Presbyterian
Medical Center between the years 1942–1946 is shown in Table 97.
Resectability based on the ratio of the number of tumors removed
to the number of patients actually explored was 83.9 per cent. The
over-all mortality was 8.4 per cent: 7.5 per cent for "curative" resections and 12.5 per cent for palliative operations. In the period

TABLE 96

END-RESULTS IN RESECTION OF THE COLON FOR CARCINOMA
(COLUMBIA-PRESBYTERIAN HOSPITAL, GRINNELL—1947)
1916–1941

Resections	Survivors of opera-tion	Untraced Cases	Five-Year Survivals
Right Half of Colon........	85	4	46 (54.1 per cent)*
Left Half of Colon..........	210	14	106 (50.5 per cent)
Total Cases..............	295	18	152 (51.5 per cent)

    * If deaths are not excluded the percentages of 5-year cures are 42.6, 39.8, and
40.9, respectively for the three categories.

TABLE 97

SUMMARY OF RESULTS IN CASES OF CARCINOMA
OF THE RECTUM AND RECTOSIGMOID
(COLUMBIA-PRESBYTERIAN HOSPITAL, GRINNELL—1947)

A—Total number of patients seen (1942–1946)......................... 248
    Admitted to the hospital...................................... 247
    No operation advised............................. 10
    Palliative operation advised......................... 3 13

B—Operation for cure advised...................................... 234
    Patient refused operation..................................... 11

C—Operated on for cure.. 223
    Inoperable at exploration..................................... 36

Resection completed.. 187
Resectability rate in relation to "A" (75.4%); to "B" (79.9%); to "C" (83.9%)

Type of Operation	Cases	Hospital Mortality
Resections for cure*	187	14 (7.5 per cent)
Abdominoperineal resection	151	9 (6.0 per cent)
Colostomy & perineal excision	2	0 (0 per cent)
Hartmann operation	7	2 (28.5 per cent)
Anterior resection	18	3 (16.7 per cent)
Local excision	9	0 (0 per cent)
Palliative operations**	40	5 (12.5 per cent)
Total operations	227	19 (8.4 per cent)

* In the period 1916–1941 there were 249 abdominoperineal operations with 52 deaths, or a mortality of 20.9%; 56 colostomy and perineal excisions with 12 deaths, or a mortality of 21.4%.
** Palliative resections not included.

1916–1941 there were 249 abdominoperineal resections with 52 deaths, or a mortality of 20.9 per cent; between 1942–1946 the mortality in 151 cases was 6 per cent. End-results are shown in Table 98.

TABLE 98

END RESULTS IN RESECTION OF THE RECTUM FOR CARCINOMA
(COLUMBIA-PRESBYTERIAN HOSPITAL, GRINNELL—1947)
1916–1941

Resections	Survivors of operation	Untraced Cases	Five-Year Survivals
Abdominoperineal	196	3	119 (60.1 per cent)*
Colostomy & perineal excision	45	2	14 (31.1 per cent)

* If deaths are not excluded, the percentages of 5-year cures are 48.0 and 25.5 respectively for the two categories.

Colon.—In 1943, Zinninger and Hoxworth reviewed the 45 cases of resection of the colon for cancer performed during the five-year period 1938 to 1942. In 1947, Hoxworth and Mithoefer reviewed a total of 144 patients in whom a diagnosis of carcinoma of the colon had been made; 87, or 60.4 per cent, were resectable. Of these resections, 16 were undertaken as palliative procedures. Resectability in the charity (public ward) cases was 45 per cent (45 out of 100) and was 95 per cent (42 out of 44) in the private patients. Resectability for the various segments of the bowel was as follows: right colon (45 cases) 53.3 per cent; transverse colon (22 cases) 72.7 per cent, and, left colon (77 cases) 61 per cent.

The over-all operative mortality for 87 resections was 6.9. Resection and immediate anastomosis is the method of choice of the authors. Twenty-three of the right colon resections were of this type and 61 of the 63 resections of the left half of the colon.

Rectum.—In 1947, Hoxworth reported the ten-year experience of members of the surgical staff, Cincinnati General Hospital and Christian R. Holmes Hospital, with 167 cases of carcinoma of the rectum. Table 99 compares resectability and mortality in the 106

TABLE 99

CARCINOMA OF THE RECTUM: COMPARISON OF RESECTABILITY
AND MORTALITY IN CHARITY AND PRIVATE PATIENTS
(HOXWORTH—1947)

	Holmes Hospital*		Cincinnati Gen. Hospital		Total	
	No.	%	No.	%	No.	%
Patients seen............	61		 106		 167	
Resectable...............	43	77	 51	49	 98	59
Mortality...............	3	6	 11	21	 14	14

* Private patients.

charity cases with 61 private cases. In the period 1936 to 1940 the mortality in both hospitals was 33 per cent as compared to 10 per cent in the 1941 to 1945 period. In the later period the figure was 17 per cent at the General Hospital and 4.5 per cent at the Holmes Hospital (private). Of the 98 cases resected, the Miles operation was used in 90 instances and in six cases a two-stage abdominoperineal resection of the Lahey type was performed. One Hochenegg and one Lockhart-Mummery procedure were performed. Follow-up data was too meager to be any significance.

TEMPLE UNIVERSITY HOSPITAL STATISTICS

In 1947, Babcock, in a discussion of radical single-stage extirpation for cancer of the large bowel, with perineal anus, made the following statement in regard to resectability and hospital mortality which we quote in full:

"In a personal experience of 617 radical operations for cancer of the large intestine the mortality has markedly decreased with experience, improvements in technique, and the routine use of antibiotics. Of the last 300 patients entering my service, 97 per cent (aged from 21 to 87 years) have had radical intestinal resection. A number of these had a previous colostomy without extirpation of the cancer. Three per cent had disease so advanced that even a

TABLE 100

TYPES OF OPERATION AND MORTALITY IN CARCINOMA
OF THE SIGMOID AND RECTUM
(TEMPLE UNIVERSITY HOSPITAL—BACON—1946)

	No. Cases	Deaths	Percentage
Abdominoperineal proctoidectomv—Babcock....	236	15	6.3
Abdominoperineal excision, 1-Stage—Miles......	51	2	3.9
Abdominoperineal excision, 2-stage—Lahey.....	6	1	16.6
Sigmoidectomy—multiple stage—Mikulicz......	27	2	7.4
Sigmoidectomy—primary anastomosis..........	24	2	8.3
Perineal excision, Lockhart-Mummery..........	14	1	7.1
Anterior resection—Hartmann................	9	0	0
Perineo-abdominal excision—Turner...........	2	0	0
Perineal excision, Cuneo-Seneque.............	2	0	0

palliative operation was considered of no advantage. Ninety-seven per cent, about one-third with advanced and ineradicable malignancy, had a radical resection of the cancerous bowel, with a hospital mortality of 9 per cent. However, in the series there were 66 consecutive radical operations with one death, and in a rather recent series of 100 admissions for carcinoma of the large bowel, two were found to have disease too extensive for resection or colostomy, with one hospital death. Ninety-eight had radical resection, including 18 with palpable metastatic carcinoma of the liver and 13 with cancerous invasion beyond the bowel. Three with carcinoma of the anus had perineal resection with perineal colostomy, without mortality. Forty-four had the abdominoperineal operation with retained anus, with two hospital deaths (one with advanced carcinoma of the liver), a mortality of 4.5 per cent; 51 had one stage, abdominal, aseptic, end-to-end resections, with two hospital deaths (3.9 per cent), one from coronary occlusion, one from peritonitis. Sixteen of these 51 end-to-end resections were for cancer of the rectum, 22 for cancer of the sigmoid or descending colon, and 13 for cancer of the right or transverse colon."

Bacon, in 1946, reported the combined experience of Babcock and himself with 461 malignancies of the sigmoid, rectosigmoid, rectum and anus over a period of five years.

There were 424 operations performed, or an operability rate of 91.9 per cent. There were 371 resections, or a resectability rate of 80.4 per cent, based on all cases seen, or 81 per cent based on total operative cases. There were 25 deaths in the 424 operations, or a mortality of 5.8 per cent. The mortality for the group of 371 resections was 6.1 per cent. On the basis of total operations performed (506) the mortality is 4.9 per cent. The types of operations performed in this series of cases and the mortality rate in each group are shown in Table 100. The end-results of this series

TABLE 101

END-RESULTS FOLLOWING PROCTOSIGMOIDECTOMY
(BABCOCK AND BACON—1943)

Name	Year Reported	No. Cases	Resectability Cure or Relief %	Mortality Rate %	Survival No. Cases to 144 Traced	
					%	Years
Babcock and Bacon (10)..	1943	414	93	6.6	81	1 to 3
					38	5 to 10

Abdominoperineal proctosigmoidectomy..................... 6.6
Perineal proctosigmoidectomy.............................. 4.0

was not given. In Table 101, however, is revealed the three- and five-year survivors in a series of 144 traced cases treated by abdominoperineal and perineal proctosigmoidectomy and which was reported by Babcock and Bacon in 1943. Thirty-eight per cent survived five or more years. The marked difference between this figure and that of 81 per cent for three-year survivals further emphasizes the appreciable percentage who develop recurrences in the fourth and fifth year after operation.

ROOSEVELT HOSPITAL STATISTICS

In 1944, White and Amendola reported that at Roosevelt Hospital, during the years 1939 to 1943, they operated upon 110 patients with cancer of the colon, exclusive of those with tumors of the rectum and rectosigmoid. Resections were performed in 85, or 77.3 per cent, of the group. The various procedures employed and the attendant mortality are summarized in Table 102. A closed

TABLE 102

CARCINOMA OF THE COLON: TYPES OF OPERATION
AND MORTALITY (WHITE AND AMENDOLA—1944)

Procedure	Number	Deaths	Per Cent Mortality
Cecostomy only.	6	3	50
Enterocolostomy without resection.	5	3	60
Abdominal exploration only.	2	1	50
Peritoneal drainage only.	2	2	100
Colostomy only.	8	3	37.5
Colocolostomy without resection.	2	0	0
Balfour resection.	2	1	50
Mikulicz-type resection.	18	4	22.2
Right enterocolectomy.	29	6	20.6
Colon resection, end-to-end.	36	4	11.1
Total.	110	27	24.5%

type of anastomosis was performed in all but one of 29 right entero-
colectomies and in all but eight of 36 resections of the left colon.

DUKE UNIVERSITY HOSPITAL STATISTICS

Unpublished statistics prepared in 1947 by Postlethwait show
that at Duke Hospital during the fifteen-year period, 1931 to 1945,
441 patients with malignancy of the large intestine were observed.

TABLE 103

TYPES OF OPERATION IN 316 CASES OF CARCINOMA
OF THE COLON AND RECTUM
(DUKE HOSPITAL-POSTLETHWAIT—1949)

	Operation	Rectum	Recto-Sigmoid	Right Colon	Left Colon	Total
Palliative	Colostomy.	53	5	0	17	75
	Ileostomy.			1		1
	By-pass.			10	4	14
	Resection.	2	1	1	6	10
	Exploratory Only.	6	3	9	8	26
	Total.	61	9	21	35	126
Prelim.	Colostomy.	8	2	0	11	21
	Cecostomy.				4	4
Curative	Resection & Anastomosis.	1	3	40	25	69
	Exteriorization.	0	2	0	24	26
	Abdominoperineal.	72	6	0	3	81
	Miscellaneous.	5	1	0	1	7
	Total.	78	12	40	53	183

TABLE 104

OPERATIVE MORTALITY IN CARCINOMA OF THE COLON
AND RECTUM (Duke Hospital—Postlethwait—1949)

Year	31–35	36–40	41–45	Total
Palliative operations......	21	50	55	
Deaths.................	3 (14%)	8 (16%)	9 (16%)	15.9%
Preliminary operations....	3	11	12	
Deaths.................	1 (33%)	3 (27%)	4 (33%)	30.7%
Curative operations.......	22	51	100	
Deaths.................	7 (32%)	8 (16%)	14 (13%)	15.9%
Total mortality........	24.4%	17.2%	15.4%	18.0%

The disposition of all patients is shown in Table 9. Three hundred and ninety-eight, or 90 per cent, were admitted to the hospital. Of these 316 were subjected to one or more major operations; 198, or 62.7 per cent, were resectable, and 183, or 58 per cent, were operated upon for cure (42 per cent of the total group; 46 per cent of patients admitted to the hospital). The types of operations performed are shown in Table 103; resectability is considered in detail in Table 10.

Fifty-seven, or 18 per cent, of the 316 patients who were operated upon died. The mortality for palliative, preliminary and curative operations are shown separately by five-year periods in Table 104. During the total fifteen-year period the gross postoperative mortality rate was reduced from 24.4 per cent to 15.4 per cent, whereas the rate for operations performed for cure decreased from 32 per cent to 13 per cent. The resectability rate during this time increased from 51 to 67 per cent. In the same period the non-preventable mortality rate increased from 2.2 per cent to 9.1 per cent, while the preventable mortality rate decreased from 22.2 per cent to 6.5 per cent.

TABLE 105

THE FIVE YEAR SURVIVALS FOR RESECTIONS PERFORMED
1931 THROUGH 1940 (Duke Hospital—Postlethwait, 1949)

	Total Resections	Died in Hospital	5-Year Survivors		
			Living	Dead	%
R.............	26	3	11	4	57.7
RS............	8	3	3	0	37.5
S.............	10	4	5	0	50.0
DC...........	7	2	2	0	28.6
SF............	4	1	1	0	25.0
TC...........	2	0	1	0	50.0
HF...........	5	0	1	1	40.0
AC...........	6	0	1	0	16.6
C.............	9	3	3	0	33.3

A follow-up study determined the status of 95.3 per cent of the 441 patients with malignant tumors of the colon and rectum. The five-year survivors of operations which were performed with a view to cure during the period 1931 to 1940, inclusive, are recorded in Table 105.

Colon.—Of the 149 major operations performed on the colon, 93 were undertaken with a view to cure; 40 were for lesions of the right colon and 53 were for lesions of the left colon. Primary anastomosis was performed in 65 instances and obstructive resection in 25 (Table 103). The highest resectability for the entire series was for tumors of the ascending colon (83.3 per cent). Resectability in the other segments was, hepatic flexure, 79.2 per cent; transverse colon and splenic flexure, each 62.5 per cent; descending colon, 57.9 per cent; sigmoid flexure, 56.4 per cent; and, cecum, 55.5 per cent.

Twenty-eight, or 18.4 per cent, of the patients operated upon for lesions of the colon died (Table 106). The mortality in the group of 93 patients operated upon for cure was 16.1 per cent; for the 53 operations on the left colon, the mortality was 20 per cent and for the 40 operations on the right colon it was 10 per cent.

Rectum and rectosigmoid.—Of the 167 major operations performed on the rectum and rectosigmoid, 90 were done with a view to cure. The resectability rate was 54.5 per cent, being identical for both the rectal and the rectosigmoidal groups. The types of operative procedure undertaken are shown in Table 103. Seventy-eight, or 86.6 per cent, performed with a view to cure were abdomino-perineal resections. Four primary resections with immediate anastomosis were done. Twenty-nine, or 17.5 per cent, of the 167 patients died postoperatively. Fifteen, or 16.6 per cent, of the 90 pa-

TABLE 106

SUMMARY OF POSTOPERATIVE MORTALITY
DUKE HOSPITAL—POSTLETHWAIT—1949

	Pallia-tive Opera-tions	Post-operative Deaths	Pre-liminary Opera-tions	Post-operative Deaths	Resec-tions	Deaths
R.........	61	7 (11%)	8	4 (50%)	78	12 (15%)
RS.......	9	2 (22%)	2	1 (50%)	12	3 (25%)
S.........	22	2 (9%)	8	2 (25%)	31	6 (19%)
DC.......	7	3 (43%)	7	1 (14%)	12	2 (17%)
SF........	3	0	1	0	5	1 (20%)
TC.......	3	1 (33%)	—	—	5	1(20%)
HF.......	3	1 (33%)	—	—	10	0
AC.......	2	0	—	—	10	0
C.........	16	4 (25%)	—	—	20	4 (20%)
Total...	126	20 (15.9%)	25	8 (30.8%)	183	29 (15.8%)

tients who had curative operations died. The mortality for the entire series of cases by five year periods is shown in Table 104. The mortality by segment of bowel involved is revealed in Table 106.

THE MASON CLINIC STATISTICS

In 1944, Baker presented an analytical review of 111 patients requiring major surgery for lesions of the pelvic colon and rectum. Ninety-nine of these were carcinoma (Table 107). Sixty-seven resections were undertaken, excluding the three who had "curative" diathermization and including two moribund patients operated upon, the resectability in the series, as determined by Baker, was 66 per cent. The surgical mortality was 5 per cent overall, 3.8 per cent for those resected. Of the 49 combined resections there was but one death, or a mortality of 2.04 per cent.

TABLE 107

MORTALITY IN CANCER OF THE PELVIC COLON AND
RECTUM (MASON CLINIC—BAKER—1944)

No. of Pts.	Type of Operation	Patient Mortality
21...............	Palliative colostomy	2 (cachexia)
6...............	Exploration only	0
2...............	Palliative diathermy	0
3...............	"Curative" diathermy	0
67 { 40..........	Combined abdominoperineal resection	1 (embolus)
7..........	Colostomy and posterior resection	0
9..........	Anterior resection with anastomosis	1 (embolus)
2..........	Anterior resection with colostomy	1 (heart)
99..........	....	5 (5.05%)

HINES VETERANS HOSPITAL STATISTICS

In 1947, Vynalek, Saylor and Schrek made a statistical analysis of the 486 cases of carcinoma of the colon seen at Hines Veterans Hospital, Hines, Illinois, in the 15-year period from 1931 to 1945 inclusive. During this period there were admitted to the hospital 16,097 patients with carcinoma, of which number 1330 were diagnosed carcinoma of the colon, rectosigmoid and rectum. The close similarity in the frequency of the sites of involvement in these patients and those reported by others is shown in Table 108. In the term resectable are included only those cases in which a cure can reasonably be anticipated following removal of all gross carcinomatous tissue. The authors explain their very low resectability rate on the basis that a number of veterans with malignant lesions of the large bowel still in a favorable stage for surgery have been operated upon successfully elsewhere. A large proportion of unfavorable cases have been sent to Hines Hospital for "palliative irradiation" and terminal care. All patients who had undergone surgery elsewhere, either with successful resections or hopeless explorations, were excluded. All other patients, regardless of the extent of the disease, are included in the total regarded as candidates for possible resection. Three hundred fifty-four operations were performed and 126 were operated upon with a view to cure. This is a resectability of 35.6 per cent. Resectability for the early period was 33.16 per

TABLE 108

A COMPARISON OF THE ANATOMIC DISTRIBUTION OF
CARCINOMA OF THE LARGE INTESTINE IN
PATIENTS OF THREE TUMOR CLINICS
(VYNALEK, ET AL., 1947)

	Hines Veterans Hospital 1931–1945	Lahey Clinic 1936–1944	Mayo Clinic 1907–1928
No. of cases	1330	1457	3542
Involved sites and percentages			
Cecum	7.7%	6.52%	5.95%
Ascending colon	4 } 15.9%	3.30 } 17.1%	} 16.99%
Hepatic flexure	2	2.94	
Transverse colon	4.1	4.51	
Splenic flexure	2	2.40	
Descending colon	3.8	3.97	
Sigmoid	13.0	12.42%	13.55%
Rectosigmoid and rectum	63.5	62.79%	62.84%

cent; for the late period, 38.13 per cent. Actually 48.44 per cent were resectable in the latter group but this includes 16 "non-resectable" cases with distant metastasis.

The over-all mortality for the 15-year period was 23 per cent. Mortality was based on those patients who died within 30 days of operation. There was a decrease from 35.9 per cent in the 1931–1945 period. The authors do not believe that chemotherapy alone is responsible for this considerable reduction in mortality. They believe that "much of the mortality in the early period was due to the erroneous tendency to diagnose complete obstruction, which is very uncommon, operate immediately, and then do too much in an acute obstruction of marked degree."

Follow-up studies were made of the group in which resections were done between 1931 and 1940. Of the 281 cases admitted in this first period, 193 candidates were left for possible resection. In 64, resection was performed with a view to cure, and 21, or 32.8 per cent, of these survived five or more years. However, of those who survived resection, 51.2 per cent were alive over five years.

CONNECTICUT STATISTICS

In 1947, Ottenheimer published an analysis of cases of cancer of the rectum occurring in Connecticut during 1935–1945. In 1935, a plan was inaugurated in this state whereby duplicate copies of hospital records of patients with cancer were made available to the Division of Cancer Research of the Connecticut Department of Health. This was a joint undertaking sponsored by the Tumor Committee and the Association of Tumor Clinics of the Connecticut State Medical Society, the general hospitals of the state, and the State Department of Health.

Ward as well as private patients are included in the survey. The patients were treated by many surgeons in both large and small

TABLE 109

RESECTABILITY ACCORDING TO YEAR OF ADMISSION
(OTTENHEIMER—1947)

Year	Resections	Proved Cases	Resectability of Proved Cases %	Total Cases	Total Resectability %
1935–1940.......	237	515	46.0	735	32.2
1941...........	66	139	47.5	172	38.4
1942...........	65	119	54.6	143	45.5
1943...........	78	130	60.0	182	42.9
1944...........	93	149	62.4	191	48.7
1945...........	82	136	60.3	187	43.9
Totals........	621	1188		1610	
Averages......			52.3		38.6

hospitals. Complete follow-up data were obtained in over 97 per cent of cases. In the eleven-year period 1610 patients were admitted to hospitals with the diagnosis of cancer of the rectum. Of these cases, 1188 were proved microscopically, and in 422 the diagnosis was made clinically. The incidence of proved cases rose from a low of 58.7 per cent in 1935 to a high of 83.3 per cent in 1942.

Resectability.—Ottenheimer states that in evaluating the resectability rates shown in Table 109 consideration should be given the fact that no one surgeon in the entire state has had an opportunity to do a large series of cases. The rate rose from 46 per cent for the years 1935–1940 to 62.4 per cent in 1944. The resectability rate in hospitals with more than 100 cases was 7 per cent higher for proved cases.

Choice of procedure.—The procedures undertaken in the microscopically proved cases are presented in Table 110. A careful study of the records revealed that approximately 25 per cent of the 275 who had palliative colostomies seemed to be in good condition on admission and, therefore, suggests Ottenheimer, radical resection might have been attempted in bolder and more skillful hands. Of the 105 patients for whom no treatment was recommended, 45 per cent were over seventy years of age, about 50 per cent were

TABLE 110

PROCEDURES IN MICROSCOPICALLY PROVED CASES
(OTTENHEIMER—1947)

Treatment	No. of Cases		Percentage	
Resection.................	621		52.3	
One-stage.............		463		74.6
Two-stage.............		158		25.4
Colostomy................	275		23.1	
None....................	105		8.9	
Miscellaneous............	76		6.4	
Local excision............	49		4.1	
X-ray and radium.........	32		2.7	
Refused treatment.........	30		2.5	

considered to be in poor general health, and over 21 per cent had remote metastasis on admission. The average duration of life from the first symptom to death for this group was 21.3 months.

Of the 621 resections, 74.6 per cent were one-stage abdomino-perineal operations, and 25.4 per cent were performed in two stages,

TABLE 111

DISTRIBUTION OF RESECTIONS
(OTTENHEIMER—1947)

Year	One-Stage Procedures	Two-Stage Procedures	Totals
1935–1940........	131 (55.3%)	106 (44.7%)	237
1941.............	48 (72.7%)	18 (27.3%)	66
1942.............	51 (78.5%)	14 (21.5%)	65
1943.............	71 (91.0%)	7 (9.0%)	78
1944.............	87 (93.5%)	6 (6.5%)	93
1945.............	75 (91.5%)	7 (8.5%)	82
Totals.........	463 (74.6%)	158 (25.4%)	621

either by the Lahey method or by perineal excision following colostomy. There was a striking increase in the frequency of one-stage resection (Table 111). In the last three years of the survey, over 90 per cent of resections were performed in one stage.

Operative mortality.—The rising resectability rate has been accompanied by a lowering of operative mortality (Table 112). In the period 1935–1940, resections were performed in 237 cases, with

TABLE 112

OPERATIVE MORTALITY FOLLOWING RADICAL RESECTION
(OTTENHEIMER—1947)

Year	One-Stage Resections	Operative Deaths	Two-Stage Resections	Operative Deaths	All Resections	Operative Deaths
1935–1940...	131	33 (25.2%)	106	26 (24.5%)	237	59 (24.9%)
1941........	48	8 (16.7%)	18	5 (27.8%)	66	13 (19.7%)
1942........	51	5 (9.8%)	14	3 (21.4%)	65	8 (12.3%)
1943........	71	16 (22.5%)	7	1 (14.3%)	78	17 (21.8%)
1944........	87	15 (17.3%)	6	3 (50.0%)	93	18 (19.4%)
1945........	75	11 (14.7%)	7	4 (57.2%)	82	15 (18.3%)
Totals....	463	88 (19.0%)	158	42 (26.6%)	621	130 (20.9%)

an average mortality of 24.9 per cent. Between 1941 and 1945 resections were done in 384 cases, with a mortality of 18.4 per cent.
Similarly, in the period of 1935–1940 one-stage resections were
done in 131 cases, with a mortality of 25.2 per cent. In the last five
years, one-stage resections were performed in 332 cases, with a
mortality of 16.5 per cent.

Results.—In reviewing the literature on cancer of the rectum in
the past ten years, one is impressed with the lack of uniformity in
reporting end results. This makes for ambiguity of interpretation
and difficulty of comparison. In this series the method of computing
five-year cures suggested by Martin was employed. Strict and logi-

TABLE 113

SURVIVAL AND CURE RATES ON THE BASIS OF COMPLETE
AND SELECTED TOTALS IN GENERAL USE
(OTTENHEIMER—1947)

Basis of Estimate	Total Cases	Five-Year Survivals		Five-Year Cures	
		No.	Per-centage	No.	Per-centage
Total admissions....................	735	94	12.8	58	7.9
Total proved cases.................	515	85	16.5	58	11.2
Proved cases with known results.....	503	85	16.9	58	11.5
Total resections....................	237	60	25.3	37	15.6
All resections except cases with remote metastases.......................	214	57	26.6	37	17.3
All survivals.......................	178	57	32.0	37	20.8
Survivals without remote metastases..	161	57	35.4	37	23.0

cal criteria are established for determination of cure, and accurate
follow-up study in over 90 per cent of cases is necessary. With the
view of advocating the adoption of a standard method of reporting
end results, the estimate was revised (Table 113). The variety of
results that may be claimed, depending on the basis used for calcu-
lation, is apparent.

Beginning with a five-year-cure rate of 7.9 per cent based on all
cases and a five-year survival rate of 12.8 per cent, there is a pro-

gressive rise to an optimistic figure of 35 per cent as different denominators are used. Statistics thus computed show the possibilities of accomplishment in selected cases, but tend to obscure the total picture.

REFERENCES

1. ABEL, A. L.: Five year cures of cancer of the rectum by the radial abdominoperineal excision. *Surg., Gynec., and Obstet.*, **60**: 481–482 (Feb.), 1935.
2. ALLEN, A. W.: Carcinoma of the colon. *Surgery*, **14**: 350–365 (Sept.) 1943.
3. ALLEN, A. W., WELCH, C. E., DONALDSON, G. A.: Carcinoma of the colon. *Ann. Surg.*, **126**: 19–30 (July), 1947.
4. BABCOCK, W. WAYNE: Radical single stage extirpation for cancer of the large bowel, with retained functional anus. *Surg., Gynec., and Obstet.*, **85**: 1–7 (July), 1947.
5. BACON, H. E.: Evolution of sphincter muscle preservation and re-establishment of continuity in operative treatment of rectal and sigmoidal cancer. *Surg., Gynec., and Obstet.*, **81**: 113–127 (Aug.), 1945.
6. BACON, H. E.: Abdominoperineal proctosigmoidectomy for cancer of the rectum: conclusions based on 5-years' experience. *Am. Jour. Surg.*, **71**: 728–742 (June), 1946.
7. BAKER, JOEL W.: Surgery of the pelvic colon and rectum. *Surg., Gynec., and Obstet.*, **79**: 92–102 (July), 1944.
8. BRINDLEY, G. V.: Carcinoma of the colon. *South. Med. Jour.*, **35**: 171 (Feb.), 1942.
9. CATTELL, RICHARD B.: Carcinoma of the colon and rectum; a report of 503 patients treated at the Lahey Clinic 1938–1941, inclusive, *Surgery*, **14**: 378–386 (Sept.), 1943.
10. COLCOCK, BENTLEY P.: Prognosis in carcinoma of the colon and rectum; a 10 year follow-up of 337 patients. *Surg., Gynec., and Obstet.*, **85**: 8–13 (July), 1947.
11. COLIGHER, J. C.: The operability of carcinoma of the rectum. *Brit. Med. Jour.*, **2**: 393–397 (Sept. 20), 1941.
12. COLLER, F. A., and RANSOM, H. K.: The one stage procedure for the treatment of carcinoma of the rectum. *Ann. Surg.*, **104**: 636–650 (Oct.), 1936.
13. COLLER, F. A., and RANSOM, H. K.: Carcinoma of the rectum. Conclusions based on 12 years experience with combined abdominoperineal resection. *Surg., Gynec., and Obstet.*, **78**: 304–315 (Mar.), 1944.
14. COLLER, F. A., and VAUGHAN, H. H.: The treatment of carcinoma of the colon. *Ann. Surg.*, **121**: 395–411 (April), 1945.
15. COLLER, F. A.: Personal communication.
16. DIXON, C. F.: Anterior resection for malignant lesions of the upper part of the rectum and lower part of the sigmoid. *Tr. Am. Surg. Assoc.*, **66**: 175–192, 1948.
17. DUKES, CUTHBERT E.: Quoted by Gabriel (18).
18. GABRIEL, W. B.: The principles and practice of rectal surgery. 3rd Ed. Springfield, Charles C Thomas, 1945, 432 pp.
19. GILCHRIST, R. K., and DAVID, VERNON, C.: A consideration of pathological factors influencing five year survivals in radical resection of the large bowel and rectum for carcinoma. *Ann. Surg.*, **126**: 421–438 (Oct.), 1947.
20. GRINNELL, ROBERT S.: Personal communication.

21. Hoxworth, Paul I.: Cancer of the rectum. *Cincinnati Jour. Med.*, **28:** (1947).

22. Hoxworth and Mithoefer: Personal communication.

23. Jones, D. F.: End-results of radical operations for carcinoma of rectum. *Ann. Surg.*, **90:** 675–691 (Oct.), 1929.

24. Jones, D. F.: Carcinoma of the rectum and colon. *South. Med. Jour.*, **29:** 339–344 (April), 1936.

25. Jones, T. E.: Treatment of cancer of colon. *Surg., Gynec., and Obstet.*, **62:** 415–419 (Feb.), 1936.

26. Jones, T. E., Newell, E. T., and Brubaker, R. E.: The use of alloy steel wire in the closure of abdominal wounds. *Surg., Gynec., and Obstet.*, **72:** 1056–1059 (June), 1941.

27. Jones, T. E.: The modified Mikulicz resection for carcinoma of the colon. *Surg., Gynec., and Obstet.*, **76:** 236–238 (Feb.), 1943.

28. Jones, T. E.: Consideration of elective procedures in various segments of the colon. *Surgery*, **14:** 342–349 (Sept.), 1943.

29. Jones, T. E.: Personal communication.

30. Lahey, F. H., and Cattell, R. B.: A two-stage abdominoperineal resection of the rectum and rectosigmoid for carcinoma. *Am. Jour. Surg.*, **27:** 201–213 (Feb.), 1935.

31. Mayo, C. W., and Lovelace, W. K.: Malignant lesions of the cecum and ascending colon. *Surg., Gynec., and Obstet.*, **72:** 1056–1059 (March), 1941.

32. Mayo, C. W.: Carcinoma of the right (proximal) portion of the colon. *Surg. Clinics N. Am.*, **27:** 875–884 (Aug.), 1947.

33. McKittrick, L. S.: Principles old and new of resection of the colon for carcinoma. *Surg., Gynec., and Obstet.*, **87:** 15–25, 1948.

34. Miles, W. E.: Cancer of the rectum. London, Harrison and Sons, Ltd., 1926, 72 pp.

35. Miles, W. E.: The present position of the radical abdominoperineal operation for cancer of the rectum in regard to mortality and postoperative recurrence. *Proc. Roy. Soc. Med., Sect. Surg., Subsect. Proct.*, **24:** 989–991 (May), 1931.

36. Newman, George: Great Britain Ministry of Health Report on Public Health and Medical Subjects. London, Bulletin, 46, 1927.

37. Ochsner, Alton, and Hines, M. O.: Carcinoma of the colon: Analysis of 113 cases. *South. Surgeon*, **13:** 269–288 (Nov.), 1946.

38. Ottenheimer, E. J.: Cancer of the rectum; an analysis of cases occurring in Connecticut during 1935–1945. The *New England Jour. Med.*, **237:** 1–7 (July 3), 1947.

39. Pemberton, J. de J., Dixon, C. F., Waugh, J. M., and Black, B. M.: Annual report of surgery of the large intestine. Proceedings of the Staff Meeting of the Mayo Clinic, **19:** 605–612 (Dec. 27), 1944.

40. Pemberton, J. de J.: In discussion of Coller and Vaughan (14).

41. Postlethwait, R. W.: Personal communication.

42. Postlethwait, R. W.: Malignant tumors of the colon and rectum. *Ann. Surg.*, **129:** 34–46 (Jan.), 1949.

43. Raiford, T. S.: Carcinoma of the large bowel.
    Part I: The colon, *Ann. Surg.*, **101:** 863–885 (March), 1935.
    Part II: The rectum, *Ann. Surg.*, **101:** 1042–1050 (April), 1935.

44. Rankin, F. W.: The choice of operation in cancer of colon; not including the rectum. *Jour. Am. Med. Assn.*, **83:** 86–90 (July 12), 1924.

45. RANKIN, F. W.: Surgery of the colon. New York, D. Appleton and Co., 1926, 336 pp.
46. RANKIN, F. W.: Colostomy and posterior resection for carcinoma of rectum. *Jour. Am. Med. Assn.*, **89**: 1961–1966 (Dec. 3), 1927.
47. RANKIN, F. W.: Mortality following colostomy for carcinoma of the large bowel. *Ann. Surg.*, **89**: 62–70 (Jan.), 1929.
48. RANKIN, F. W.: A review of surgery of the colon and rectum at the Mayo Clinic for the year 1929. *Internat. Clin.*, 3, 1930.
49. RANKIN, F. W.: The curability of cancer of the colon, rectosigmoid, and rectum. *Jour. Am. Med. Assn.*, **101**: 491–495 (Aug. 12), 1933.
50. RANKIN, F. W.: Resection of the rectum and rectosigmoid by single or graded procedures. *Ann. Surg.*, **104**: 628–635 (Oct.), 1936.
51. RANKIN, F. W., and JOHNSTON, C. C.: Surgical treatment of cancer of the rectum and rectosigmoid. *Jour. Am. Med. Assoc.*, **136**: 371–375 (Feb. 7), 1948.
52. RAVDIN, I. S., ZINTEL, H. A., and BENDER, D. H.: Adjuvants to surgical therapy in large bowel malignancy. *Ann. Surg.*, **126**: 439–447 (Oct.), 1947.
53. STONE, H. B., and McLANAHAN, S.: Resection and immediate anastomosis of the colon. *Jour. Am. Med. Assoc.*, **120**: 1362–1366 (Dec.), 1942.
54. WANGENSTEEN, O. H.: Primary resection (closed anastomosis) of the rectal ampulla for malignancy with preservation of sphincteric function. *Surg., Gynec., and Obstet.*, **81**: 1–24 (July), 1945.
55. WANGENSTEEN, O. H., and TOON, R. W.: Primary resection of the colon and rectum with particular reference to cancer and ulcerative colitis. *Am. Jour. Surg.*, **75**: 384–404 (Feb.), 1948.
56. WAUGH, J. M., and CUSTER, M. D.: Segmental resection of lesions occurring in the left half of the colon with primary, end-to-end aseptic anastomosis. *Surg., Gynec., and Obstet.*, **81**: 593–598 (Dec.), 1945.
57. WAUGH, J. M.: Personal communication.
58. WAUGH, J. M.: In discussion of Wangensteen and Toon (55).
59. WHIPPLE, ALLEN O.: Surgery of the terminal ileum, cecum, and right colon. *Surgery*, **14**: 321–327 (Sept.), 1943.
60. WHITE, W. C., and AMENDOLA, F. H.: The advantages and disadvantages of closed resection of the colon. *Ann. Surg.*, **120**: 572–581 (Oct.), 1944.
61. VYNALEK, W. J., SAYLOR, L. L., and SCHREK, ROBERT: Carcinoma of the colon: a statistical study. *Surg., Gynec., and Obstet.*, **84**: 669–676 (April 15) 1947.
62. ZINNINGER, M. M., and HOXWORTH, P. I.: Cancer of the colon. *Surgery*, **14**: 366–377 (Sept.), 1943.

CHAPTER X

PREOPERATIVE AND POSTOPERATIVE TREATMENT

It is well to bear in mind that the standard of efficiency in extirpation of lesions of the colon and rectum is, in the hands of the average operator, the percentage of resectability rather than the percentage of mortality and to increase the resectability and at the same time reduce the mortality, measures of rehabilitation and decompression are the most essential factors to be observed. A great many of these patients, perhaps a majority of them, on admission are in a state of lowered resistance; they frequently are dehydrated as a result of obstruction and its concomitant toxemia and of lowered physiologic equilibrium. Many of those who at first appear inoperable because of general debility or chronic diseases, such as diabetes, tuberculosis, cardiovascular or urinary, will respond so well to measures of rehabilitation in the preoperative period that they will withstand radical surgical treatment without untoward incident. It seems unreasonable to us to eliminate arbitrarily patients as inoperable merely because they are elderly, or because their less robust organs are potentially the sites of postoperative complications. Such a decision would deprive of the hope of cure a large percentage of those suffering from carcinoma of the large intestine. Of course with inclusion of these cases the burden of responsibility becomes decidedly increased. Nevertheless, a reasonable mortality can be maintained while at the same time the horizon of resectability is extended, if the following factors of safety are adhered to closely: (1) Careful attention to the details of preoperative treatment; (2) the selection of an operation for the patient rather than attempting to standardize maneuvers to fit all cases; (3) care in the choice of an anesthesia; (4) employment in properly selected cases, of operation in multiple stages; and (5) rigid adherence to a standardized postoperative regime.

PREOPERATIVE PREPARATION

As a rule, patients should be hospitalized during the full period of preliminary preparation. Rarely can adequate care be secured in the home, as it is essential during this period that the patient be closely observed by both surgeon and physician, that irrigations be administered by one especially skilled in such procedures, that the diet be carefully planned and prepared by a capable and co-operative dietitian, and that accurate estimates of the functional ability of the various organs be obtained with the aid of laboratory methods, such as tests of renal function, blood counts, blood typing, electrocardiographs, roentgenographic studies, and so forth. It has been our tendency, in recent years, to prolong the preoperative period, until now we seldom undertake the more formidable procedures under seven days of preparation, often not until ten days have elapsed. That this must be accomplished frequently with disregard of the economic situation of the patient, and of the protests of both patient and physician, is unquestionable, and yet experience has shown that the success or failure of radical extirpative measures in dealing with cancer of the large intestine is dependent in great measure on adequate preliminary preparation of not only the intestinal tract but of the patient as a whole.

Obstruction.—The first and foremost consideration is one of obstruction which unquestionably is present in a vast majority of cases of carcinoma of the large bowel at some time during their existence, varying in degree from the chronic variety to acute stenosis, the relative instance of which has been discussed in detail in the chapter on symptoms and diagnosis. As a rule, obstruction is slow and progressive, and with the exception of a small group of patients who present themselves with acute intestinal obstruction, cancer of the colon and rectum may be relegated, so far as their surgical treatment is concerned, into the category of chronic ailments. This is of not inconsiderable significance in that it allows time to institute the preliminary measures which we have listed above. By medical measures we have found it possible, in about 90 per cent of the cases, to reduce the obstruction, even of the subacute variety, to a point at which the bowel is flat and satisfactory for segmental resection at the time of operation.

Obstruction of the thin-walled colon, and ulceration which frequently accompanies it, increase enormously the permeability of the attenuated wall; consequently extravasation of organisms of considerable virulence into the pericolonic tissues takes place and this is the process from which lethal peritonitis most often develops. It is not sufficient, therefore, that increased intracolonic pressure alone be relieved; the bowel wall itself must be restored to a more healthy state and this necessitates, in the more advanced cases, an extension of the preparatory period.

If a barium enema is used in the diagnosis of the lesion, a thin mixture should be employed, and as soon as the roentgen examination has been made, it should be removed thoroughly with repeated irrigations. One of the greatest difficulties, perhaps, and one which should not occur, is the removal of a barium medium which has been administered by mouth. It is now generally agreed by roentgenologists that for an examination of the colon the most satisfactory method of visualization is by administration of opaque medium by rectum. Its oral administration cannot be too heartily condemned; it is a positive menace if incomplete obstruction exists, since not infrequently an acute obstruction is thus superimposed on a chronic one.

The medical measures employed to overcome chronic obstruction consists of initial purgation, repeated irrigations of the colon, and a diet of foods which have a minimum of residue.

Purgation should be practiced with considerable caution and a careful selection of cases. If patients are markedly obstructed, with considerable distention, and irrigations produce no results, the employment of a purgative is more apt to produce harmful effects. However, in a majority of instances, patients tolerate well the administration of fluid extract of senna, milk of magnesia, or a mild saline cathartic. We have rarely found it necessary or advisable to prolong the period of purgation beyond the first forty-eight hours. To do so might promote marked irritability of the colon, which would interfere with the proper cleansing of the bowel, in our opinion the more important procedure. Moreover, these patients are more or less dehydrated and prolonged use of purgatives only aggravates this condition which at best is difficult to overcome quickly.

Irrigations of the colon with a warm solution of physiologic saline not only rid the bowel of its content but secondarily they reduce the infection and inflammation around the growth and in the wall of the obstructed colon. It is essential that these irrigations, which are repeated every twelve hours until twenty-four hours before operation, should be done with considerable care and thoroughness. It has frequently been noted that failure to obtain satisfactory results is due to carelessness or inexperience on the part of one conducting the irrigation. Consequently we have found it advantageous to train nurses and orderlies whose special duty it is to care for these patients during the preoperative period. Ordinarily the irrigations are conducted with patients on their sides, but at times this is best accomplished with the knee-chest position assumed.

When irrigations fail to secure decompression of the colon in instances of carcinoma of the rectum, it is often worth while to pass a catheter through the lumen of a stenosed growth, by direct vision through a proctoscope. One of us (Graham) has employed this procedure on occasions in recent years, in the face of acute obstruction in patients who constituted grave surgical risks. In each instance deflation of the markedly distended colon was almost instantaneous on passage of the catheter beyond the obstructed lumen. Evidently the stenosed bowel had become suddenly plugged with a seed or other foreign body. The greatest difficulty encountered, particularly in lesions at the rectosigmoid, is in preventing the catheter from being ejected by peristalsis. However, this can be overcome by attaching a piece of wire to the catheter, several inches from its tip, by means of adhesive tape. On removing the proctoscope the wire is held in position against the buttock with strips of adhesive, and in this manner irrigations may be carried

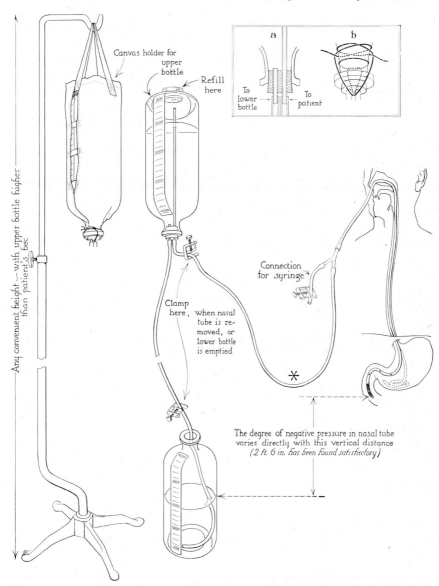

FIG. 70. Suction apparatus for gastro-duodenal siphonage. A trap-bottle is always used when the fluid returns are large. (Transactions, Western Surgical Association, 1931, and West J. Surg. 40: 1, 1932.)

out over a period of days, at frequent intervals, and with little inconvenience. It should be understood that we do not advocate attempts at decompression of an acutely obstructed colon by other than surgical methods, except in unusual circumstances such as we just cited. If on the passage of a catheter through a constricting rectal growth relief is not promptly secured, then cecostomy should be resorted to without further delay.

When the colon is filled with an enormous quantity of inspissated material, irrigations with solutions of normal saline are of little avail. In such instances we resort first to a mixture of magnesium sulphate, glycerine and water, and if not effective then to solutions of 50 per cent hydrogen peroxide. If there is also a marked stenosis of the bowel lumen cecostomy is indicated, for attempts at medical decompression of the bowel under the circumstances would be futile.

Suction siphonage, described by Wangensteen, is less useful in obstruction of the colon than in simple mechanical obstruction of the small intestine for which it was primarily devised. However, lesser grades of colonic obstruction may be satisfactorily decompressed by suction applied to an inlying duodenal tube. This procedure, which is illustrated in figure 70, is contraindicated in acute obstruction of the colon with enormous distention in which the ileocolic sphincter limits the distention to the large intestine.

Some surgeons, notably Whipple (1940) and Ravdin (1947), employ the Miller-Abbott tube regularly, feeling that the advantages of an operative decompression measure are thereby provided. Wangensteen and many other surgeons, including ourselves, have found that suction applied to an ordinary indwelling duodenal tube preliminary to, during, and constantly after operation for a period of three to five days will, in most instances, preclude the occurrence of intestinal distension as satisfactorily as the Miller-Abbott tube. A survey made by us in 1947 revealed that the long tube decompression method has not been generally adopted by surgeons as an adjuvant to surgery of the colon and rectum.

The principal disadvantages of this method as applied to the colon are that a competent ileocecal valve will in many instances prevent decompression of an obstructed colon and owing to the considerable distance the tube must traverse, the process will require the continued attention of the surgeon or a highly competent assistant over a long period of time and will necessitate repeated fluoroscopic studies of the position of the tube. Wangensteen states that in patients with the greatest distension, in which quick intubation of the duodenum is most important, the greatest difficulty is had, almost invariably. It has, he states, taken days to get the tube out of the stomach.

For a detailed consideration of acute obstruction the reader is referred to the original contributions of Wangensteen, cited in the references.

Measures of rehabilitation.—These are directed toward overcoming dehydration, malnutrition, anemia and hypoproteinemia with which many patients enter the hospital. This is accomplished by feeding the patient food of high caloric value but low in residue, forcing the intake of fluids orally; and when necessary, by the subcutaneous or intravenous route, transfusions when needed, and special measures as indicated.

Diet.—A diet in which the residue content is materially reduced must necessarily consist principally of carbohydrates, and although most patients will tolerate such a diet, many are in the late years of life when tolerance for carbohydrate is more or less reduced. If preparation for operation requires only three or four days there is rarely cause for concern, but when this period is extended, as has been our tendency in most cases in recent years, the problem increases in importance. With this in mind we have attempted to alter the basic allowance of 2,000 to 3,000 calories of carbohydrate, proposed by Bargen and Victor, by the addition of proteins which are relatively low in residue as follows:

LOW RESIDUE PREOPERATIVE DIET

BREAKFAST	Strained fruit juice, sweetened. Pablum or strained well-cooked oatmeal gruel; rice cereals. Heavy cream. Eggs. Bacon, thin and crisp. Butter. Butter-thins or arrowroot crackers, 2 or 3. Coffee or tea.
DINNER AND SUPPER	Essence of beef or chicken to which butter is added. Beefsteak, rare, to be chewed but not swallowed. Scraped tender beef, occasionally. Rice with gravy, strained tomatoes, butter, or added to broths. Eggs. Egg custard, jello, soufflées, with cream. Heavy cream in ginger ale. Strained fruit juices, sweetened.
BETWEEN MEALS	Sweetened fruit drinks. Candy (pure sugar candy or milk chocolate without nuts)

The size of the portions served and the relative percentage of carbohydrate, protein, and fat will vary with the caloric need of the individual. Admittedly this diet offers very little variety yet it is far more liberal, and much less insipid, than the initial diet so commonly employed in the treatment of peptic ulcer. A competent and interested dietitian can serve this diet for periods up to two weeks to the complete satisfaction of a majority of patients.

Pablum is a pre-cooked cereal of high nutritive value which has been vitamin and mineral enriched. The approximate protein content is 15 per cent, and analysis reveals that it contains less than 1 per cent residue. Probably the most important addition which we have made to the low residue diet has been beefsteak in liberal quantities, which the patient is only permitted to chew. Tender cuts, properly prepared and served, stimulate gastric secretion and provide an excellent substitute for broth, of which most patients tire quickly. In regard to the latter, it is not sufficient that one merely orders "broth" as a part of the diet. Our observation has been that the usual broth served in hospitals is, perhaps, little more that a secretagogue. Only essence of beef or chicken should be employed, since from these considerable nourishment is obtained. When these substances are not available, owing either to scarcity or prohibitive expense, it is possible to materially increase the protein intake by the ingestion of one of the several palatable digests now available, or the administration of a protein hydrolysate by tube feedings into the stomach or jejunum.

Eggs constitute the main source of protein in this diet. Unless co-operation is sought from the dietitian, patients will invariably receive soft-boiled eggs and therefore will soon tire of them. Formerly we encountered difficulty when patients were asked to consume six or eight ounces of heavy cream each day, yet this is often necessary in order to supply the caloric need of the individual. Although still a problem at times, it has been found that most patients will take cream in ginger ale with no objections. A common error is to permit patients on a low residue diet to have milk, ice cream, and the general run of cereals, all of which contain a relatively high percentage of residue. Butter-thins and arrowroot crackers fit into the same category, but because of their small weight, two or three are allowed at each meal. In the event patients are unable to ingest sufficient food to maintain caloric needs, intravenous administrations of protein hydrolysates along with solutions of dextrose (d-glucose) are resorted to.

On restricted activities, patients gain weight on such a diet as we have outlined; yet the bowel remains comparatively empty. Sugar rarely will appear in the urine, but there is usually a slight elevation of the blood sugar within normal limits.

Dehydration, anemia and hypoproteinemia.—One will often encounter dehydration in cases of carcinoma of the distal segment of the bowel and evidences of profound anemia when lesions are situated in the proximal segment. Many of these patients, regardless of the location of the lesion, will show evidences of malnutrition, a circumstance brought about chiefly by an insufficient intake of food or the impaired digestion and absorption of protein, and the loss of protein in the stool during periods of diarrhea. It is our practice routinely, upon admission of these patients to the hospital, to determine the variation from normal of the blood chemistry (non-protein nitrogen, chloride, plasma protein and the CO_2-combining power), to obtain a complete blood count and concentration of hemoglobin. At the same time the patient's blood is typed and cross matched.

Dehydration, once decompression is commenced, can often be overcome simply by increasing the fluid intake by mouth. However, when desiccation is marked and the chlorides of the blood are depleted, or when fluids taken orally are not well tolerated, dextrose in a physiologic solution of saline or Ringer's solution is administered intravenously. Fortunately, marked changes in blood chemistry, such as noted in pyloric and small bowel obstruction, are rarely encountered when lesions are situated in the large intestine.

Anemia is combated by repeated blood transfusions. It has long been our belief that it is not necessary to wait for a profound anemia before blood transfusion is utilized. We have felt that the administration of blood, even when the hemoglobin estimate is relatively normal, has been an advantageous factor in many cases. Tremendous benefits from the liberal use of blood transfusions noted in World War II have only strengthened these convictions.

Hypoproteinemia, or plasma protein deficiency, is indicative of a serious reduction in the 'labile' or reserve stores of body protein. For a detailed consideration of this important and somewhat complex state, the reader is referred to the comprehensive reports of Ravdin and his co-workers, Lund and Leverson, Elman, Binkley, Abels and Rhoads, Ariel, et al., Co Tui, et al., Meyer and Kozoll, Lyons and Mayerson, and G. H. Whipple, which are only a few selected from a vast literature on the subject.

When accompanied by anemia, hypoproteinemia presents a complex situation. It has been shown by G. H. Whipple that when the body needs both plasma protein and hemoglobin the protein flow favors hemoglobin, which under these circumstances is produced in more abundance than the plasma protein. It is therefore highly important that strenuous efforts be made to correct existing anemia first when confronted with a patient in whom there exists both a hemoglobin and plasma protein deficiency. This frequently calls for a number of transfusions of 500 cc. of blood each.

Although protein reserves may appear to be approximately sufficient prior to operation it should be borne in mind that a considerable demand will be placed on these reserves at the time of operation as a result of hemorrhage and serum loss, and following operation owing to increased protein catabolism during a period when food cannot be ingested, and to infection and suppuration. Ample evidence indicates that depletion of the protein reserves results in delayed wound healing, wound separation, edema at the sites of anastomosis, decreased production of antibodies, and a reduced resistance to local and generalized infections. Ariel found a greater fall in plasma protein in patients with cancer of the gastro-intestinal tract than in other patients. Meyer and Kozoll found a drop of 25 per cent of the plasma protein after operations for carcinoma of the colon and for intestinal obstruction. Binkley, Abels, and Rhoads found the incidence of hyperproteinemia in patients with carcinoma of the rectum and colon to be 36 per cent. The incidence was increased to 86 per cent after operation.

Various methods have been employed in an attempt to sustain or reinforce the protein stores of the body either before or after operation. All investigators, however, are in agreement that when no contraindication exists, the ideal method is oral feedings of a diet that appeals to the patient. In the case of malignancy of the large bowel accompanied by obstruction maintenance of nitrogen balance is difficult of accomplishment owing to the high residual content of foods rich in proteins. Ravdin states that there is no beneficence in feeding hydrolysates unless there is evidence of faulty digestion. Feeding of mixtures of polypeptides and amino acids, he states, may result in an absorption rate of amino acids which is more rapid than can be resynthesized by the liver, especially when the function of this organ is not normal. Our own experience with the use of protein hydrolysates by tube feedings into the stomach or jejunum has been somewhat discouraging owing chiefly to diarrhea which has usually occurred when adequate amounts were fed in this manner. Palatable protein digests for oral administration, recently made available, have, on the other hand, proved to be valuable sources of protein when used to supplement diets consisting mostly of carbohydrates. There are occasions, both preoperatively and postoperatively, when intravenous solutions of hydrolysates produced either by the enzymatic or acid hydrolysis method, and reinforced with dextrose, are indicated. Nitrogen balance has been maintained in man for periods of more than two weeks by such solutions administered in adequate quantities. Weinstein has recently (1948) emphasized the simplicity, rapidity and safeness with which protein hydrolysate may be administered intramuscularly. Whole blood is not an economical source of proteins in hypoproteinemia. Transfusions of plasma are also expensive since 250 cc. of plasma supplies only 14 or 15 gm. of protein. Moreover, as Ravdin has demonstrated, a practical contraindication to the use of large amounts of plasma or albumin intravenously is that the greatly increased blood volume which occurs under such circumstances may so increase the circulating volume as to lead to cardiac embarrassment.

Lyons and Mayerson have recently (1947) suggested that under a program proposed by them of blood volume restoration through transfusions of whole blood until total correction of blood hemoglobin deficits has been accomplished, it is unnecessary to utilize other methods of protein replacement in order to withstand the trauma of surgical procedures. As the two cardinal features of their concept are the reduced blood volume and the therapeutic response to whole blood transfusions, the syndrome has been designated as chronic shock. These authors state that it has been learned that both blood transfusions and early surgical intervention are important in resuscitation in hemorrhagic shock; an analogy, they state, exists in the nutritional resuscitation of the patient with chronic shock due to protein deficiency.

Vitamin therapy is of particular importance in the pre- and postoperative preparation of patients with lesions of the large intestine both for the reason that many of these patients will show evidences of vitamin deficiency and because drugs of the sulfonamide class, when given orally in the preparation of patients for resection of the colon or rectum, require an increase in the intake of certain vitamins. Najjar and Holt have demonstrated that thiamine is synthesized in the intestines as a result of bacterial metabolism and that succinylsulfathiazole given orally promptly reduced both bacterial growth and the synthesis of thiamine. Ravdin referred to studies which demonstrated that oral sulfonamide therapy may also result in a definite reduction in the synthesis of vitamin K in the intestines with a resulting hypoproteinemia and hemorrhage at the suture line.

It is our practice to administer to all patients taking oral feedings vitamin capsules containing larger than ordinary quantities of vitamins A, D, ascorbic acid, thiamine, riboflavin and nicotinic acid. Those patients sick enough to require intravenous feeding, alone or as a supplement, are given intravenously or intramuscularly water soluble vitamins in approximately the following doses: vitamin C 500–1000 mg., thiamine 20–40 mg., riboflavin 20–40 mg., and niacine 150–300 mg.

Chemotherapy.—The importance of chemotherapy as an adjuvant to the pre- and postoperative care of patients with carcinoma of the large intestine is attested by the abundant literature favorable to its employment. In a survey conducted by us in 1947 all but eight of 50 surgeons contacted stated that they used chemotherapeutic agents routinely in connection with surgical procedures on the large intestines. Sulfasuxadine (succinylsulfathiazole) or sulfathalidine (phthalylsulfathiazole) was employed preoperatively by 79 per cent. Five used streptomycin orally and four used sulfa-diazine orally or by the intravenous route. Fifteen signified regular use of sulfa compounds within the peritoneal cavity. Penicillin intramuscularly was employed postoperatively for five to ten days by 22, or 52 per cent (Table 31).

Ravdin has recently (1947) reported on the use of streptomycin. He stated that although the oral sulfonamides have been useful in reducing the total bacterial population, their action on the intestinal bacteria is highly selective and in the occasional patient the usual or even larger, doses are without marked effect. Streptomycin on the other hand, was found to be effective in part at least against all the common pathogens. When given by mouth in a dosage of 0.25 gm. every six hours the feces are free of streptococcus fecalis in eight days and there results a marked reduction in the coliform group and the anerobic organisms of the Welchi type. In the immediate postoperative period he administers both streptomycin and penicillin. He quotes Zinsser and Zintel, now preparing data soon to be published, as having found these two antibiotics to be more useful in preventing spreading peritonitis following peritoneal soiling than any other chemotherapeutic combination.

Valuable as these chemotherapeutic agents have proved to be it should, nevertheless, be emphasized that their employment does not warrant any compromise with sound surgical principles such as adequate decompression of an obstructed bowel, care in the conservation of blood supply, prevention of gross soiling and accurate approximation of the bowel edges.

Urinary tract.—It is well to know in advance of any operation the status of the urinary tract; in lesions of the rectosigmoid and rectum such knowledge is particularly important. Probably the most frequent and constant complication of abdominoperineal resections of the rectum is a disturbance in the urinary tract. This will occur in a high percentage of cases in the absence of preoperative disease in this tract; it is a great deal more likely to occur if patients are elderly men with hypertrophied prostates and residual urine. We prepare these patients just as if they were to undergo a prostatectomy and in a few instances have instituted suprapubic drainage preliminary to excision of the rectum. Admittedly these patients constitute graver risks than the average patients but it is often striking, once they pass through the period of vesical dysfunction incident to the excision, the manner in which their former symptoms disappear completely or else become milder.

Patients suffering with diabetes or cardiorenal disease are placed under the strict surveillance and supervision of clinicians who are especially trained along those lines. These patients, as well as all others, are observed carefully during the period of preoperative treatment in an effort to estimate surgical risk and to determine the procedure suitable for the individual case. Diabetes *per se* is not a contraindication to resection of a lesion of the large intestine, nor is hypertrophy of the prostate or nephritis; each case must be decided on its individual merits and an operative procedure must be selected to suit the case.

Anesthesia.—Tremendous strides have been made during the past decade in the development of new anesthetic methods and in the improvement of old ones. While spinal anesthesia has many advantages to the surgeon and to the patient as well, we are inclined to favor in most instances the use of cyclopropane or ethylene administered through an intratracheal tube, supplemented by intravenous injections of curare if relaxation is not adequate. If curare is not employed the gas is reinforced by ether vapor sufficient to produce relaxation. Inhalation anesthesia administered through an intratracheal tube provides completely unobstructed respiration, controlled ventilation, and markedly improved relaxation, even when curare is not used. Curare affords relaxation comparable to that obtained with spinal anesthesia, yet the patient may be carried under very light general anesthesia or intravenously administered pentathol sodium. Although we prefer to employ this drug in conjunction with intratracheal anesthesia, we do not hesitate to use it in the absence of an intratracheal tube provided the anesthetic mask fits properly and the anesthetist can inflate the lung by bag pressure. Prostigmine, which is a satisfactory antidote in case of a small overdose of curare, is always kept readily available, although its use has never been found necessary by us.

Continuous spinal anesthesia has proved highly satisfactory in the experience of one of us (Graham) in carefully selected cases, including combined abdominoperineal resections of the rectum, since he routinely employs the dorsal lithotomy position in undertaking the perineal portion of the operation. We are, however, in complete accord with Wangensteen in the belief that spinal anesthesia is not invariably indicated in instances of complete obstruction. Our experience in the surgical management of acute intestinal obstruction, like that of Wangensteen, has failed to substantiate the contention of R. R. Graham and W. E. Brown that "a surgeon who operates upon a patient suffering with acute intestinal obstruction using inhalation anesthesia, if adequate facilities for spinal anesthesia are available, is guilty of malpractice." The employment of constant suction to an indwelling duodenal tube before and during operation has eliminated the hazard of regurgitation which might occur during the administration of inhalation anesthesia.

POSTOPERATIVE TREATMENT

In the average run of general surgical cases, if the operation has been skillfully performed and the patient leaves the operating room in a satisfactory condition, the surgeon has little reason for concern as to the details of the postoperative care, which to a great extent he can leave to assistants. Such, however, is not true where resections of the colon and rectum have been undertaken. We are thoroughly convinced, if a low morbidity and mortality is to be maintained in these cases, that either the surgeon himself must closely supervise the postoperative treatment, including personal attention to many minute details, such as removal of packs, irrigations of wounds, manipulation of clamps, and so forth, or else it will be necessary for him to carefully train not only competent assistants but also nurses and orderlies.

Immediate postoperative care.—Before leaving the operating room the patient's condition is carefully appraised. If the procedure has been a formidable one we invariably give a citrated blood transfusion on the operating table, the blood of the patient, in every instance, having been grouped and cross-matched with the blood of relatives or a professional donor during the preoperative period. The patient's bed is adjusted to a moderate Trendelenburg position which is maintained for a period of twelve to twenty-four hours, regardless of the type of anesthesia administered. This position serves a two-fold purpose: first, it helps to forestall or relieve shock; and second, it is believed this position is helpful in reducing the incidence of pulmonary complications (Call, and Coleman).

The following regime is instituted after the majority of operations on the large intestine, and is carried out for at least the initial forty-eight hours: (1) continuous suction applied to indwelling duodenal tube (Wangensteen method); (2) penicillin, 50,000 units intramuscularly every three hours; (3) intravenous administration of 5 or 10 per cent dextrose in normal saline or Ringer's solution, 2,000 to 3,000 cc. in twenty-four hours; (4) opiates in liberal doses sufficiently large to allay pain; and (5) strict oral hygiene in an effort to prevent parotitis.

Duodenal suction is continued until flatus is freely expelled, either spontaneously, or on the insertion of a rectal tube into the bowel. Strict observance of this rule has, in our experience, meant greater freedom from abdominal distention and gas pains. Maintenance of fluid balance, by which is meant the ratio between the total intake of fluids (orally, intravenously, and subcutaneously) and the total excretion of fluid (by skin, lungs, kidneys, bowel, or by a fistula), is a vital factor in the successful outcome of patients operated on for cancer of the large intestine.

The absorption of normal saline by hyperdermoclysis (used when large quantities of fluids intravenously are contraindicated) is greatly facilitated if a 10 per cent dextrose solution is given intravenously at the same time; or if absorption is markedly retarded this may be quickly overcome by the intravenous injection of a 50 per cent solution of glucose, given into a small vein near the wrist in order to avoid sclerosing the larger veins higher up. Ordinarily we prefer to give a 5 per cent solution of dextrose, which is isotonic. This solution tends to maintain the water balance, supply calories, serve as a prophylactic agent in shock, and tends to promote diuresis. It is said that if dextrose is injected more rapidly than 0.35 gm. per pound of body weight per hour, sugar is secreted in the urine. For a person of average weight two hours will be required to administer 1,000 cc. of a 10 per cent solution, an hour and a half if a 5 per cent solution is employed.

The danger of overnarcotizing the patient has never given us cause for concern; the real danger of shock and hemorrhage that results from physical suffering and restlessness is of far greater significance.

Patients who have been adequately prepared in the preoperative period seldom experience distention and are remarkably free of gas pains. Enemas are avoided during the first five or six days, for during this period there is often a physiological cessation or retardation of peristalsis. At times a glycerine suppository will suffice to stimulate evacuation. Daily rectal examinations are made in order to rule out the formation of a fecal impaction. If the bowel has been sutured following resection as in ileocolostomy, a rectal spool or catheter is inserted as a precaution against increased intracolonic pressure, unless the rectal sphincters have been fully dilated under anesthesia.

Decompressive measures.—These measures consist of cecostomy, ileostomy, and colostomy.

Cecostomy and ileostomy.—The fecal discharge from both cecostomy and ileostomy is liquid and in the early stages is very likely to be irritating to the skin. The indwelling catheter, in both instances, is connected at once with rubber tubing which permits drainage into a bottle beside the bed. The cecostomy tube alone will require irrigating, and then only when the colon is filled with inspissated feces as a result of long standing obstruction. In such instances it will usually be necessary to employ a solution of magnesium sulphate, glycerine, and water, or 50 per cent hydrogen peroxide.

The most significant consideration in the postoperative care of these patients is one of water balance. The natural function of the right half of the colon is the absorption of fluids from the fecal current. Rowntree has estimated the daily amount of water excreted into the gastro-intestinal tract by the salivary glands, stomach, liver, pancreas and the small intestine to be between 7,500 and 10,000 cc. Under normal circumstances this would be returned to the circulation by the colon, but ileostomy diverts the entire fecal current and cecostomy a considerable portion of it. Until the physiologic equilibrium is re-established, that is, until the ileum begins to assume the function of the proximal half of the colon, the patient with ileostomy invariably loses weight and to a certain extent becomes dehydrated, even when receiving 4,000 to 5,000 cc. of fluid a day. During this period a chart should be kept of the fluid intake and output, the chemical constituents of the blood (chlorides, CO^2-combining power, and nonprotein nitrogen) should be studied frequently and dehydration and salt depletion be combated by the administration of adequate quantities (based on the intake-output chart and estimates of invisible fluid losses) of normal saline solution, by hyperdermoclysis, and intravenously. The Hendon continuous intravenous drip of 5 per cent glucose in normal saline is particularly advantageous here.

Drugs such as paregoric, bismuth, and kaolin have proved of little or no value in checking the liquid fecal discharge during the first five to seven days, but after this kaolin in doses of one or two teaspoonsful three or four times a day, and continued over an indefinite period, is definitely beneficial. Kaolin, made into a paste with olive oil, is also employed to protect the skin about the iliac stoma from the excoriating action of the intestinal discharges during the first two weeks. After that, when there is no longer a catheter in the ileum, and the wound has healed sufficiently to permit use of an ileostomy bag, zinc oxide and paraffin "washers" are employed. These are made from three- or four-inch squares of soft cloth in which a hole sufficiently large to encircle the ileac stoma is cut in the center. Placed in containers in piles of twenty-five or more, paraffin of a relatively low melting point is poured into one, while into the other is poured a mixture of glycerine and zinc oxide. A zinc oxide square is applied next to the skin which previously has been cleansed with pledgets of cotton and normal saline solution; the paraffin square, which should be a little larger, is applied directly over the other. The bag may be applied directly to the paraffin washer with little likelihood of leakage unless the patient is very emaciated or the ileac stoma is situated too near the crest of the ileum. An ideal ileostomy bag has yet to be designed, but of those available, the Grenfeld pouch has proved to be the most satisfactory.

Diet apparently has little influence on the discharges during the first two weeks. Hypermotility of the entire gastro-intestinal tract often exists and nourishment taken orally will soon pass out of the stoma undigested. Eventually patients can resume their normal manner of eating, but at first they are given a constipating type of diet of which boiled milk and cheese are important items; raw fruit and vegetables are eliminated. The fluid intake by mouth is limited considerably and usually restricted to meal times. The stool practically never becomes formed but a semi-solid passage is the rule within a period of six to ten weeks. Complete rehabilitation following ileostomy seldom can be expected in less than three months and if resection of the colon is to be undertaken subsequently an interval of five or six months should be allowed.

Cave in 1946 made a valuable contribution to the study of ileostomy function at different periods after its establishment. Fifty patients were personally interviewed and examined. Thirty-one had been operated on four or more years previously. Many patients had gained more than 100 pounds; the average weight-gain was 45 pounds. There was found to be a surprising adaptability in the care of ileostomy. Forty were at work. They included laborers, a bank clerk, police detective, dentist, insurance agents, college professor, and a number of housewives who had resumed all their household activities. Many played golf, tennis and base-ball. Those patients who had had ileostomy from five to ten years were questioned closely to see if they could suggest a diet which would be helpful in reducing to a minimum the number of discharges from the ileostomy. No conclusion could be reached as to what is the most suitable diet for all patients with ileostomy. These patients can eat practically everything, except spinach, uncooked fruits and vegetables, and they cannot drink fruit juices, but they can drink in moderation, alcoholic beverages. Of the 38 patients with ileostomies, 19 had no trouble from irritation of the skin around the ileal stoma; eight had slight or moderate excoriation and the remaining 11 suffered considerably from this constant burning annoyance. It is significant that all of the 19 patients, devoid of irritation, used Fuller's earth (kaolin) around the stoma. The 11 who suffered most all used some sort of greasy application, either zinc oxide ointment, aluminum paste or vaseline. There were three striking instances of repeated collapse from sudden salt deprivation, on account of unexplained abrupt and profuse diarrhea from the stoma.

Loop colostomy.—Seldom is it necessary to open a loop colostomy for forty-eight hours, and frequently it need not be opened for a matter of five to seven days. It is not uncommon for gas to pass over the loop easily without discomfort, and in a great many cases, if the fecal column is semi-solid or liquid, the bowels will move over the loop quite easily. When distention occurs and it becomes necessary to decompress the colon, this is easily done by puncturing the top of the loop with a cautery, after which a catheter is inserted into the proximal loop. After five or six days the colon is divided through its anterior two-thirds with a cautery or scalpel whether the colostomy is to be temporary or permanent; later, about the tenth day, the bowel is cut completely across, if the colostomy is to be a permanent one. This separates the two ends for a matter of one-half to one inch, and prevents the fecal current from pouring down into the distal segment. By postponing the opening of the bowel, as described, it has been possible to avoid gross infection in the subcutaneous tissues about the colostomy in most instances and this is decidedly worth while. Prolonged purulent drainage means postponement of the second stage of the operation, if resection of the rectum is to follow, possible extension of the infection to the peritoneal cavity, and greater likelihood of a ventral hernia subsequently. Care of these wounds is considered later.

It is impossible to outline a diet which will be suitable for every colostomy case, but in the main more or less constipating foods should be the basis of the early diet. Raw fruits and vegetables are usually prohibited at first but most patients soon learn what foods are best for them; few find it necessary to alter the diet to which they have been accustomed. If stools are loose in spite of strict adherence to a constipating type of diet, which has included boiled milk, milk-toast, and cream cheese, kaolin in doses of one or two teaspoonfuls are given two or three times a day. Paregoric is reserved for diarrhea of a severe nature. When bowel movements have become regular, patients are advised in case of diarrhea, the result of indiscretion of diet or food poisoning, to remain in bed and permit the intestinal tract to empty itself before resorting to drastic measures of control. Irrigations of the proximal loop of bowel with warm saline solution is usually beneficial on such occasions.

As for apparatus to be used over the colostomy, the simpler the more satisfactory they are. We have long since abandoned all the cumbersome bags and cups, and believe that a simple corset-like, lightly constructed belt with a removable rubber inner section which may be cleansed frequently is the most satisfactory of all the types of apparatus (Figs. 71 and 72). With a properly manufactured colostomy so long as the stool is formed, the care is relatively simple and easy; and the individual is comfortable. Regardless of the type of colostomy, where it is placed, or by whom it is manufactured, when the patient develops a diarrhea, the only recourse left is to stay at home and care for the condition. Liquid stools make any colostomy intolerable, but are largely the result of indiscretion of diet and in the large majority of cases can be avoided.

Some patients find it advantageous to irrigate the proximal loop of the colostomy at a definite hour each day or every other day in order to insure regular habits; such irrigations are entirely harmless provided a solution of normal saline is used. In most instances the patient finally determines upon a regime suited to his individual circumstances and inclinations.

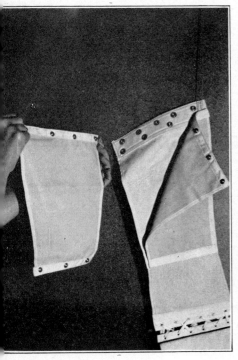

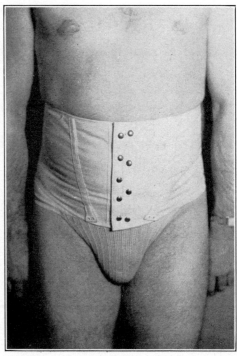

Fig. 71. Simple elastic girdle with removable rubber attachments which fits over the colostomy opening.

Fig. 72. Colostomy belt in place.

Wounds.—These wounds require frequent, minute inspection and considerable painstaking care. Our regime for the care of wounds of patients on whom operations for carcinoma of the large bowel has been performed is based on the following measures: (1) strict preliminary precaution against contamination; (2) exposure of all drainage wounds to infra-red-rays twice daily; and (3) irrigation of all infected wounds at frequent intervals with a warm solution of normal saline or a 1:5,000 solution of iodide of mercury.

Wounds made for purposes of exploration are very likely to become contaminated as a result of undue manipulation of an infected,

obstructing growth. In cases in which unusual opportunity for contamination is present, we have been inclined to practice delayed
closure as originally advocated by Finney, Gamble and others for
peritonitis secondary to appendicitis and which was subsequently
recommended by Coller and Valk for use in abdominal wounds that
were contaminated by the contents of the gastro-intestinal tract.
The need for either drainage of the abdominal wound or the practice of delayed closure has been practically eliminated through the
routine employment of sulfathaladine or sulfasuccidine in the preoperative period, a closed technic of intestinal anastomosis, and
penicillin intramuscularly in the postoperative period. A number
of surgeons, notably Babcock and T. E. Jones, have reported re-
ductions in mortality and in wound morbidity following the routine use of buried alloy steel sutures in operations for gastrointestinal malignancy. A detailed report by Jones is discussed in the chapter on mortality and end-results.

Drainage operations (cecostomy, ileostomy, colostomy, and obstructive resection) necessarily increase the hazard of contamination in both the wound which contains the loop of bowel and the
larger exploratory incision. Nevertheless, this danger can be reduced to a considerable degree if preventive measures are instituted
promptly. The initial dressing applied to ileostomy or colostomy incisions is an important part of this plan. Dry gauze is placed
next to the incision; over this and around the protruding bowel are
applied heavily vaselinized wide gauze strips. If the vaseline is of
a thick, tenacious quality, the gauze strips will become closely adherent to the bowel and serve as an efficient protection for the incision after the bowel is opened. The exploratory incision should
then be carefully separated from the drainage wound. This is accomplished by placing heavy dressing pads that cover separately
the two incisions. These pads are made to swing laterally along a
line halfway between the two where they are joined by the wide
strips of adhesive tape. This arrangement affords ready access to
both wounds.

Perineal wounds.—These wounds, the result of posterior excisions or abdominoperineal procedures, are usually more or less infected. Removal of the packing need not be an ordeal to the patient
if at the operation one thrusts a square sheet of oiled silk or rubber
dam into the hollow of the pelvis and then packs gauze tightly into
it. Several purposes are accomplished by this procedure: venous
oozing is controlled (this is particularly important if spinal anesthesia has been used and the blood pressure is very low on completion of the operation); support is afforded the newly made pelvic
floor; and, by use of the oiled silk or rubber tissue, the pack may be
removed (forty-eight hours) with great ease and freedom from pain.

Irrigations of the wound are instituted the third day and are conducted once or twice daily in this manner: with the patient on his side a catheter is inserted to the upper extent of the wound, into the hollow of the sacrum. A sterile two-liter irrigation can is suspended from a standard beside the patient's bed, the rubber tubing from which is connected with the catheter and four to six liters of very warm solution are allowed to run into the wound. Normal saline solution is used in the early stages and mercuric iodide in a 1:5,000 solution later. This latter agent, which has been employed by Terrell with such satisfactory results in the postoperative care of rectal fistulas and other proctological conditions, is non-irritating yet is strongly bacteriocidal, and keeps the wound free of unhealthy granulation tissue. Sitz baths may be resorted to when the patient's condition permits, but it is believed carefully conducted irrigations are more satisfactory in the majority of cases.

We have no hesitation in removing all retaining sutures if a virulent type of infection with profuse purulent drainage develops. As a matter of fact, when the wound is left wide open, fewer late complications such as osteomyelitis of the sacrum, abscesses in the upper extent of the wound, and persistent draining sinuses are encountered.

Urinary tract infections.—Probably the most frequent and constant complication of abdominoperineal resection of the rectum is a disturbance in the urinary tract; it is a great deal more likely to occur if patients are elderly men with hypertrophied prostates and residual urine. However, vesical disfunction will occur in a high percentage of cases, even in the absence of preoperative disease in the urinary tract, due to the trauma incident to resection. Controversy still exists concerning the mechanism of this complication. Hill (1937), T. E. Jones (1942), Bacon and McCrea (1947) and many others are convinced that injury to the nerve supply to the bladder is entirely responsible for the bladder disturbances. Bacon and McCrea from a study of 244 patients subjected to proctosigmoidectomy concluded that vesical dysfunction is due to the inadvertent removal of the inferior hypogastric or pelvic plexus. There were 7 instances in their series in which normal micturation was impossible at the time of discharge from the hospital. Of these 7 cases, 5 returned to normal voiding and are without residual urine. One committed suicide and the other had just recently been operated upon. They considered the best procedure to maintain normal musculature is to keep the bladder at rest through continuous drainage with a catheter. Jones is in agreement with these investigators as to the cause of bladder dysfunction. He discontinues continuous drainage, however, twenty-four hours after operation. The patient is then catheterized every eight hours until he voids spontaneously. Despite various methods he has employed to increase bladder tone, Jones concluded that "the bladder regains its tone at its own rate, and nothing yet tried seems to hurry the process." This has also been our experience.

Coller (1942) and his associates, and more recently Marshall, have stated that endoscopic examinations and cystograms disprove the neurogenic theory of vesical dysfunction following resection of the rectum. Marshall found that the percentage of patients with severe urinary difficulty (8 per cent lasting over three months) are approximately the same whether combined abdominoperineal or posterior resection only was done. They concluded that the dysuria is due to a sag of the bladder, bladder neck and prostate resulting from the dissection at the base of the bladder and removal of the support of the rectosigmoid colon with consequent alteration of the arrangement of the urethra and external sphincter of the bladder.

We have systematically tried out various postoperative regimes in the care of these patients, often with the co-operation of urologists who have given considerable thought to the problem but we are now back to about where we commenced. Our present regime is as follows: (1) maintenance of a high urine output by forced fluids, including the intravenous administration of a 5 per cent dextrose solution; (2) prevention of bladder distention by frequent catheterizations or the installation of a retention catheter; and (3) frequent, thorough irrigations of the bladder until there is no longer residual urine. The so-called urinary antiseptics, if given in quantities sufficient to kill bacteria in the urinary tract, will usually cause gastro-intestinal disturbance. Moreover, we are far from convinced that they often serve the purpose for which they are intended, in which opinion we find many urologists of experience in agreement.

Regardless of the regime adopted, once vesical dysfunction becomes manifest, one can be certain that it will continue to a greater or less degree for a period of between six weeks and three months. Yet it is comforting to know that practically without exception, barring previous disease such as prostatic hypertrophy or cystocele, the residual urine disappears as the tonus of the bladder returns, and that in no instance has permanent damage been observed.

REFERENCES

1. ARIEL, I. M., REKERS, P. E., PACK, G. T., and RHOADS, C. P.: Metabolic studies in patients with gastrointestinal cancer: XI, Postoperative hypoproteinemia and relationship of serum protein fall to urinary nitrogen excretion. *Surg., Gynec.,and Obstet.*, **77**: 16–20 (July), 1943.
2. BABCOCK: Quoted by Jones (16).
3. BACON, H. E., and MCREA, L. E.: Abdominoperineal proctosigmoidectomy for rectal cancer. The management of associated vesical dysfunctioı. *Jour. Am. Med. Assoc.*, **134**: 523–526 (June), 1947.
4. BARGEN, J. A., and VICTOR, SISTER M.: Diet in intestinal disorders. *Jour. Am. Med. Assn.*, **97**: 151–153 (July 18), 1931.
5. BINKLEY, G. E., ABELS, J. C., and RHOADS, C. P.: The treatment of postoperative hypoproteinemia in patients with cancer of the colon and rectum. *Ann. Surg.*, **117**: 748–753 (May), 1943.
6. CALL, MANFRED: Quoted by Coleman.
7. COLEMAN, C. C.: Management of unconscious patients with special reference to posture in treatment. *Virginia Med. Monthly*, **61**: 270–276 (Aug.), 1934.
8. COLLER, F. A.: In discussion of Jones (15).
9. COLLER, F. A., and VALK, W. L.: The delayed closure of contaminated wounds. *Ann. Surg.*, **112**: 256 (Aug.), 1940.
10. CO TUI, WRIGHT, A. M., MULHOLLAND, J. S., CARABBA, V., BARCHAM, I., VINCI, V. J.: Studies on surgical convalescence. *Ann. Surg.*, **120**: 99–122 (July), 1944.
11. ELMAN, R.: Acute starvation following operation or injury, with special reference to caloric and protein needs. *Ann. Surg.*, **120**: 350–361 (Sept.), 1944.
12. GRAHAM, A. STEPHENS: Unpublished material.
13. GRAHAM, R. R., and BROWN, W. E.: Spinal anesthesia in abdominal surgery. *Ann. Surg.*, **110**: 863 (Nov.), 1939.
14. HILL, M. R.: Vesical dysfunction following abdominoperineal resection of carcinoma of the rectum. *Jour. Am. Med. Assn.*, **109**: 1194 (Oct. 9), 1937.
15. JONES, T. E.: Complications of one-stage abdominoperineal resection of rectum. *Jour. Am. Med. Assoc.*, **120**: 104 (Sept. 12), 1942.
16. JONES, T. E., NEWELL, E. T. JR., and BRUBAKER, R. E.: The use of alloy steel wire in the closure of abdominal wounds. *Surg., Gynec., and Obstet.*, **72**: 1056–1059 (June), 1941.
17. LYONS, CHAMP, and MAYERSON, H. S.: The surgical significance of hemoglobin deficiency in protein depletion. *Jour. Am. Med. Assoc.*, **135**: 9–11 (Sept. 6), 1947.
18. MARSHALL: Quoted by Rosser (24).
19. MYER, K. A., and KOZOLL, D. D.: Protein deficiency in surgical patients. *Surg., Gynec., and Obstet.*, **78**: 181–190 (Feb.), 1944.
20. NAJJAR, V. A., and HOLT, L. E. JR.: The biosynthesis of thiamine in man; and its implications in human nutrition. *Jour. Am. Med. Assoc.*, **123**: 683–684 (Nov. 13), 1943.
21. NEWTON, F. C., and BLODGETT, J. B.: *Surgery*, **18**: 200–206 (Aug.), 1945.
22. RAVDIN, I. S., and ABBOTT, W. O.: The use of the Miller-Abbott tube in facilitating one-stage resection of the small bowel. *Clinics of N. Am.*, **1**: 179, 1940.
23. RAVDIN, I. S., ZINTEL, H. A., and BENDER, D. H.: Adjuvants to surgical

therapy in large bowel malignancy. *Ann. Surg.,* **123**: 439–447 (Oct.), 1947.

24. ROSSER, CURTICE: In discussion of Bacon and McRea (3).
25. ROWNTREE, L. G.: Normal water balance and its regulation. *Oxford Med.,* Vol. I.
26. TERRELL, EMMETT H.: Personal communication.
27. WANGENSTEEN, OWEN: Intestinal obstructions. Springfield and Baltimore, Charles C Thomas, 1937, 250 pp.
28. WEINSTEIN, JACOB J.: Intravenous, subcutaneous, and rapid intramuscular infusions of "protein hydrolysate." *Surg., Gynec., and Obstet.,* **87**: 93–107 (July), 1948.
29. WHIPPLE, A. O.: The use of the Miller-Abbott tube in surgery of the large bowel. *Surgery,* **8**: 289–293 (Aug.), 1940.
30. WHIPPLE, G. W.: Hemoglobin and plasma protein: their production, utilization, and interrelation. *Am. Jour. Med. Sc.,* **203**: 447–489, 1942.

PART III

OPERATIVE PROCEDURES

CHAPTER XI

HISTORICAL CONSIDERATIONS

Surgery of the large intestine, like most things pertaining to the art and science of medicine, can be traced to the earliest antiquity, but, in the main, such facts as have been found are little more than hazy traditions that strongly suggest a mythical origin. Probably the earliest allusion to surgery of the rectum was a description by Aristotle of a calf born at Perinthus with imperforate anus and of attempts to relieve the condition by incising the intact membrane. There is no doubt that minor operations on the rectum were practiced during the period in which Hippocrates lived. These procedures consisted chiefly in ligation and subsequent strangulation of hemorrhoids, cauterization of hemorrhoids, their excision with scalpel, and incision of fistulous tracts. Of actual instances of such surgical procedures we have little evidence, but that such knowledge was had and practical application probably made of it, is witnessed in this ancient commentary circulated with the books of Hippocrates: "The intestinum rectum may be cut, and repeatedly cut, may be sewed up, may be burnt with actual or potential cauteries, and may be sloughed away afterwards, and yet, notwithstanding these things, may seem so very violent, they will have no mischievous consequences." Early in the seventeenth century there was considerable interest exhibited in the disorders of the rectum, as a considerable literature attests, but aside from minor operations and Morgagni's suggestion that the rectum be excised in cases of malignant involvement, there was little progress in surgery of this organ. It was not until near the close of the eighteenth century that real progress began.

The history of colostomy from its inception as a decompressive measure to its present-day acceptance as a necessary part of a radical maneuver for extirpation of cancer of the lower gastro-intestinal tract is an intriguing saga. Unquestionably, the medical profession was preceded by our veterinary colleagues in the performance of this operation, since the latter are recorded from remote ages as having stabbed the colon of a sheep or horse suffering from obstruction, and with frequent relief.

In the ancient writing of Aurelianus it is recorded that Praxagoras, 400 years before Christ, annoyed at the unsuccessful means of treating ileus, had opened the belly and incised the bowel to evacuate its contents and then closed the bowel. There is no available record of the success of this operation.

Dinnick quotes Fine, of Geneva, who in 1797 made a contribution to colostomy in the transverse colon, as observing that it was the custom to open the stomach to remove knives which had been accidently swallowed, and praising the incision of a strangulated hernia to evacuate the bowel contents. Littre is given the credit for performing the first colostomy in 1710. As a matter of fact, Littre observing the dead body of an infant with maldevelopment of the rectum suggested an operation to overcome this by incising the abdominal wall and making either an anastomosis between the two ends of the bowel or bringing the proximal end to the surface of the belly where the anus could function. This idea, important as it was, rested for 66 years until Pillore, of Rouen, performed a cecostomy for cancer of the rectum.

After Littre and Pillore, DuBoise performed Littre's operation for an imperforate anus in 1783; but the patient, a small child, died on the tenth day. Duret, ten years later for the same lesion performed a left iliac colostomy, thus establishing the modern type of colostomy, nearly a century and a half ago. It is true that he did this for a case of imperforate anus; thus the principle was not recognized in cases of cancer of the rectum for nearly a century. Callisen, after him (1796), utilized lumbar colostomy without enthusiasm.

Amussat, an excellent French surgeon, in 1839 was actually responsible for colostomy assuming its real place in surgery. Observing a death from obstruction due to rectal cancer, he urged colostomy as a routine and humanitarian measure. A great anatomist, his contribution to the anatomy of the lumbar spaces and its relationship to the mesocolon demonstrated that lumbar colostomy, both in adult and infant subjects, was possible. He performed both right- and left-sided decompressive operations and advanced this maneuver no little.

It is interesting to note that he approved of colostomy a century ago in these words, "an artificial anus it is true is a grave infirmity, but it is not insupportable." Following Amussat we find Baudens, 1842, Keyworth, 1848, Phillips, 1850, all making technical advances in the performance of colostomy; but in 1865 Nathaniel Ward, twenty-five years after Clements had done the first colostomy in England, urged that lumbar colostomy for rectal cancer be performed as a routine upon the recognition of the cancer.

Following Ward, Bryant and Allingham (1870 and 1874) began their contributions to rectal surgery which were landmarks in the advance to its present day status. During the last twenty-five years while the majority of surgeons have recognized the importance of accepting colostomy as a part of the plan for excision of rectal cancer, a great many attempts, versatile it is true, but uniformly futile, have been made to manufacture control of a colostomy by the use of the abdominal wall muscles. All of these have failed without exception. The acceptance of colostomy as a part of the operation, however, has permitted the development of multiple procedures which have ranged far from the anal amputation of the 1880's to the present day combined abdominoperineal resection.

To Allingham, Reeves, and Cripps chiefly should go credit for abandonment of lumbar colostomy. In the twenty-five years ending in 1900 the trend toward inguinal colostomy was so definite that by the end of the century the lumbar procedure was almost completely discarded. Allingham pointed out that in most instances it was impossible to open the lumbar segment of the colon without injury to the peritoneum, consequently the operation was not safer as regards peritonitis than that of the anterior colostomy, and further, that the lumbar situation was inconvenient for the patient.

Temporary by-passing of the fecal current was first suggested by Schede in 1887. In the older procedures, closure of colostomy necessitated resection of that portion of bowel involved in making the stoma. This operation proved more fatal than the original procedure; consequently surgeons hesitated to recommend colostomy except for incurable conditions.

Operations for cancer of the rectum date back to the proposal of Morgagni early in the eighteenth century and the first attempt by Faget in 1739. The earlier procedures were all variations of a posterior type of proctectomy, leaving an uncontrollable sacral anus. The perineal method of resection usually is attributed to Lisfranc in 1826, little being known of Faget's earlier attempt in 1739. Lisfranc's first successful operation was done in 1826 and reported in 1832, and meanwhile his pupil, Pinault, published a thesis in 1829 reporting nine cases. The operation was merely a circular amputation of the anal canal. Following this, however, Dieffenbach and Velpeau modified these earlier procedures. Heavy mortality followed all these procedures and surgery of the rectum languished somewhat for lack of enthusiasm among surgeons.

The modification of this operation largely revolved around whether or not to remove the coccyx, or a portion of the sacrum and the coccyx, Amussat being the first to practice coccygectomy. Verneuil, in 1873, adopted this modification routinely as giving better exposure. In 1876 Kocher took away the coccyx and a portion of the sacrum. Kraske, in 1885, made his epoch-making presentation before the Fourteenth Congress of German Surgeons. He not only removed the coccyx and a portion of the sacrum, but he suggested the preservation of the perianal skin and the external sphincter with a division of the peritoneum close to the bowel as Kocher favored. This sacral operation immediately gained popularity and maintained it for a quarter of a century. In the 1890's Kraske's operation was again modified by Hochenegg, Bardenheuer, Billroth, Rehn, Rydygier, and many others who took away more of the sacrum even to the point of making osteo-integumental flaps. These procedures gained no popularity nor did the various V- and H-shaped incisions of Schelky, in 1892, DePage, in 1893, or the lateral incision of Hartmann, in 1892.

It should be noted that all of these operations might be performed with or without a preliminary colostomy and that the more conservative surgeons preferred the posterior type of excision which did not open the peritoneum and left a sacral anus, while others more daringly opened the abdomen, making a colostomy and subsequent excision. Probably the first surgeon to perform preliminary colostomy was Adams, in 1882, and its most ardent advocates were Allingham and Kelsey. There was little difference in the percentage of recurrences in the operations of this date, and the more conservative type could be performed with a lower mortality.

Von Volkmann, in 1887, may be said to have envisaged the so-called combined abdominoperineal operation, and he published his method in a work on the removal of carcinoma of the rectum, but Czerny, in 1883, unintentionally performed an operation of this type. He was attempting to do a posterior type of excision without exploration. The growth evidently was at the rectosigmoid juncture where the majority of them are, and he was unable to bring it down so that he could resect it. Consequently, this bold and daring pioneer opened the abdomen, ligated the blood supply of the lower sigmoid, and removed the whole segment transperitoneally. Unfortunately, the attempt was unsuccessful, but a principle had been established.

At the beginning of the present century Miles began to practice this combined abdominoperineal resection of the rectum, and over the ensuing years has established it firmly as the fundamentally correct operation for cancer here. Nevertheless, it has been borne in upon the medical profession that all cancers of the rectum are not of a piece, and that individualization and versatility in the matter of selection of operation is as essential here as elsewhere. Consequently, the work of Lockhart-Mummery, Paul, Gordon Taylor, and many other surgeons of the British Empire, as well as Jones, David, Stone, and other American surgeons, has established the fact that the radical operation, desirable as it is in one stage, may be utilized advantageously by a graded type of maneuver occasionally, and that the less radical but useful operation of colostomy and posterior excision still has definite indications.

This huge progress over the period of years in rectal surgery is a monument to these pioneers whose untiring efforts, sturdy courage, and maintenance of the highest tradition of the profession, forced progress in a field not too favorably looked upon by general surgeons as a whole because of an unwarrantably high mortality, unpleasant, and prolonged and complicated convalescence.

Surgery of the colon proper necessarily awaited its development until the era of asepsis warranted a bold invasion of the peritoneal cavity. The ancients, however, recognized wounds of the gastro-intestinal tract as well as invented ingenious appliances and types of sutures for their repair. In the Book of Judges of the Holy Writ it is recorded that Ehud, a left-handed warrior, stabbed the king of the Moabites "and his dirt ran out and he died." Similar wounds observed by Hippocrates, Celsus, and others led to the conclusion that nature was perhaps the best physician under such circumstances, and Celsus, while mentioning intestinal suturing, disparaged it.

Traumatic ileostomy, engaging as it did the surgeon's attention frequently, is beautifully described by William Hildani in his works done in 1644. He pictures a wound of the small bowel with prolapse of a large amount of the intestine and complete severance of the continuity of the gastro-intestinal tract, on which he made many important physiological observations.

Military surgeons observing these bizarre and deadly injuries frequently began to cast around for methods of repair and in 1730 we find Purman advocating suture with linen or catgut immersed over night in wine. Abulkasim recommended the jaws of large ants for apposing wounds and also referred to the use of catgut made from the intestines of sheep. Roger, Jamerius, and Theodoric, of Cervia, in about 1739, inserted into the bowel a hollow cylinder of elder over which the wound was sutured. Wilhelmus V. Saliceto used segments of dried animal intestine with the same object in view, and later stated that he preferred the dried trachea of a goose or some larger animal.

Samuel Sharp, in 1769, passed a needle through the lips of the wound from within outward so as to leave a length of thread at both ends to hang out of the incision, and pull the bowel so as to get adhesions. Du Verger (beginning of the eighteenth century) modified suturing over a cylinder by including the cylinder in the suture in a manner not practiced by earlier surgeons. Sabatini substituted for the trachea a cylinder of cardboard smeared with sweet oil, while Watson advised a cylinder of fish glue. Von Walther preferred to use a tube of India rubber.

Reybard, in 1823, after experimenting on dogs, resected a portion of the sigmoid flexure in a human for cancer and performed an end-to-end anastomosis. The patient, a twenty-nine-year-old man, lived one year to succumb to recurrence. Unfavorable comment by his colleagues resulted in this operation lying fallow until Thiersch, in 1843, twenty years later, resected the colon again, this time for acute intestinal obstruction.

As late as 1880 only 10 resections of the large bowel were recorded, 7 of which had failed, but in the next decade the total number grew to 48 and the mortality decreased to 45 per cent. It would be difficult to attribute any particular procedure to any one surgeon prior to 1885. However, a few brief instances must be noted. Billroth, in 1879, did a resection with closure of the distal end of the bowel, bringing the proximal end out as a colostomy. Schede, in 1879, brought out both ends of the bowel from the wound when he found it impossible to approximate them, and thus unintentionally performed the first graded resection of the colon. Marshall, in 1882, did Billroth's operation but made an additional stab wound incision in the left iliac region through which he made a colonic stoma. Resection of the cecum was first attempted by Kraussold in 1879, and Maydl, in 1883, performed the first successful right colon resection in two stages; Billroth accomplished the one-stage operation in 1884. Weir was the first American surgeon to do a successful resection of the colon. Exclusion of a segment of the bowel was first practiced by Maisonneuve while Trendelenburg and many others between 1880 and 1890 performed ileosigmoidostomy and colocolostomy.

From all this ingenuity came the gradual evolution of intestinal surgery and while many of the old surgeons observed and recorded spontaneous recovery from complete transverse wounds of the intestine by adhesion of the ends to the external wound and consequently delayed operation, they were inevitably led to attempt many methods to imitate nature. The Lambert suture is the result of the discovery that adhesion took place rapidly when serous surfaces were approximated, and a new era in intestinal surgery resulted from this single fact.

Gradually accumulated experience, buttressed by the arrival of anesthesia and asepsis forged forward through the evening of the past century to give birth to modern operative surgery. Between 1890 and 1900 many ingenious devices for intestinal suture were evolved, notably among which were Magraw's elastic ligature, in 1891, and Murphy's button in 1892. The Murphy button may be said to have revolutionized all gastro-intestinal procedures.

Around 1900 a new principle in colonic surgery was firmly established as being highly desirable, largely through the efforts of Mikulicz; that is, exteriorization of the colon with its offending growth, and graded resection with subsequent reestablishment of the bowel lumen. While Block was the first man to do the so-called exteriorization operation in 1892, its association with Mikulicz's

name in this country is very common because of the latter's
championing it in 1902. Block did an exteriorization operation in
that year for acute obstruction and decompressed the colon with
a tube in the proximal loop. This was a local type of operation
which was subsequently modified by Hochenegg in an effort to remove the regional lymphatics, and McGraw, Allingham, and others followed a similar procedure. Paul's operation was different from
that of Block and Hochenegg in that he excised the exteriorized
portion at the time of the operation and sutured large tubes into
the two limbs, the subsequent closure being made after destroying
the spur after the method of Dupuytren. This exteriorization procedure reduced the high mortality which had followed colon surgery all down the years, from around 40 to 50 per cent to approximately 15 per cent.

The operation of Block, or the exteriorization procedure, was
in reality the second attempt at graded resection of the colon, a
principle which now is recognized as equaling in importance preoperative decompression, Schede, in 1879, having brought both ends
of the bowel out of the wound when he found it impossible to approximate them, and thus unintentionally, as has so often been the
case, established a fundamental in colonic surgery.

It is unquestionably true that the necessity of preliminary decompression of the obstructed large bowel has not been duly appreciated until the past decade. A quarter of a century ago it was
recognized that slow decompression of an obstructed bladder was
necessary in the treatment of prostatism. An obstructed stomach
from a cicatrizing duodenal ulcer likewise was advantageously
treated by preliminary decompressive measures, and obstruction
elsewhere in the body was granted this preliminary emptying. With
the colon it is no less desirable that the decompressive measures
be instituted before any radical attempt at removal be made, slow
as has been the recognition of this fact.

It is not too arbitrary, we think, to express the opinion that
decompression preliminary to extirpation, whether it be medical or
surgical, is among the most important fundamental principles in
the removal of rectal and colonic cancers.

The present-day concept of the surgical management of malignancies of the large bowel and rectum is the result of the gradual
evolution of operative maneuvers throughout the years. The acceptance of the graded operation in many cases, and of decompression as of primary importance in all cases, has been a great step
forward in establishing a satisfactory routine. It is now definitely
recognized that not only should patients who are not acutely obstructed be isolated for a period of preliminary preparation and
decompression, but that individualization of patients and the selec-

tion of operation for each patient on its merit, rather than selection of the patient for operation, is of paramount importance.

Consequently, a lowering of the hospital mortality with a widening of the operative scope has taken place to a point where surgery of the large bowel and rectum—while it may be considered a special field—has influenced standardization to the end that the principles are established and satisfactory end-results following radical surgery outbalance those of other portions of the gastro-intestinal tract.

REFERENCE

RANKIN, F. W.: How surgery of the colon and rectum developed. *Surg. Gynec,* *and Obst.*, **64**: 705–710 (March), 1937.

CHAPTER XII

PROCEDURES FOR OVERCOMING OBSTRUCTION

In operations on the large bowel, the urgent necessity demanding operations in multiple stages for benign or malignant conditions usually revolves around obstruction, acute or chronic, or subacute perforation or fixation to adjacent structures or organs. Combating either of these conditions to allow as near a return to normal physiological equilibrium as possible, and to raise the threshold of safety, while extending the opportunity for radical removal of the lesion and gland-bearing tissues in immediate juxtaposition to it, if the lesion is malignant, approaches the most desirable achievement. To accomplish this the surgeon must often resort to measures of decompression such as cecostomy, colostomy, ileostomy, or appendicostomy. We believe that the employment of one of these measures is always indicated for acute obstruction or chronic obstruction unrelieved by medical measures and occasionally as an additional safeguard in resections of the left half of the colon followed by immediate anastomosis. Determining the necessity for such procedures is discussed in detail under "Choice of Operation" and "Preoperative Preparation."

Decompression may precede resection by days or weeks, according to the degree of obstruction present, or it may be accomplished at the time of resection as an additional precaution. In instances of complete obstruction from a malignant growth, for which these procedures are chiefly used, the operation should be performed without exploration; manipulation of the colon under the circumstances is highly dangerous, for, as Herrmann has pointed out, obstruction and ulceration increases enormously the permeability of the bowel wall and consequently extravasation of the infective organisms into the pericolonic tissues takes place. This is the process from which peritonitis most often develops.

CECOSTOMY

Although a most valuable and often urgently needed measure, cecostomy is nevertheless not completely satisfactory in diverting the fecal current and placing the colon at rest unless the cecum, at its juncture with the ascending colon, is brought completely out on the abdominal wall as in the establishment of a colostomy elsewhere. Cecostomy, as usually performed, may be consummated by one of several methods, as that of Hendon, Gibson, Witzel, or Kader, with excellent likelihood of subsequent spontaneous closure. We prefer the exteriorization (colostomy) method in most instances for preliminary decompression, but one of the above as a complement to resection of a well decompressed bowel.

Exteriorization technic.—Through a right rectus or a McBurney incision the ascending colon at its juncture with the cecum is mobilized and delivered into the wound in quite the same manner as described for colostomy, established in the proximal sigmoid. If necessary to facilitate mobilization, the avascular lateral parietal peri-

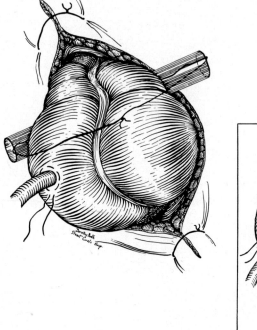
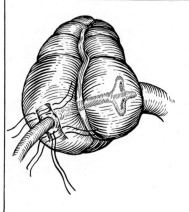

FIG. 73. Exteriorization type of cecostomy with temporary catheter drainage as safeguard against early wound infection.

toneum close to the bowel is incised. A small rent is then made in the mesocolon with the aid of a pointed forceps. A rubber tube is pulled through and retained for traction on the bowel during the remainder of the procedure, at the completion of which a glass tube is substituted for the tubing (Fig. 73). Ordinarily no suturing is required, but the wound is packed with iodoform gauze, over which, and in close proximity to the bowel, are placed strips of generously vaselinized gauze in order to lessen the likelihood of contamination if early decompression of the colon is indicated. In such event a purse-string suture is placed, and in the center of the area enclosed by the suture a small incision is made through which a catheter is inserted into the cecum. Subsequently, usually in about forty-eight hours, the colon is incised sufficiently to permit the complete side-tracking of the fecal current. Even then it will often be found advantageous to retain in the cecal opening a catheter which is connected by tubing with a drainage bottle. If the catheter is of sufficient diameter (we prefer a 28 or 32 F) discharges of liquid feces on to the abdomen can be avoided. This is important for several

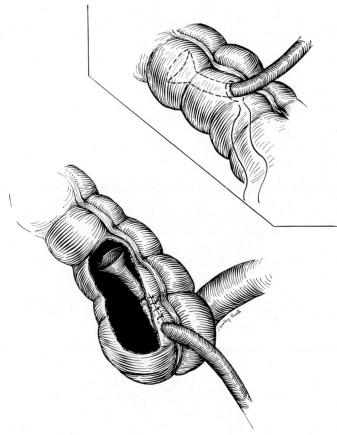

Fig. 74. Witzel cecostomy employing a Pezzer catheter (Hendon) from which the top of the mushroom portion has been cut.

reasons: excoriation of the skin of the abdomen is thus prevented, the possibility of wound infection is lessened, and accurate determination of the ratio of intake to output, so important in preventing a serious degree of alkalosis in these cases, is permitted.

Spontaneous closure seldom is obtained in this type of cecostomy, but the advantages of the method easily compensate for the necessity of an additional surgical procedure (see "Closure of Colostomy").

Catheter technic.—This type of cecostomy can be accomplished satisfactorily by one of several popular methods, as that of Witzel, Gibson, or Kader, which are also employed in performing gastrostomy and enterostomy. Our preference is a combination of technics, based on the employment of a Pezzer or wing catheter, as suggested by Hendon, which is Witzelerized. Through a McBurney or a right rectus incision the cecum is delivered into the wound, and a portion is fixed by a rubber-covered clamp after it has been emptied of its contents by compression with the hand. After the surrounding tissues have been carefully protected with moist gauze packs to prevent soiling, a purse-string suture is placed, and in the center area enclosed a small incision is made. Through this opening a large (28–32 F) Pezzer or wing catheter is inserted into the cecum and the suture is tied as the mucosa is being inverted. The catheter is then buried by the Witzel technic (Fig. 74). As applied to the cecum, this procedure is adequately covered in a description of the Witzel type of ileostomy. Occasionally this is difficult to accomplish because of inability to deliver sufficient bowel into the wound when the latter is of the McBurney type. A satisfactory alternative in such cases is the Gibson procedure in which two layers of sutures extend from the tube up and down the bowel, so as to form a broad surface that will adhere to the peritoneum and will tend to produce inversion of the wall of the cecum when the tube comes out. We have modified Hendon's technic in that the top of the mushroom portion of the Pezzer catheter is cut off in order to insure more adequate drainage, leaving a wide, cuff-like structure at the end of the catheter, which insures against the tube coming out before the desired time. If there is difficulty in removing the tube it may be cut off flush with the skin, and the short, remaining portion may be pushed into the lumen of the bowel.

APPENDICOSTOMY

This procedure no longer enjoys its early popularity. As in the case of cecostomy, as generally performed, appendicostomy does not exclude the large bowel and put it at rest; nor does it afford adequate access to the colon for purposes of decompression. It is even less efficient than cecostomy because catheters of small calibre, seldom larger than an 18 F, must be employed. This procedure frequently is not available because the appendix is absent, retrocecal, short, or obliterated.

The technic consists simply of delivering the appendix through a McBurney incision as in appendectomy and closure of the wound in layers about the exteriorized organ, care being taken to maintain its blood supply. If an immediate opening seems imperative the appendix may be divided at once with a cautery and a catheter inserted, otherwise, a delay of forty-eight hours is advisable.

ILEOSTOMY

This procedure is usually employed preliminary to total colectomy but also on rare occasions as a means of decompressing an obstructed colon when the establishment of a cecostomy is judged impossible or too hazardous because the cecum is completely retrocecal, tightly fixed by adhesions from an old inflammatory process, or because of marked distension and hypertrophy in a very sick individual. Ileostomy not only puts the colon completely at rest but offers satisfactory access to the interior of the cecum for purpose of irrigation, medication, and decompression if this is desired. However, the most satisfactory type of ileostomy is that which results in a single-barreled stoma and in the absence of obstruction in the colon is the type generally employed by us. This stoma is more easily and efficiently cared for by the patient, and hernia is less likely to occur. Irrigations, when needed, can be carried out with ample satisfaction by means of rectal injections. In instances of generalized polyposis or chronic ulcerative colitis, for which ileostomy most frequently is done, we seldom have considered that irrigation of the colon was advisable. The postoperative care of these cases, which has been described in detail, is very important.

Single-barreled technic.—The abdomen is opened through a McBurney incision and the terminal portion of the ileum, 10 to 15 cm. from the cecum, is delivered into the wound. Ordinarily it will be found necessary to ligate only a few of the terminal branches of the mesenteric vessels just before they enter the intestinal wall. By avoiding the larger vascular branches and therefore disturbance to the circulation of the bowel, the technic is simplified and time is saved in that the necessity for removing a segment of bowel is eliminated. Two clamps are applied at the selected site in opposite directions and close together, and between the two the ileum is divided with a cautery. The distal end is inverted and dropped back into the abdomen whereas the proximal end is brought out of the wound which is closed snugly about it, the peritoneum being fixed to the ileum by interrupted sutures of fine catgut. The muscle, fascia, and skin are approximated in the usual manner. We no longer keep the lumen occluded by a clamp during the first twenty-four hours after operation. On closure of the wound a purse-string suture is placed around the bowel just beneath the clamp (Fig. 75). After carefully protecting the wound with strips of well-vaselinized gauze the clamp is removed, a Pezzer or wing catheter inserted into the ileum, and the purse-string tied. The catheter is promptly connected with a drainage bottle by additional tubing. The simplicity of the procedure and the small likelihood of contamination during operation are the features that chiefly commend it.

General abdominal exploration should not be done because in the case of multiple adenomatosis it gives one little information and in the case of chronic ulcerative colitis it is contraindicated because of the fear of rupturing a concealed perforation, or otherwise damaging the fragile colon to cause leakage and peritonitis.

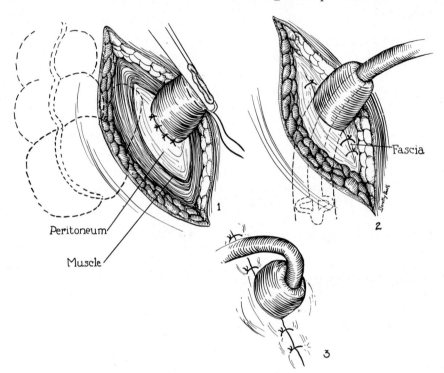

Fig. 75. Technic of ileostomy. The terminal portion of the ileum is divided between clamps with a cautery, the distal end being inverted and dropped back into the abdomen. 1. Purse-string suture is placed about the proximal clamped end of ileum; 2. Winged catheter is inverted into ileum after closure of fascia, and the purse-string suture is tied; 3. Wound closed, the catheter is connected by tubing with a drainage bottle.

Double-barreled technic.—The foregoing procedure may be readily modified in order to establish a double-barreled ileostomy. Instead of dropping the inverted cecal end of ileum back into the abdomen it may be fixed into the abdominal wound just as is the proximal end, being thus made readily available for purpose of irrigation by single puncture with a cautery point. If early access to the cecum is desired it will be more expedient to leave the clamp on the distal segment of ileum than to invert it.

John Young Brown technic.—The technic for this procedure can be carried out as has been described above for the single-barreled ileostomy. In addition to ileostomy, however, a cecal stoma is also established, the tube of which is brought out through a stab wound. When it is desired to re-establish continuity of the intestinal current the cecal stoma is closed, the ileac fistula is excised, and the proximal end of the ileum is implanted end-to-side into the cecum or ascending colon. By modifying this procedure, Stone has been able to circumvent the necessity of the latter step.

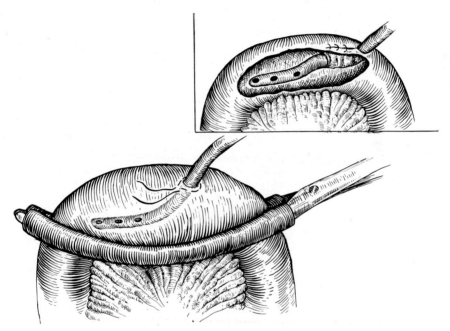

Fig. 76. Witzel enterostomy. Catheter is introduced into the bowel through an opening encircled by a purse-string suture. Insert shows purse-string suture tied and catheter buried by row of interrupted sutures.

Witzel technic.—As an adjunct to surgery of the colon, enterostomy serves its chief function in preventing distention by gas which would produce pressure on the line of suture, and possibly leakage and peritonitis. It is not intended as a measure that diverts all the fecal current, consequently it is not a suitable substitute for the foregoing types of ileostomy or for the exteriorization type of cecostomy.

The loop of ileum selected will depend on the purpose of enterostomy: if employed as a safety-valve in connection with an anastomosis between terminal ileum and colon, it is placed 25 or 30 cm. proximal to the suture line; if the objective is decompression of an obstructed colon, it is situated a similar distance from the ileocecal valve. The elected segment is brought out of the wound and isolated from the rest of the abdomen by gauze packs; a rubber-covered clamp, which includes both limbs of bowel, is applied unless the ileum is well deflated and relatively empty. A purse-string suture is placed and in the center of this a small opening is made, (Figs. 76 and 77) either with a knife, or cautery (Long). The latter possesses the advantage of preventing bleeding and the tendency

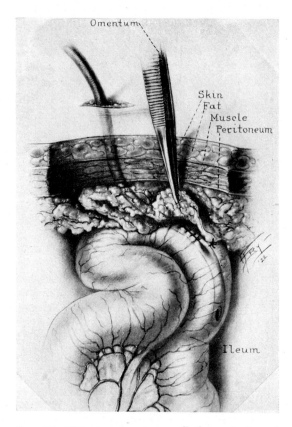

Fig. 77. Witzel enterostomy. Catheter is forced through the omentum and brought out through a stab wound.

of the mucosa to evert when incised. A catheter of small calibre (the primary object of enterostomy is deflation and not drainage of content of the bowel) is inserted into the lumen of the bowel and the purse-string suture is tied. The operation can be completed simply by further inversion of the bowel wall with another purse-string suture placed around the first. Hendon, Pfeiffer, and Levering, and others have reported complete satisfaction with such a procedure; the ease and rapidity with which it may be accomplished recommends it.

In the Witzel technic, the catheter is buried for a distance of about 3 cm. from its point of entrance into the ileum, by folds of bowel wall which are approximated over the tube with interrupted sutures of catgut. Where possible the catheter is passed through the omentum, after which it is brought through a stab wound or else out of the end of the wound; the ileum is attached to the edge of the peritoneum with a suture or so, and the wound is closed in the usual manner. Seldom have we found it necessary to close a fistula following removal of the catheter.

COLOSTOMY

Formerly an artificial opening in the colon, whether temporary or permanent, was termed "colotomy," from the two Greek words meaning "colon" and "cutting." However, at about the turn of the present century, owing chiefly to the efforts of Petit, the term colotomy was dispensed with and henceforth surgeons spoke of temporary or permanent colostomy. A detailed record of the development of colostomy, from the date of its proposal by Littre, in 1710, to the beginning of this century may be found in the chapter devoted to history of surgery of the large intestine. Shortly before the close of the last century there was a decided trend away from the time-honored conviction that colostomy should be used in cases of malignancy of the large bowel, merely as a palliative measure, and in favor of colostomy, either temporary or permanent, in conjunction with resection. The struggle for a general acceptance of colostomy by the profession was, however, by no means over. Only in recent years have a majority of surgeons ceased to employ procedures for the extirpation of the rectum which entail the establishment of a perineal anus.

That some members of the medical profession have adopted a pessimistic attitude toward colostomy as a step in the radical cure or comfort of a patient with cancer of the rectum is unfortunately true. Nor can it be denied that occasionally a physician is willing to go so far as to advise a patient with cancer of the rectum against operative maneuvers which have as one of the stages the manufacture of an artificial anus. Consequently it is easy to understand the average patient's abhorrence of colostomy, and while it may be due in a large majority of cases to the ability to view the artificial anus, it is unquestionably in part due to the prejudice handed down from the earlier days by both laymen and surgeons. It seems impossible for any member of the present-day profession longer to justify himself in refusing to accept colostomy as a part of the necessary procedure for the radical removal of a rectal growth because of statistical data available to prove incontrovertibly that thousands of persons in every walk of life are comfortable and contented and little handicapped by the artificial opening. To justify the assertion that operative relief or cure of cancer of the rectum entails the performance of a colostomy in a large percentage of cases is easily provable to one of open mind. In fact, it is our belief that colostomy is a basic part of any operation which offers the best chance of longevity to the individual suffering from cancer of the rectum or rectosigmoid.

The type of operative measure employed in colostomy varies somewhat according to the personal inclination of the surgeon, but certain procedures, proved essential by experience, establish the advantages of one or two maneuvers. In performing colostomy, either as a palliative procedure or as a part of an extirpative procedure for cancer, it is important that exploration of the abdomen, liver, regional lymph nodes, and finally the neoplasm should be carried out through a low mid-line incision. The exact location of the artificial anus on the abdominal wall is still being debated by surgeons, the three main locations being: first, through a stab wound in the left groin; second, in the middle or upper portion of a low mid-line incision; and third, at the site of the umbilicus, which has been removed.

There are various advocates of all of these locations, and reasons advanced for utilizing each. Hirschman, of Detroit, is a staunch advocate of removing the umbilicus and utilizing its location for the site of the colostomy. Jones, of Cleveland, prefers to put the colostomy in the upper part of the mid-line incision, leaving the umbilicus. In our experience, the most satisfactory position has been a left inguinal colostomy through a small stab wound.

The type of procedure which does not bring the loop outside but sutures it to the peritoneum and subsequently punctures it is entirely undesirable for many reasons: first, it allows part of the fecal column to pass into the lower loop; second, it has a tendency to close up; and third, it is frequently accompanied by a tendency of the mucous membrane to prolapse, usually from above downward, but occasionally from below upward.

In regard to the portion of the bowel that should be selected for permanent colostomy, it is generally agreed that the sigmoid flexure is the most advantageous point, although occasionally the transverse colon is advocated.

Fecal control following colostomy has been the object of ingenious procedures directed toward manufacture of a sphincter muscle, but almost invariably is the result unsatisfactory. With a properly constructed colostomy, so long as the stool is formed, the care is relatively simple and easy, and the individual is comfortable. Regardless of the type of colostomy, where it is placed, or by whom it is made, when the patient develops diarrhea, the only recourse left

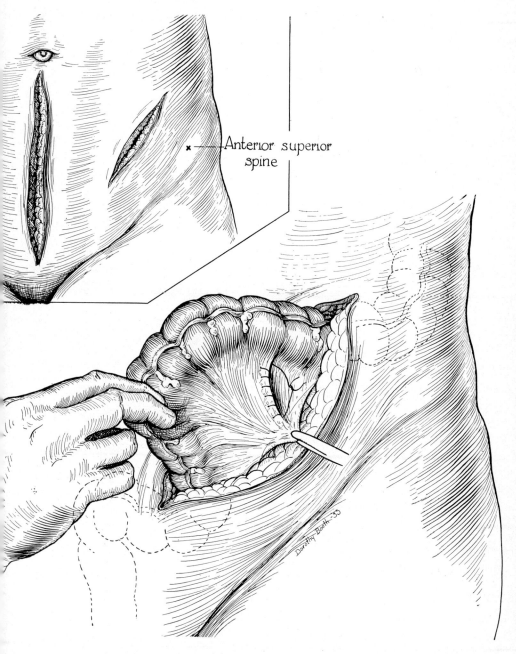

Anterior superior spine

78. Left inguinal colostomy. In the upper corner of the picture is shown the low mid-line incision exploration, and lateral to it the stab wound for bringing out the colostomy. In the lower part of picture is shown the placement of the suture which shuts off the space between the mesentery he bowel and the lateral peritoneum.

is to stay at home and care for the condition. Liquid stools make any colostomy intolerable, but are largely the result of indiscretion of diet, and in the large majority of cases may be avoided. As for apparatus to be used over the colostomy, the simpler it is the most likely the patient is to find it satisfactory. Our patients are taught to control their movements by a diet that tends to cause constipation, in conjunction with daily irrigation of the bowel at the same time each day, until regular habits are acquired. As a consequence of this education it has seldom been found necessary for patients to resort to cumbersome cups or pouches which tend to promote herniation about the stoma and from a psychological standpoint often appear to affect the patient unfavorably. Instead, they use a simple, corset-like, lightly constructed belt which exerts just sufficient pressure to insure closure of the stoma. Usually these patients eventually experience a high degree of continence (see "Postoperative Treatment").

Left inguinal type.—After exploring the abdomen through a low, right paramedian incision, a left inguinal stab wound is made (Fig. 78). The sigmoid is brought out of the latter incision until its most fixed point, close to its juncture with the descending colon, is reached. Simultaneously the sigmoid distal to this point is fed back into the abdomen. In this manner herniation of the mucous membrane of the proximal loop is prevented. There is generally a fold of peritoneum running off from the lateral parietal peritoneum onto the mesentery of the upper portion of sigmoid. A simple pursestring suture placed around this obliterates the foramen and prevents obstruction from a loop of small bowel slipping through it (Fig. 79). We have encountered such a complication on only two occasions, but Gabriel in 1928 reported five cases. A small opening is made in the mesosigmoid with the aid of a pointed forceps just in front of this purse-string suture. A rubber tube is pulled through and retained for traction on the bowel during the remainder of the procedure, at completion of which a glass tube is substituted for the tubing (Fig. 79). A glass tube has the advantage over a glass rod of being less liable to break; moreover the tube is more easily retained in place since it can be threaded with suture material, the ends of which may be tied over the bowel. The peritoneum at the center of the incision is brought under the bowel, through the rent in the mesentery of the sigmoid, and sutured to the peritoneum of the opposite side. In permanent colostomy skin is similarly pulled through the rent in the mesosigmoid and sutured to skin, with silk-worm catgut or equisitenne. Ordinarily the only additional sutures required are one or two interrupted catgut sutures in the fascia of the external oblique muscle and one stay suture at each end of the wound for reinforcement in the event of infection. Sutures are never placed in the bowel itself. This is important, because there is ample proof that with distention of the colon the sutures have torn large openings in the bowel which have resulted in abscesses and fatal peritonitis. As a final step the epiploic tags are removed

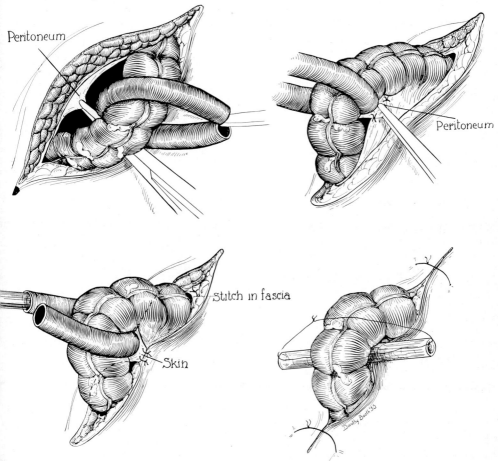

. 79. Left inguinal colostomy. Above: The bowel is shown brought out of the incision and the itoneum is being pulled under it and sutured. Below: The fascia is closed snugly around the bowel l the skin is pulled under the loop. Sutures are not placed in the bowel itself. On completion of the ration a glass tube is substituted for the rubber one (see Figures 71 and 72).

from the exposed loop since they have a tendency to slough, and to make subsequent division of the bowel more difficult. After forty-eight hours,[14] unless the patient is markedly undernourished and anemic, the natural reparative powers of the tissues seal off the peritoneal cavity and it is safe to open the bowel for colostomy. This, however, is best postponed for six or seven days if discomfort from gas and distention does not render it impossible. Postponement for such a period of time has in our experience markedly reduced the incident of wound infection and subsequent herniation. Simple puncture with the hair-pin cautery point and insertion of a small catheter which is retained often suffice to relieve early painful distention. For permanent colostomy, eventual complete division of the bowel is usually advisable.

Temporary colostomy.—Temporary colostomy differs from permanent colostomy in that ordinarily sutures are not taken except to fix the peritoneum beneath the bowel. Skin is not pulled under. The bowel is divided through the outer third of its diameter and the spur is maintained by virtue of the glass tubing beneath the bowel.

Single-barreled type.—The establishment of a single-barreled inguinal stoma is an essential part of the radical operations of the abdominoperineal type, and in our experience is the most satisfactorily managed of any artificial anus. The technic is described in conjunction with the combined abdominoperineal operation in two stages. It is technically even less complicated than simple left inguinal loop colostomy. The stoma is made through a stab wound in the left flank, which is small and fits snugly around the bowel, and the liability to hernia or prolapse is considerably less common than in association with loop colostomy. Moreover, the disagreeable features of a blind segment of bowel, incident to loop colostomy, are avoided.

Transverse colostomy.—This procedure was favored by Allingham, and more recently has been advocated by Devine, Gurd, and by Heyd as a temporary, "disconnecting" type of colostomy and by Dennis, Fallis and Wangensteen as a simple loop colostomy for purposes of decompressing an acutely obstructed colon. Objections to permanent colostomy in the transverse colon are several: first, herniation is prone to occur; second, there is a tendency of the bowel content to maintain its semi-solid nature and make control over the colostomy less complete than when it is established in the sigmoid; and third, colostomy in the transverse colon, preceding resection, leaves a long, blind pouch of colon, which is apt to fill with fecal material despite most earnest measures for washing it out. Resulting discomfort is the rule rather than the exception.

A high, right rectus incision permits adequate exploration and the establishment of a colostomy in the transverse colon, which is loosened from the great omentum. Some prefer excision of the umbilicus and utilization of this site. Wangensteen, Fallis and Dennis advocate decompression of the acutely distended colon through a high, short, transverse right rectus incision.

Defunctionalization of colon and rectum.—According to Devine, who in 1938 described a method of defunctionalizing the colon, "a

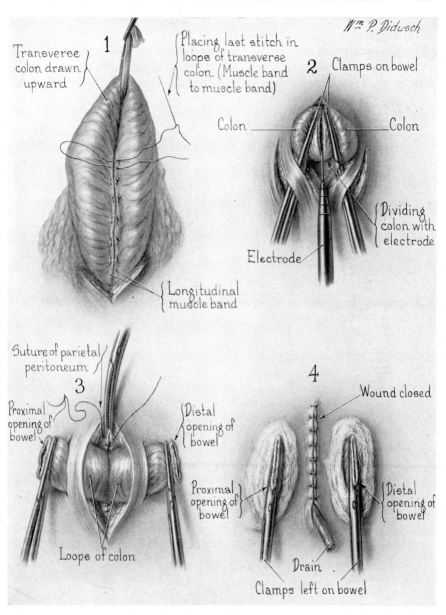

Wm. P. Didusch

1 — Transverse colon drawn upward / Placing last stitch in loops of transverse colon. (Muscle band to muscle band) / Longitudinal muscle band

2 — Clamps on bowel / Colon — Colon / Dividing colon with electrode / Electrode

3 — Suture of parietal peritoneum / Proximal opening of bowel / Distal opening of bowel / Loops of colon

4 — Wound closed / Proximal opening of bowel / Distal opening of bowel / Drain / Clamps left on bowel

Devine Colostomy

Fig. 80 (No. 1) Approximation of white bands by suture.
Fig. 81 (No. 2) Bowel segments clamped and colon divided by cautery.
Fig. 82 (No. 3) Exit of the proximal and distal loops.
Fig. 83 (No. 4) Final appearance of wounds of a Devine colostomy.
(From Heyd: courtesy of *Annals of Surgery*)

defunctionalized colon is one which has been completely disconnected from the alimentary canal so that it cannot be soiled in any way by even the smallest quantity of feces; one from which the fecal contents have been washed out and one which has been allowed to remain functionless until such time as the bacterial content has been considerably reduced; reduced on the principle that

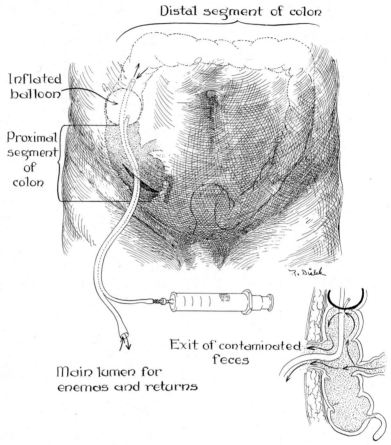

Fig. 84. Berman Method of defunctionalizing the colon. (From Berman: courtesy of *Surgery, Gynecology and Obstetrics*.)

if, experimentally, a segment of bowel be completely isolated and thus deprived of its function, it will lose most of its bacterial content." We have felt that the Devine type of "disconnecting" colostomy is an unnecessarily complicated procedure and are in agreement with Dennis, Fallis, Wangensteen, Allen and others who have expressed the belief that satisfactory defunctionalization as well as decompression can be obtained by a simple loop colostomy.

A detailed discussion of the merits and description of the technic of this measure are to be found in a recent, exceptionally well illustrated (Figs. 80, 81, 82, 83) article by Heyd, one of the foremost proponents of the Devine colostomy in this country.

Berman has recently described a simple method by which the colon may be defunctionalized. Through a temporary cecostomy or colostomy opening there is inserted a special double lumen tube to which an inflatable balloon is attached (Fig. 84). The tube is placed so that the balloon will be 4 to 5 inches distal to the opening in the bowel. The balloon is then inflated with the amount of air previously determined to obstruct the bowel, after which the segment of colon distal to the balloon may be cleansed by repeated irrigations. Allen, in 1947, credits his associate, Millet, with having devised a similar method which utilizes a Miller-Abbott tube that is inserted through a rent in a large cecostomy tube. Allen considers "this method to be so simple and thorough that preliminary transverse colostomy may be rarely needed in the future."

Division of colostomy.—This can be done in the patient's room with little inconvenience and practically no discomfort. The cautery is quite satisfactory in most instances but incision with a scalpel is simpler and avoids the odor of burning flesh and edema of the mucosa, particularly of the posterior wall, which so frequently follows employment of the cautery. Seldom is it necessary to ligate more than two or three small vessels when the scalpel is used, the remainder of the bleeding being readily controlled by hot wet compresses made of sponges. Even when employing the cautery it is frequently necessary to resort to ligatures, particularly in the presence of considerable fat.

REFERENCES

1. ALLEN, A. W., WELCH, C. E., DONALDSON, G. A.: Carcinoma of the colon. *Ann. Surg.*, **126**: 19–30 (July), 1947.
2. BERMAN, EDGAR F.: A new simplified method of defunctionalizing the colon. *Surg., Gynec., and Obstet.*, **79**: 419–426 (Oct.), 1944.
3. DENNIS, C.: Treatment of large bowel obstruction; transverse colostomy— Incidence of incompetency of ileocecal valve. *Surgery*, **15**: 713–734, 1944.
4. FALLIS, L. S.: Transverse colostomy. *Surgery*, **20**: 249 (Aug.), 1946.
5. HENDON, G. A.: Simple enterostomy technic. *Ann Surg.*, **94**: 156 (July), 1931.
6. HERRMANN, S. F.: Experimental peritonitis and peritoneal immunity. *Arch. Surg.*, **18**: 2202–2215 (May), 1929.
7. HEYD, C. G.: The increasing usefulness of the Devine colostomy in left colon and rectal surgery. *Ann. Surg.*, **116**: 913–923 (Dec.), 1942.
8. HIRSCHMAN: Quoted by Rankin.[7]
9. JONES, T. E.: Quoted by Rankin.[7]
10. LONG, J. W.: Enterostomy: a perfected technic illustrated. *Tr. South. Surg. Assn.*, **29**: 59–64, 1916.

11. RANKIN, F. W., and GRAHAM, A. STEPHENS: Surgery of the colon: chapter in Cyclopedia of Medicine. Philadelphia, F. A. Davis Co., 1932.
12. RANKIN, F. W.: Concerning colostomy. *South. Med. Jour.*, **29**: 130–139 (Feb.), 1936.
13. RANKIN, F. W.: The value of cecostomy as a complementary and decompressive operation. *Ann. Surg.*, **110**: 380–388 (Sept.), 1939.
14. SLIVE, A., SHOCK, D., FOGELSON, S. J.: Healing of the abdominal wall after loop colostomy. *Surg., Gynec., and Obstet.*, **78**: 525–526 (May), 1944.
15. WANGENSTEEN, O. H.: Intestinal obstruction, ed. 2, Springfield, Ill., 1942, Charles C Thomas, Publisher.

CHAPTER XIII

PROCEDURES FOR EXTIRPATION OF LESIONS OF THE COLON

Development of surgery of the colon is treated historically at the beginning of Part III. The factors determining selection of a procedure in the two halves of the colon are considered under "Choice of Operation." Before deciding on any type of operation in any portion of the colon, exploration of the abdomen should be carried out in the following order: the liver, the aortic glands, glands of bifurcation of the mesenteric vessels, the pelvis, and the growth and its adjacent structures. The growth itself must be palpated last, and it should be done carefully and gently. The information one obtains from palpation of the growth concerns complications, such as formation of abscess, its extent, its mobility, and the presence or absence of enlarged lymphatic structures in the vicinity, which may or may not be malignant, the determination being possible only by microscopic examination. Gentleness is essential since should an abscess be present, one might easily and unsuspectingly insert a finger into it. This will make another complication, and will force resection at an undesirable moment. Likewise, as is easily demonstrated, infection is spread from the primary growth throughout the peritoneal cavity by the examining hand because of the number and virulence of organisms in and around the growth.

Technical maneuvers for the removal of cancer of the colon differ in their application to the two halves because of the type and pathological processes present, the presence or absence of obstruction, and the local complications, such as fixation, abscess formation, and attachment to adjacent viscera, but the principle of radical extirpation of the gland-bearing tissues in juxtaposition to the growth is of paramount consideration. A better understanding of preoperative and postoperative mesaures, improvement in anesthetic methods, and the advent of chemotherapeutic agents permit the more frequent employment of primary anastomosis, with or without antecedent or simultaneous proximal drainage, by cecostomy or transverse colostomy. Graded operations, nevertheless, still are occasionally indicated.

RESECTION OF THE RIGHT HALF OF THE COLON

The factors which influence selection of a procedure in one or two stages are considered in detail under "Choice of Operation." In operating on the right half of the colon, it is our feeling that ileocolostomy between the teminal ileum and the transverse colon, followed by resection of the right segment at the same stage or a subsequent one, is the procedure of choice. The employment of the end-to-side anastomosis rather than lateral anastomosis is preferred in this particular instance because of the desirable feature which end-to-side method possesses over the lateral, in side-tracking the fecal current and allowing as much reduction of local inflammatory reaction around the growth as possible. Moreover, Cannon and Murphy and others have demonstrated by animal experimentation that lateral anastomosis is an unphysiologic procedure. The stasis that tends to develop at the new juncture and the concomitant attempt on the part of the normal segment of bowel proximal to this point to overcome the obstacle probably accounts for the upper abdominal discomfort frequently mentioned by patients in whom lateral anastomosis has been established. At the time this anastomosis is made, and we prefer the closed method which employs the Rankin clamp (Fig. 85), one may decide

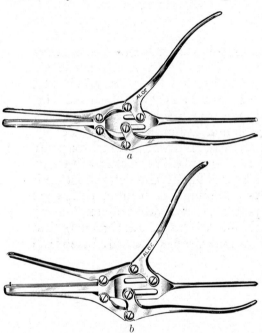

Fig. 85. The Rankin clamp for closed intestinal anastomosis and obstructive resection: *a*, narrow blade for intestinal anastomosis; *b*, wide blade for obstructive resection.

whether to do the resection, making the operation complete in one stage, or to abandon the procedure and extirpate at a subsequent stage the segment which harbors the neoplasm. This is a decision which must be made at the operating table in each case, on its own merits. Except for those cases in which subacute perforation or marked obstruction is encountered, a single-stage resection may be safely undertaken. The depleted and severely anemic patient can be readily rehabilitated preoperatively. In contemplating any method of anastomosis between two segments of bowel one must take into consideration certain important technical factors such as ability to approximate accurately the bowel edges, adequacy of blood supply, liability to obstruction from stricture formation

or excessive diaphragm, probability of hemorrhage, and danger
from contamination or subsequent leakage at the line of suture. In
our opinion, the end-to-side procedure (when the union is between
the colon and ileum), is attended by fewer technical difficulties in a
greater number of cases, and by less danger, than is the end-to-end
anastomosis, notwithstanding the general impression that the converse is true. One frequently encounters considerable disparity in
the diameters of the ends of bowel about to be united, even after
an attempt is made to compensate for this difference by dividing
the ileum at an angle. Further compensation must be made at the

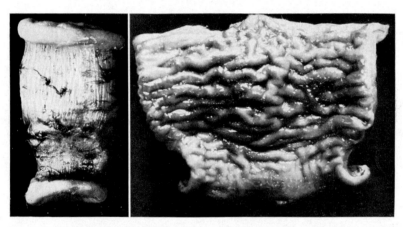

FIG. 86. (left) End-to-end anastomosis, Rankin clamp method. Specimen
unopened. Absence of bulging was observed at operation due to unequality
in size of bowel.
FIG. 87. (right) Specimen open. Complete absence of diaphragm at site of
operation.

expense of accurate approximation by continually taking wider
bites on the colonic side and in this manner produce a sort of pleat-
ing effect throughout its circumference. Not only does this tend to
prevent accurate union but it would seem to enhance the opportunity for contamination and subsequent leakage at the line of
suture. In well over 250 cases of end-to-side ileocolostomy by the
Rankin clamp technic, which include in addition to our own those
cases that have been reported to us by other surgeons, there has
not occurred a single postoperative hemorrhage. In our first 60
cases, which we reported on in 1932, there was no obstruction
at the site of the anastomosis, yet in only 3 instances was an
enterostomy established proximal to the anastomosis. Infection at
the site of union and subsequent leakage must be extremely rare
since it did not occur in our series, although two patients died and
one revealed evidences of peritonitis. In the latter cases there was
no evidence of leakage at the anastomosis on postmortem examina-

tion, but the growth in the cecum was large and infected, with evidences of subacute perforation. It is energetic palpation of such growths at the time of exploration that will more often be the cause of a fatal peritonitis than leakage about the line of suture. The good clinical results, we believe, bear out the experimental advantages demonstrated by one of us (Graham) in Mann's laboratory. The closed methods of anastomosis have been called fanciful procedures, aseptic in name only, but such disparagement and the theoretical objections advanced cannot stand in face of practical

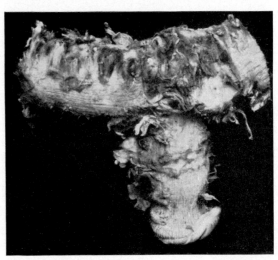

FIG. 88. End-to-side anastomosis, Rankin clamp method. Specimen has not been opened.

results. It is not our contention that our clamp method or the other so-called aseptic technics are actually aseptic from a strictly (Figs. 86 to 87) bacteriologic standpoint, but there is little question that the cleaner the anastomosis, the less likelihood of subsequent contamination. If resection is postponed to a second stage, experience dictates that the interval should be at least three weeks and often as long as five weeks.

Ileocolostomy by the Rankin clamp method.—Selection of an incision presents a real problem. The opinion generally expressed is that an abdominal wall is probably stronger after two incisions made at intervals through the same site, than after two incisions in close proximity. Formerly it was our custom, when it could be determined in advance that the contemplated resection would not be attempted at the initial operation, to make a left rectus incision which centered on the umbilicus. The current trend, however, of undertaking on most occasions a single-stage procedure has influenced us to discontinue this practice. We now make an upper right rectus incision in practically every instance. The terminal portion of the ileum, about ten to fifteen centimeters from the ileocecal valve is brought into the wound. Ordinarily it will be found necessary to tie but a few of the terminal branches of the mesenteric vessels just before they enter the intestinal wall. By avoiding the larger vascular branches and therefore disturbance to the circulation of the bowel, the technic is simplified and time is saved in that the necessity for removing a segment of bowel is eliminated. In order to secure as large an opening in the intestine as is possible

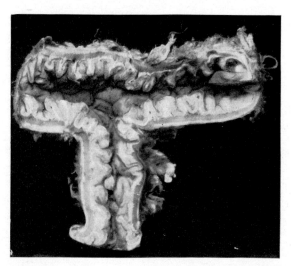

Fig. 89. Sagittal view of end-to-side anastomosis. Complete absence of diaphragm at site of anastomosis.

the special clamp is applied to the ileum at about an angle of 45°. A Payr, or any other suitable clamp, is applied distal to the first and as close to it as is possible, and the bowel between them is divided with a cautery; the cecal end is inverted and dropped back into the abdomen, to be removed with the colon (Figs. 90 to 93). Probably the simplest method of accomplishing this invagination is by crushing the ileum with a clamp, ligating with catgut at the crushed point and inverting the stump beneath a purse-string suture; in this way gross soiling is avoided. A site is now selected on the anterior surface of the transverse colon, ordinarily at about the juncture of the proximal and middle thirds unless the growth is at the hepatic flexure, in which case a more distal point is chosen. Allis forceps are then applied to the colon sufficiently far apart to assure an opening midway between the longitudinal bands, comparable in size to the diameter of the ileum, and with these forceps elevated the selected segment of colon is fixed by the free blade of the special clamp, one blade of which already contains the proximal portion of ileum (Fig. 91). The elliptical piece of colon which protrudes above the closed blade of the clamp is removed with a cautery, leaving the cauterized edges of the two pieces of bowel occupying positions exactly opposite each other.

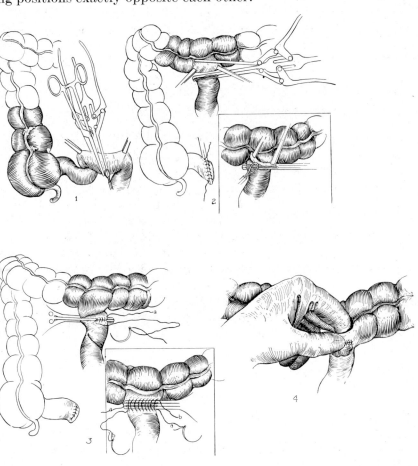

Fig. 90. (No. 1) Ileocolostomy, Rankin clamp technic: application of clamp to ileum. The blood supply in the mesentery has been tied off and the special clamp is applied at an angle so as to obtain a wider lumen for anastomosis. The bowel is divided with cautery.

Fig. 91. (No. 2) Ileocolostomy, Rankin clamp technic: The clamp is shown being applied to a point selected on the transverse colon for the colonic end of the anastomosis. Insert shows an elliptical portion of the colon being removed by cautery and the small bowel is shown approximated at this point. The cecal end of the divided ileum is being inverted.

Fig. 92. (No. 3) Ileocolostomy, Rankin clamp technic: Posterior layer of suture anastomosing the ileum and transverse colon. Insert shows clamp turned back to its original position and the anterior layer of sutures applied. (a) Posterior suture; (b) anterior suture.

Fig. 93. (No. 4) Ileocolostomy, Rankin clamp technic: The fingers introduced through the anastomosis to break up the agglutination which forms a diaphragm.

The clamp and the mobility of the transverse colon permit easy manipulation in establishing the anastomosis. The clamp is now turned completely over so as to bring the posterior side of the bowel into view. This permits accurate approximation of the peritoneal coats of the bowel on the under surface of the anastomosis because here the two arms of the bowel are in juxtaposition (Fig. 92). A continuous suture (our preference is chromic catgut to which a curved needle is welded) is employed and it is tied at one end locked at the other; the two ends are left long in order that the ends of the anterior suture may be tied to them after removal of the clamp. The clamp is now turned back to its original position and starting with a new suture (this should be an invariable rule) the anterior line of suture is applied by means of a continuous Cushing stitch which passes over the upper surface of the clamp; ties are not made at either end at this stage since to do so would defeat the purpose of this inverting type of suture. Preparations are now made for removing the clamp. An assistant grasps one of the long ends of the posterior suture in order to steady the bowel, and as the operator withdraws the clamp, the blades of which have been opened slightly, the assistant draws his end of the anterior suture taut, thus commencing the process of inversion. When the clamp has been completely withdrawn, the operator draws his end of the anterior suture taut and in this manner completes the inversion. The adhesion of the two ends of the bowel under the steady pressure keeps it intact as this step is carried out. Leakage at this stage has not occurred in any of our cases. The ends of the anterior suture are now tied with the corresponding ends of the posterior suture. Another layer of sutures, either continuous or interrupted, is inserted around the entire anastomosis and tags of fat and omentum are attached at both ends as a precaution against leakage. At this stage the wall of the colon is forced ahead of the fingers until they are felt to have passed through the anastomosis, in order to break out the agglutination which forms a diaphragm. We do not, as a rule, establish an enterostomy proximal to the anastomosis, for we have found that with the institution of proper preoperative cleansing measures, supplemented by a non-residue diet, simple decompression by means of suction applied to an indwelling duodenal tube is usually adequate protection to the suture line. Decompression with the Miller-Abbott tube may also be utilized here.

If resection of the proximal colon is to constitute a second stage the abdominal wound is closed in the usual manner and without drainage. It is important in these cases always to insert a rectal spool or rectal tube, which is left in place, except for cleansing, during the first seventy-two hours in order to prevent an increase in intra-colonic pressure.

Mobilization and resection.—Resection of the cecum and ascending colon, as the second step of the Rankin clamp method, is accomplished either immediately on completion of the ileocolostomy

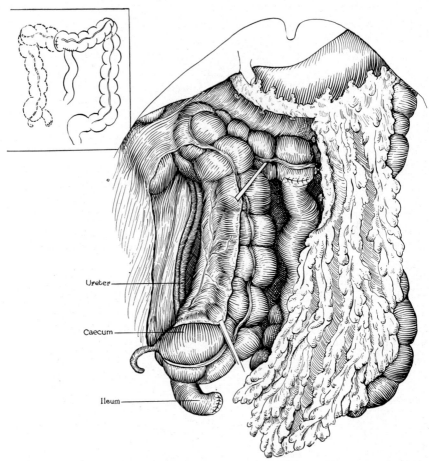

Fig. 94. Resection of the right half of the colon. Beginning mobilization of the cecum and ascending colon. An incision is made through the parietal attachment of bowel and the dissection made from without, inward. End-to-side ileocolostomy has been established (see Figures 90 to 93).

or at a second stage. Since exploration has been carried out at the first operation it is possible to proceed at once to the resection after the small intestines have been excluded from the operative field with packs. Beginning to mobilize the cecum and ascending colon, the outer leaf of the peritoneum, which is practically devoid of blood vessels, is incised and this entire segment is rotated toward

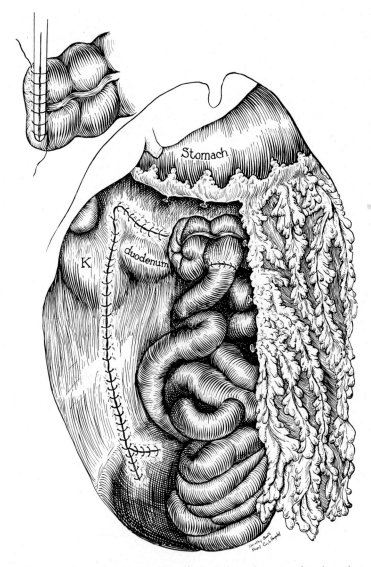

Fig. 95. Resection of the right half of the colon completed, and the raw surfaces left by the dissection have been closed by a continuous suture. Insert shows inversion of divided end of transverse colon (see Figure 88).

the mid-line, wiping inward with gauze, the fat, and lymphatic structures (Figs. 94 to 97). First the spermatic vessels and vas deferens, then the ureter, come into view as the dissection is carried upward. The former may or may not be sacrificed as seems indicated. Of more serious consideration is resection of the ureter which, fortunately, seldom is involved. When necessary, however, wide excision with ligation is preferable to anastomosis, provided the function of the other kidney is adequate. Atrophy of the kidney is the rule following ligation and if infection is present secondary nephrectomy may be necessary. The inverted terminal ileum is mobilized with its contiguous lymphatic tissue, and removed with the colon. As the hepatic flexure of the colon is freed of its attachments and rotated, the retroperitoneal portion of the duodenum appears and must be carefully avoided since injury to this structure is repaired with difficulty and carries with it a high mortality.

Up to this point the necessity for ligation of blood vessels seldom occurs, a circumstance arising from the fact that in the embryonic development of the colon it revolves around the superior mesenteric vessels as an axis and becomes attached along the lateral abdominal parites by fusion of the peritoneum of its outer layer with the lateral parietal peritoneum. The mesenteric vessels, which are entirely mesial along the whole course of the ascending colon, now come clearly into view and may be clamped and ligated as encountered. The operation can be simplified and shortened by ligating the vessels to the segment of colon involved in their central position, i.e., the ileocolic, the right colic, and the marginal arteries just proximal to the anastomosis (Fig. 17). This necessitates careful identification of vessels and may not be feasible if the patient is obese. In order to insure adequate blood supply to the transverse colon at the site of division just proximal to the ileocolostomy much care should be exercised in ligations carried out in this vicinity. Venous oozing originating in retroperitoneal structures from which fat and lymphatic tissue has been dissected is readily controlled by hot, wet gauze packs.

A satisfactory point is chosen in the transverse colon 5 to 7 centimeters proximal to the anastomosis between the ileum and colon and the bowel is divided between clamps with a cautery (Fig. 95). The clamped end of divided colon is then inverted with a catgut suture, the ends of which are left long and brought out through the end of the wound at which point the closed bowel is fixed to the peritoneum (Fig. 96). These serve as a guide for puncture of the bowel if intracolonic pressure should increase too much. Twice in a series of 46 cases a spontaneous colonic fistula developed as a result of increased pressure within the colon and in both instances closure likewise was spontaneous. This maneuver, suggested by C. H. Mayo, is an important safeguard and may well be employed routinely when the end-to-side type of anastomosis is consummated.

Peritonealization of the raw surfaces should always be practiced as a safeguard against small bowel obstruction. It is our practice to establish drainage to these cases regularly, not because of

contamination, but because serum collects in the large raw retroperitoneal spaces and, latent infection often being present, ab-
cesses form. By the use of Penrose drains with gauze and a split
rubber tube, the former of which is removed at the end of forty-
eight hours, we have been able to largely avoid this unpleasant
complication.

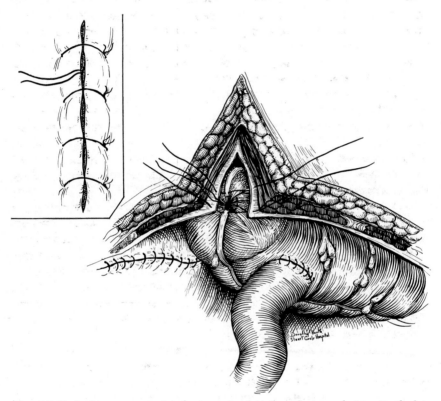

FIG. 96. End of transverse colon just proximal to ileocolostomy being attached to
the peritoneum at the upper angle of the wound (C. H. Mayo method).

Alternative procedures.—Following resection of the right half of
the colon, continuity may be restored by end-to-end, end-to-side,
or side-to-side anastomosis, which may be accomplished by the
open suture method, the closed, clamp technics, or basting-stitch
technic of Parker-Kerr.

1. The Parker-Kerr method, which in our hands has proved entirely satisfactory, is described elsewhere (p. 296).

2. The open end-to-end anastomosis is preferred by many surgeons and from the standpoint of ultimate functional results is
entirely satisfactory. However, it has been our experience that in
a number of instances a two-stage procedure is desirable. Under

such circumstances it would be necessary either to form a lateral or an end-to-side anastomosis. Moreover, one frequently encounters considerable disparity in the diameter of the ends of the bowel about to be united, even after an attempt is made to compensate for this difference by dividing the ileum at an angle. Further com-

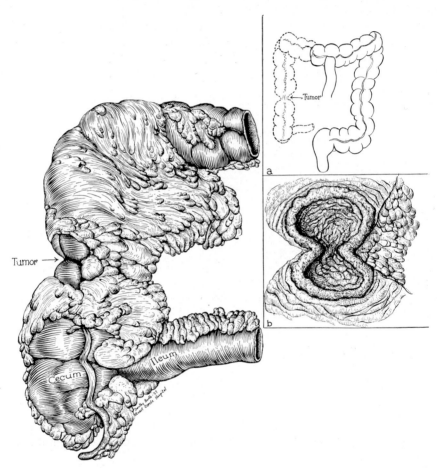

Fig. 97. Resection of the right half of the colon. Drawing of resected specimen of a carcinoma of the ascending colon. *a*, Schematic representation of the extent of the resection and the completed operation; *b*, annular ulcerating adenocarcinoma, graded 3.

pensation must be made at the expense of accurate approximation by continually taking wider bites on the colonic side. Not only does this prevent accurate union but it would seem to enhance the opportunity for contamination and subsequent leakage at the line of suture. In performing open anastomosis it is of paramount importance that the strictest possible attention be given to technical accuracy and avoidance of contamination. Division of the bowel should be extra-abdominal, after the peritoneal cavity has been carefully protected with large moist gauze packs and soft-bladed, rubber covered clamps have been applied to either limb of bowel. It should be remembered that the bacteria inhabiting the terminal ileum and colon are of considerably greater virulence than is encountered in the stomach and jejunum. In making the axial anastomosis the disparity in the size between the ileum and colon is partially overcome by incising the small bowel opposite its mesenteric border for a distance of 1 to 2 cm. and rounding off the angular flaps which are formed. The disproportion is further overcome by cutting the bowel at an angle of 45°, and at the same time a better blood supply is obtained. The anastomosis is accomplished in the usual manner. The mucosa is sutured to mucosa by a continuous suture of catgut to which is welded a straight or curved needle, as personal inclination may prompt. A second row of sutures incorporates the musculoserous coats, special care being taken at the mesenteric border because of the excess of adipose tissue usually encountered there. Moreover, in consummating a circular suture there is danger of diminishing the lumen by exerting too much tension on the suture as it is placed. In order to guard against this the left forefinger and thumb may be held in the opening, the anastomosis being made between them. Finally, interrupted silk sutures are placed, tags of omentum being incorporated in these.

Side-to-side open anastomosis possesses objectional features from the standpoint of ultimate functional results, which have been discussed fully under "Choice of Operation." Our personal experience with this method tends to bear out the experimental objections of Cannon and Murphy. However, this type of anastomosis has been advocated by a few surgeons who state that mortality is less than for end-to-end or end-to-side anastomosis, and that the vascularity of the cut ends of the bowel is more readily insured. Sufficient statistical proof of such claims is lacking. The anastomosis is accomplished by the same technic as gastro-enterostomy.

3. In addition to our closed method of anastomosis, accomplished over the narrow-bladed model of the Rankin clamp, and which has been described above, there are available a number of other clamp technics which have proved highly satisfactory in the hands of many surgeons. Clamps over which anastomosis can be made have been described by Allen, Young, Stone and Furness. The Furness clamp has been modified by Clute and again by McClure. A modification of the Stone clamp has been devised by Welch.

As advocates of closed anastomosis, we believe it is more desirable because it diminishes if it does not abolish the element of infection, and experience has shown that it may be accomplished with ease and satisfaction in the hands of most surgeons. At the same time it would be extremely dogmatic to urge that any single operative method to accomplish an objective so far outbalanced the advantages of all other methods as to make it indispensable. Elements of personality and circumstance must inevitably influence the choice of technic, and in consequence, the range of maneuvers continues wide and at the same time acceptable so long as fundamental principles are observed. The utilization of absorbable or non-absorbable materials likewise is more a matter of personal choice than of grave importance and arbitrary pronouncements, relative to the advantages of one type of anastomosis or one type of suture are rarely fundamentally sound.

RESECTION OF THE LEFT HALF OF THE COLON

In the left half of the colon, by which is meant the major portion of the transverse colon, the descending colon and sigmoid, the choice of operation is between (1) a graded procedure, such as obstructive resection, and (2) primary resection with immediate anastomosis; either procedure with or without antecedent or concomitant proximal drainage. The factors that determine selection of the one or the other are considered under "Choice of Operation." Although we are fully aware of the advantages of immediate anastomosis and consider it the procedure of election in many instances, we also recognize the merits of multistage, extraperitoneal resection and still believe it is indicated in a relatively high percentage of cases. Other surgeons who, in 1947, also hold this view are: T. E. Jones, who performs obstructive resection altogether for lesions of the distal colon; David, Lahey, Cattell and Daniel, who employ primary anastomosis only in 5 to 15 per cent of these cases; and Cole and McFee who utilize this measure in not more than 25 per cent of instances. In our experience obstructive resection accomplished with the Rankin clamp has proved to be a most satisfactory operation from the standpoint both of hospital mortality and remote mortality from metastasis. We continue to employ it in approximately 65 per cent of cases. In the remainder we perform primary resection with immediate anastomosis, usually without complementary proximal drainage.

Obstructive resection.—This multiple-stage procedure, which employs the Rankin clamp (Fig. 82), permits primary resection of the lesion and its contiguous lymph-node-bearing tissue with subsequent restoration of the lumen of the bowel. It is applicable to any portion of the colon that is mobile or mobilizable. The procedure is contraindicated in the presence of obstruction which should be first relieved by medical measures of decompression, cecostomy, or colostomy. The operation is performed in two or three stages: (1) resection of segment of bowel harboring the growth; (2) destruction

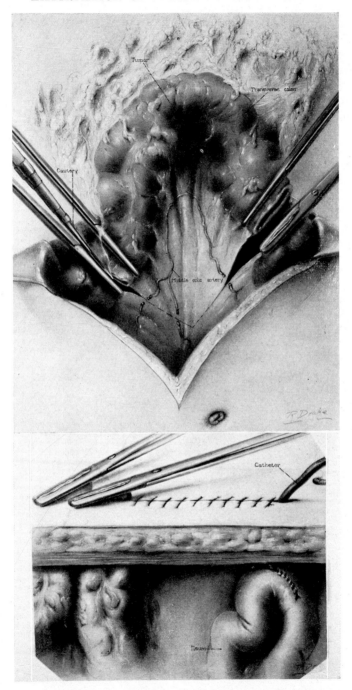

FIG. 98. Obstructive resection as originally performed and reported (Rankin) in 1924. A special clamp is now employed (Figure 85). Above, resection transverse colon; Below, clamps *in situ* and enterostomy established.

of the colostomy spur by the application of clamps; and (3) surgical closure of the colostomy stoma when this is not of spontaneous occurrence.

First stage.—This is comparable to the first two stages of the exteriorization operation (Figs. 98 to 105). An incision is made over the site of the growth and abdominal exploration is carried out in the manner described at the beginning of this chapter. If the transverse colon is the structure involved the omentum is first dissected away from the bowel. If the growth is in the sigmoid, and it most

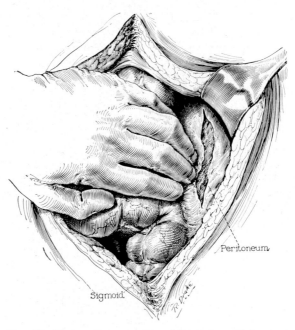

Fig. 99. Obstructive resection of the colon. Abdominal incision exposing carcinoma of the sigmoid which is mobilized by incising the avascular lateral parietal peritoneum.

frequently is, the involved segment is delivered into the wound after the parietal peritoneal attachments are severed in order to insure adequate mobility, the operating table is placed in the Trendelenburg position and the small bowel is excluded from the operative field with large moist gauze packs (Fig. 99).

The thoroughly mobilized bowel is held in such a way that the vessels can be clearly seen. These are now ligated close to the root of the mesentery and the intervening expanse of mesentery with its regional lymph nodes is widely excised (Fig. 100). The special three-bladed (Rankin) clamp, which we also employ for aseptic anastomosis, is applied to the two limbs of colon, special attention being paid at this stage to insure ample blood supply to the terminal ends of the divided colon (Fig. 85). The clamp should be applied so that the handle subsequently may rest on the abdomen. From the opposite direction, just above this clamp, another is placed and between these the bowel is divided with a cautery (Fig.

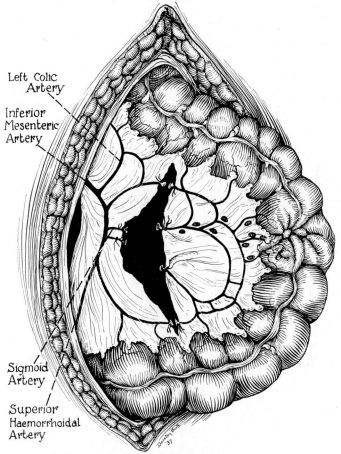

Left Colic
    Artery

Inferior
Mesenteric
Artery

Sigmoid
Artery

Superior
Haemorrhoidal
Artery

FIG. 100. Obstructive resection of the colon. The mesenteric blood vessels are ligated near their points of origin and a wide expanse of mesentery is sacrificed.

101). The divided mesentery is accurately closed without placing sutures in the bowel and lateral to the resected bowel, when the sigmoid is involved, the raw surfaces are carefully peritonealized (Figs. 102 and 103). The clamp holding the two ends of bowel is now brought out of the wound in such a manner as to leave the structures loose. The wound is now closed, layer by layer, close to the limbs of colon, and peritoneum is pulled between the two, under

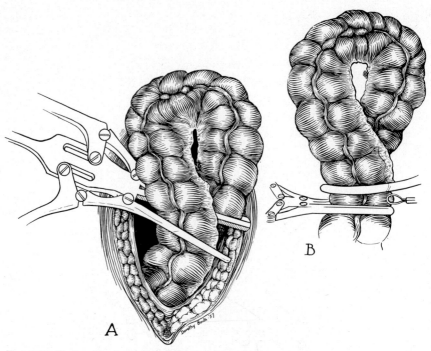

FIG. 101. Obstructive resection. Mobilization completed. *A*, The special clamp (see Figure 85) has been applied to the proximal limb of bowel and the distal limb is about to be fixed by the other blade of the clamp; *B*, shows the exteriorized segment of colon being removed with cautery.

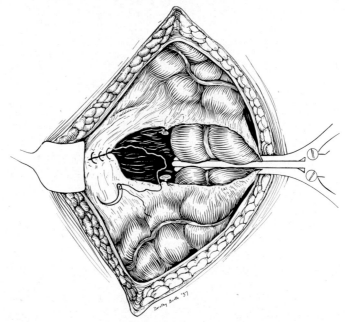

FIG. 102. Obstructive resection. The growth has been removed and the special clamp rotated laterally to facilitate closure of the rent in the mesocolon.

the clamp, to be sutured to peritoneum of the opposite side (Figs. 104 and 105). No sutures are placed in the bowel. At times when the loop of sigmoid is very short and cannot be exteriorized readily, we do not hesitate to leave the end of the clamp, grasping the bowel ends, deep in the wound. In such instances, however, iodoform gauze is wrapped around the bowel, beneath the clamp, so as to avoid contamination in case of leakage due to some technical mishap. Noting that when the bowel ends were thus left deeply placed,

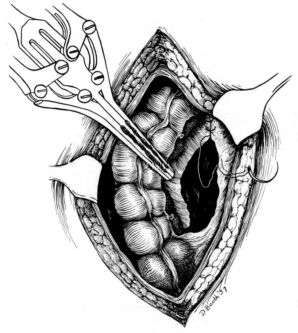

Fig. 103. Obstructive resection. The lateral raw surfaces are being peritonealized.

beneath the muscles, spontaneous closure occurred in almost every instance following destruction of the colostomy spur, we have adopted this technic even in instances of growths situated in readily mobilizable portions of the bowel.

The bowel is left completely obstructed for at least forty-eight hours and often for as long as seventy-two hours. This obstruction, however, is well tolerated if proper preoperative cleansing measures have been instituted and a low residue diet has been adhered to. In those cases of obstruction which fail to respond to such preoperative treatment cecostomy should be resorted to before obstructive resection is attempted. When it seems advisable to relieve the obstruction the proximal blade of the clamp is opened but the distal blade is left attached to the distal end of bowel, until the clamp drops off, which usually occurs about the sixth day. If the agglutinated proximal end of the bowel on release of the blade is probed opened, this should be done with great care lest the peritoneal cavity be inadvertently entered; ordinarily it is better to allow the distention from pressure of gas within the colon to force it open. Contrary to a widespread belief among surgeons, ends of the bowel brought out of the abdominal wounds for the purpose of establishing a colostomy or ileostomy do not frequently recede into the ab-

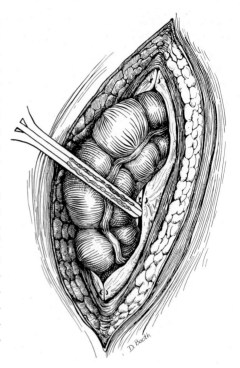

FIG. 104. Obstructive resection. The peritoneum is brought under the loop and is sutured snugly around all sides. No sutures are placed in the bowel itself.

domen. We have never observed such an occurrence, even when the ends of the bowel were left deep within the wound and despite the fact we have never sutured the peritoneum to the bowel. (For the care of these wounds, see "Postoperative Treatment.")

The principle of obstructive resection has been applied in selected cases to lesions of the rectosigmoid but very seldom in recent years.

Second stage (application of clamps to the colos-

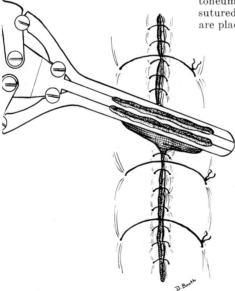

FIG. 105. Obstructive resection. The wound is closed and the clamp is *in situ*, the handle of which rests upon the abdomen.

tomy spur).—One practical point which seems worthy of emphasis is the length of time which one should wait before attempting
to cut out the spur of the colostomy. The general tendency, not
only of the patient, but of the surgeon also, is to hurry to finish
the operative procedure. When one considers the great amount
of edema which is present in and between the two loops of bowel
after the operation has been accomplished, one realizes that it
is a matter of several weeks' waiting before the spur may be safely
and deeply incised. Six weeks or two months is not too long in
the majority of cases to wait before application of clamps, and
during this time the patient returns home to a normal mode of

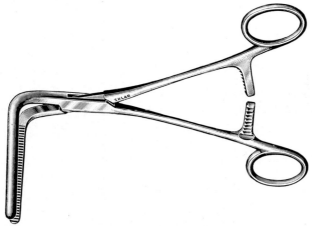

Fig. 106. Warthen enterotome for destruction of the colostomy
spur.

life and acquires a bowel habit suitable to his new colostomy sur-
roundings. As a result of this policy of delay more than one-half of
the fistulas which we have made following obstructive resection
have closed spontaneously. For those which do not close spontaneously after a reasonable length of time, or for those in which the indications seem to favor a deliberate closure of the colostomy by
suture, we have found some points in technic which are described
here and which have served us advantageously in a reasonably
large series of cases.

In our experience the Warthen enterotome (Fig. 106) has proved
to be one of the most useful of the special appliances but the long
curved Kelly-Pean forceps (Fig. 107c) is also satisfactory. Into each
of the two openings of the bowel a blade of one of these clamps
is introduced, care being taken to maneuver the tips under the
guidance of the finger away from the mesenteric border. The clamp
is closed after it has been inserted as deeply as possible to the first
notch (Fig. 107c). On each subsequent day the clamps are tightened

one notch and by pressure necrosis they slowly penetrate the spur without the fear of opening into the peritoneal cavity. Usually the septum is completely cut through in five or six days (Fig. 107d), although occasionally the clamps hang on for a matter of eight or nine days. It is safer to wait until the clamps either drop over onto the abdominal wall when the supporting dressings are removed for their daily change, than to make any pull upward to deliver them from the wound. Occasionally when the clamps stick a bit at the end of what seems a sufficient time for them to cut through, and one impatiently pulls on them, hemorrhage results which is difficult to control. The application of these clamps is not a very painful procedure and usually is satisfactorily accomplished under either a hypodermic of morphine, or some preliminary barbiturate preparation.

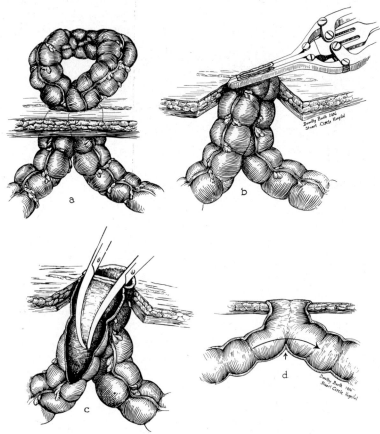

Fig. 107. Schematic representation of exteriorization procedures which necessitate reestablishment of the bowel continuity and closure of colostomy: a, The Block or so called Mikulicz type of exteriorization; b, obstructive resection employing the Rankin clamp; c, application of clamp to the septum separating the approximated loops of bowel; d, the septum has been removed and the bowel continuity restored.

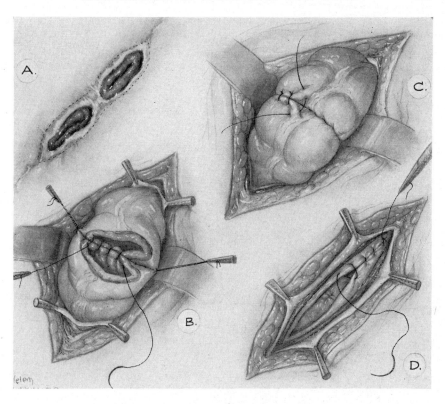

Fig. 108. Closure of colostomy (intraperitoneal): a, double-barreled colostomy; b, the ends of bowel have been entirely freed of adhesive attachments to the abdominal wall and the end-to-end anastomosis commenced; c, anastomosis being completed with interrupted non-absorbable sutures; d, the anastomosed bowel has been returned to the abdomen and the abdomen is being closed.

Third stage (closure of colostomy).—In contemplating closure of colostomy, especially if the operation has been made through the rectus muscle, preparation should be made for a formidable procedure because it is frequently necessary to repair a ventral hernia in this location in addition to a plastic operation on the bowel. Primary healing of the wound and the closure of a hernia in the face of a colostomy, in spite of the extensive dissection of the abdominal layers, is generally a pleasant surprise to the operator who finds that the rule is not an infected wound, but merely a short period of serous drainage.

The closure of the colonic stoma can usually be accomplished extraperitoneally. However, occasionally the loss of substance is more than has been figured upon, and it may be necessary to mobilize the involved segment of bowel and make what amounts to almost an end-to-end anastomosis. Moreover, an intraperitoneal end-to-end anastomosis is necessary in order to close a loop colos-

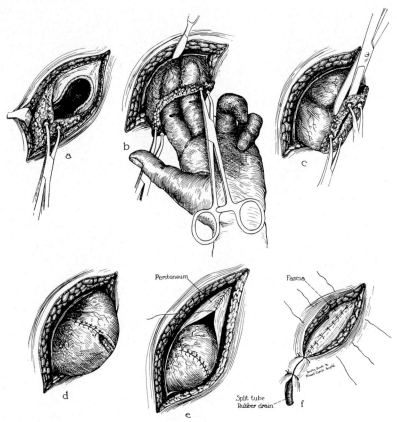

FIG. 109. Closure of colostomy: *a*, Elliptical incisions encircle the stoma and extend down through the fascia and muscle; *b*, the index and middle fingers of the left hand inserted into the two loops of bowel act as tractors and facilitate dissection; *c*, immobilization complete, the edges of the bowel ends are trimmed clean of the margin of skin; *d*, the opening in the colon is sutured with two rows of chromic catgut in the transverse diameter of the bowel; *e*, abdominal cavity, and the peritoneum sutured with catgut; *f*, the fascia is closed with interrupted sutures of catgut and wicks of rubber tissue placed down to the fascia.

tomy, the divided ends of which are separated by an inch or so of skin (Fig. 108). We have described (1937) a technic for closure of colostomy (Fig. 109) as follows: Elliptical incisions encircle the stoma and extend down through the fascia and muscle to the peritoneum. The skin border of the stoma, thus produced, is grasped by forceps which serve as tractors in elevating the limbs of the bowel. When the bowel has been opened down to the peritoneum by dissecting back on each side and exposing the fascia and muscles, we have found it particularly advantageous to insert the index and middle fingers of the left hand into the two loops of bowel, using them as tractors to lift the bowel up and thus facilitate exposure.

The practical advantages of this procedure which minimize the danger of injury to the bowel and opening into the peritoneal cavity decidedly outweigh the theoretical objections which may be offered. Immunity to infection which the tissues in the vicinity acquire makes careful preliminary closure of the stoma unnecessary, and in our feeling, undesirable. The dissection to free the loop is a cautious one, carried out by a sharp scalpel close to the bowel. When one comes down to the peritoneal cavity one may dissect it free enough to leave the peritoneum attached to where it originally adhered, but infrequently he may, with blunt gauze dissection, wipe it back carefully without opening into the peritoneal cavity. When there is considerable fatty tissue present, there is more liability to injury to the colon when dissecting through the subcutaneous layers than elsewhere. Occasionally the peritoneal attachment may be very close to the stoma and therefore limit the extent of the dissection. Fortunately, firm adhesions generally wall off the abdominal cavity so that even with the division of the peritoneum close to the bowel the general cavity is not usually entered. If accidentally a rent does occur, it should be closed at once; the operator continues to exert tension on the loop with two fingers of the left hand in the bowel while with the other hand he puts in one or two sutures and the assistant ties them quickly, thus shutting off any danger of contamination.

When the exteriorized ends are completely free of attachments down to the peritoneum, the edges are trimmed clean of the margin of skin which has been left on them and the arms are sutured together with two rows of chromic catgut in the transverse diameter of the bowel. If there is plenty of room and it seems essential, a third layer of sutures may be employed, but silk sutures are usually not desirable in this location because of the danger of contamination and prolonged drainage due to irritation of a foreign body.

Regardless of the type of colostomy, whether of the loop variety or of two divided ends, the result of resection of a segment of bowel, the necessity for suture is usually restricted to the anterior part of the bowel. If there is disparity in the size between the openings of the two ends of bowel, produced not infrequently by the distention of the proximal segment of colon as the result of long-standing obstruction, this may be overcome by splitting the entire thickness of the bowel with the smaller lumen opposite its mesentery and rounding off the angular flaps which are formed.

Before closing the abdominal wound it is flushed out with large quantities of warm saline solution, followed by ether. The fascia is closed with interrupted sutures, leaving sufficient space between to permit escape of gas and feces to prevent obstruction. Wicks of rubber tissue are placed down to the fascia, to be removed after forty-

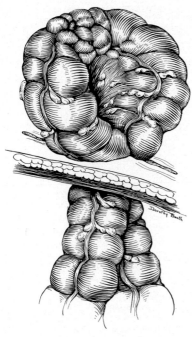

Fig. 110. Exteriorization procedure involving segment of bowel delivered through the abdominal wall (see also Figure 107).

eight hours. The edges of the skin margin are approximated loosely.

A decided improvement in the handling of these wounds has been noted during the past two years since we adopted a new postoperative regime (see "Postoperative Treatment").

Exteriorization procedure (Mikulicz type). The type of operation known popularly by the name of Mikulicz, which is a modification of the original procedures of Paul and of Block, cannot be employed in very obese individuals. It is impossible to apply it when the mesentery is short, without sacrifice of the blood supply, and once the blood supply is ligated and the bowel exteriorized, one finds at the end of forty-eight hours a foul, thick, pregangrenous tumor from which not only wound infection but actual peritonitis frequently takes place (Fig. 110). In our experience the old type of Mikulicz procedure is seldom justified but on rare occasions may be applied to a small, constricting, scirrhous growth, in a mobile segment of the colon of an elderly patient who constitutes a grave risk for an extensive operative procedure, provided the involved segment, under local or light general anesthesia, can be rapidly exteriorized without manipulation or attempts at extensive mobilization.

The technic is as follows: The involved segment of bowel is mobilized and delivered into the wound as described in the obstructive type of resection but the mesenteric blood vessels and lymphatic structures are left intact. The abdomen is now closed snugly around the exteriorized mass, which is surrounded with vaseline gauze in an attempt to prevent transplantation of carcinoma cells to the abdominal wall. The second stage, which should be delayed six or seven days if possible, consists in the excision of the exteriorized segment, flush with the abdomen. This is usually accomplished without anesthesia. The third and fourth stages correspond to the second and third stages, respectively, of the obstructive resection, described above. Formerly, it was a not uncommon practice, in cases of marked obstruction, to excise the extruded segment of bowel at once and insert a large tube (Paul method) in the proximal part of the lumen. This procedure, however, is a hazardous one; cecostomy or colostomy is far safer and more satisfactory.

Primary intestinal anastomosis.—The factors which determine selection of a multiple-stage procedure or primary resection and immediate anastomosis in the distal half of the colon have been considered under "Choice of Operation" and also at the beginning of this section. The choice of method of accomplishing the anastomosis is between an open technic (Fig. 108) and a closed, so-called aseptic technic such as described by Parker and Kerr, Furness, Frasier and Dott, Stone, Rankin, and Young,

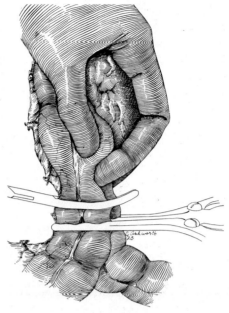

FIG. 111. End-to-end anastomosis over Rankin clamp. Segment ready for removal with cautery. One clamp above the anastomosis line catches both limbs of the bowel to be removed (see Figure 85).

all of which are satisfactory in the hands of those experienced in their employment. The simplicity of accomplishment, and the ease of adaptation to circumstances, make the Parker-Kerr basting-stitch and the Rankin clamp methods entirely satisfactory in performing resection and anastomosis with the minimum of contamination.

Rankin clamp method.—The narrow rather than the wide-bladed model should be employed for anastomosis (Fig. 85). The latter was devised primarily for employment in obstructive resection. Mobilization of the involved segment of bowel, ligation of vessels, dissection of the mesenteric lymphatic structures, and application of the clamp to the two limbs of bowel is carried out as described above under "Obstructive Resection" (Figs. 111 to 114).

Owing to the comparatively scanty anastomosis between the small terminal arteries in the wall of the colon and the greater vascular supply to the mesocolic two-thirds of the bowel, the colon should be cut at an angle (Fig. 13) in order that a greater part of vascular mesocolic portion be retained than the amesocolic third. If the colon is cut perpendicular to its axis, the incision may just include one of the long terminal branches to the amesocolic portion, thus destroying for perhaps 2.5 cm. the only supply to a naturally impoverished portion of the bowel. The blood supply is also endangered when an effort is made to clear fat from the colon, owing to the subserosal course of the long terminal arteries. In elevating and clamping fat tabs and epiploic appendages it is easy to include the long artery, especially if the colon is contracted and there is

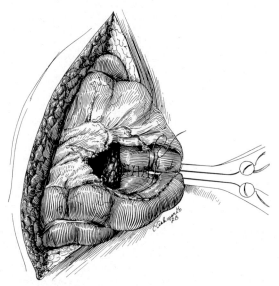

Fig. 112. End-to-end anastomosis (Rankin clamp method). The first layer of sutures being applied posteriorly. See also figures 113-114.

increased redundancy of the arteries (Fig. 15). We have found it advisable in many instances to clamp and then to cut between the two with a cautery before carrying out a similar manipulation on the distal end. This permits one to gauge the exact amount of bowel which may be sacrificed and to determine the possibility of establishing anastomosis without tension and with adequate supply of blood to the ends.

If the clamp is put on the bowel with the handle away from the operator, the posterior line of sutures is made more accessible. The clamp is rotated laterally so as to bring the posterior side of the colon into view (Fig. 112). A continuous suture (our preference is chromic catgut to which a curved needle is welded) is applied; the suture is tied at one end and locked at the other. The two ends are left long in order that the ends of the anterior may be tied to them after removal of the clamp. The clamp is turned back to its original position, and starting with a new suture (this should be an invariable rule), the anterior line of suture is applied by means of a continuous Cushing stitch which passes over the upper surface of the clamp; ties are not made at either end at this stage since to do so would defeat the purpose of the inverting type of suture (Fig. 113a). Preparations are now made for removing the clamp. An assistant grasps the long end of the posterior suture on his side in order to steady the bowel as the operator withdraws the clamp, the

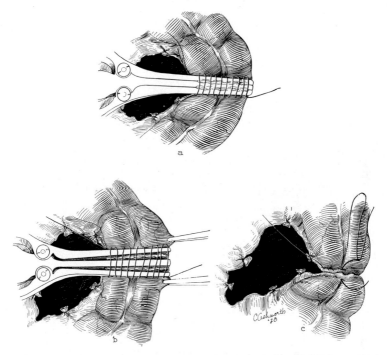

FIG. 113. End-to-end anastomosis (Rankin clamp method). Resection has been made. a, Suture applied on anterior side of the bowel with continuous peritoneal stitch; b, clamp unlocked ready to be withdrawn after which the suture will be drawn taut, inverting the end of the bowel; c, completed operation and final row of sutures being placed around the anastomosis.

blades of which have been opened slightly (Fig. 113b). Simultaneously, the assistant draws his end of the anterior suture taut, thus commencing the process of inversion. When the clamp has been completely withdrawn, the operator draws his end of the anterior suture taut and in this manner completes the inversion. The adhesions of the two ends of the bowel under the steady pressure of the clamp keep it intact as this step is carried out and leakage does not occur. The ends of the anterior suture are now tied with the corresponding ends of the posterior suture. Another layer of sutures, usually interrupted and of nonabsorbable material, is inserted around the entire anastomosis, and tags of fat or omentum are attached at both ends as a precaution against leakage. At this stage the wall of the colon is forced ahead of the fingers until they are felt to have passed through the anastomosis, in order to break out the agglutination which forms a diaphragm (Fig. 114a). The opening in the mesentery is closed with interrupted sutures of fine catgut.

Parker-Kerr basting-stitch method.—In anastomosis by this method (Fig. 115) the involved segment of bowel is mobilized, brought out of the wound, and the vessels in the mesentery ligated. Small Payr clamps are applied separately to the two limbs of bowel at levels at which adequate circulation to the divided ends will be

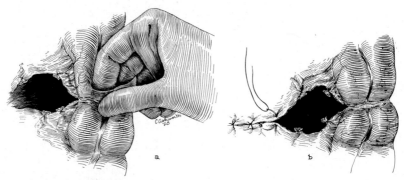

FIG. 114. *a*, Finger introduced through the anastomosis to break up the agglutination which forms a diaphragm; *b*, the operation is completed with two layers of sutures. Closure of the rent in the mesentery is made with interrupted sutures.

assured; in close apposition to these, two other forceps are applied from the tumor side and the bowel is divided by cautery between the two sets of clamps. The basting stitch is applied first to one clamped end of bowel, then the other, with the loops between the stitches passing over the clamp. The first and last stitches are placed under the clamps on the free mesenteric border of the colon, running parallel to its axis. The remaining stitches are placed at right angles to the axis of the bowel. In our experience, pressure from the crushing clamps has proved adequate in the control of hemorrhage in the wall of the colon. The free ends of the stitches are drawn taut as the clamps are opened and withdrawn. The two crushed ends of the bowel, thus inverted, are brought into apposition and held in this position by traction on the basting stitch. A continuous suture of catgut anastomoses the abutted ends of the colon, on the completion of which the two basting stitches are withdrawn. The crushed adherent ends are opened by inverting the bowel wall through the stoma with forefinger and thumb and while being held in this manner a second layer of silk or catgut is applied. The operation is complete with closure of the opening in the mesentery.

This method may be employed even where there is considerable disparity between the two ends to be anastomosed, for it is only necessary to pucker the larger end of bowel in order to secure satisfactory approximation. Axial, lateral, or end-to-end anastomosis can be accomplished by the Parker-Kerr method.

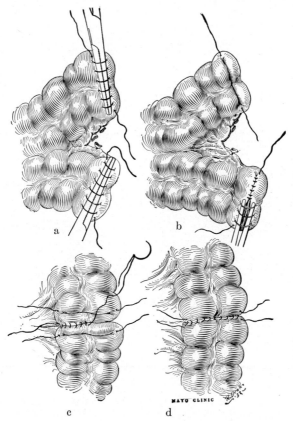

FIG. 115. Parker-Kerr basting-stitch anastomosis: *a*, The basting stitch is being applied over the clamp; *b*, inversion and peritonealization of the divided ends of the bowel are accomplished by withdrawal of the clamps and tightening the basting stitch; *c*, the anastomosing suture is being applied to the blind ends of the bowel; *d*, complete anastomosis, withdrawing the basting stitch. Reinforcing sutures may now be applied.

TOTAL COLECTOMY

The debilitation resulting from prolonged diarrhea, blood loss and chronic infection, and the pathologic knowledge of the high incidence of malignant change occurring in diffuse adenomatosis of the colon, are the factors that have made radical surgical treatment imperative. To remove a part of the involved bowel, leaving diseased segments, has proved a temporizing benefit at best. Obviously then, to be permanently free from the process, treatment had to be designed to remove the whole colon.

Colectomy when first performed was a formidable procedure and, when undertaken in one stage without considerable preparation and rehabilitation carried a high mortality. A temporary ileostomy was soon devised and its value or necessity was immediately ap-

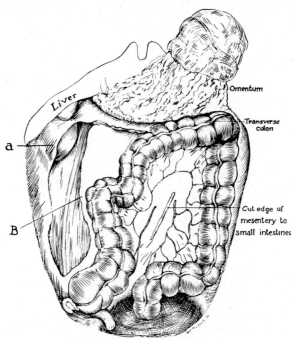

Fig. 116. Second stage of colectomy: The mobilization of the colon is shown beginning from right to left by dividing the lateral perietal peritoneal attachments of the mesentery of the bowel, saving sufficient peritoneum for covering raw surfaces. The omentum is retracted upward with the stomach and is saved (see Figure 75).

preciated. By sidetracking the fecal current in this way the associated infection subsided and the rectal discharges of blood and mucus were greatly reduced to allow for marked general improvement. The patient's weight usually registered an appreciable increase, the secondary anemia was frequently overcome without aid of transfusion, and the patient's general health was more sturdy and able to withstand the shock of a major surgical procedure. With the colon at rest and peristalsis at low ebb, the infection and some of the polyps readily subside and make the colon more easily manageable when resection is undertaken. Otherwise the thick-walled, infected bowel is difficult to suture satisfactorily and may often be the source of a fatal peritonitis when manipulated. An optimal period of about three months is desirable for an ileostomy. In addition to allowing for favorable changes in the colon, the ileum is given time for necessary adjustments vital to restoration of fluid balance. At first the substance issuing from the ileostomy is liquid and more or less continuous, but in time it is altered in consistency to a semi-solid state. Whether the ileum dilates sufficiently to take over some of the functions of the colon or whether, as Wakefield suggested, the kidneys compensate in maintaining the electrolytic balance of the body, the benefits of the procedure preceding total colectomy or subtotal colectomy are definitely established. Any artificial sto-ma of the gastro-intestinal tract will meet with objection from the patients; but when the benefits of such a procedure are enumerated their sanction is readily secured (See "Preoperative and Postopera-tive Treatment.") With recent improvement and modification in the surgical attack of diffuse adenomatosis, the rectum is more fre-quently saved than destroyed and provides a site for subsequent anastomosis of the ileum, which dispenses with the ileostomy as a permanent fixture.

At one time we did a total colectomy with removal of the rec-tum, having a permanent ileostomy in all cases. It was a bearable and often comfortable appendage which could be countenanced, but it was never as convenient as the normal mechanism with con-tinence. The introduction of surgical diathermy made possible modifications in technic, combining conservation with effective treatment and preservation of the rectal control. The rectum to the rectosigmoid juncture has come within the range of attack through the proctoscope. The polyps in this field can be destroyed by fulgu-ration and this segment of bowel with its sphincteric mechanism salvaged for anastomosis with the ileum. This can be accomplished at intervals during the existence of the ileostomy, while time is be-ing allowed for the patient's general improvement as well as reduc-tion of the infection and edema of the colon.

The removal of the colon may be undertaken by one of several steps after the ileostomy has been performed and the rectal polyps completely destroyed by fulguration. Some advocate the anasto-mosis of the ileum to the rectal stump before doing a subtotal colectomy. On the other hand, there are those who believe that a reversal of this plan by doing the colectomy first, allowing for sev-eral weeks or months to pass before anastomosing the ileum to the rectal stump, is the better procedure.

In any individual case the order may vary because of specific indications, but in a general way we prefer to do an ileostomy,

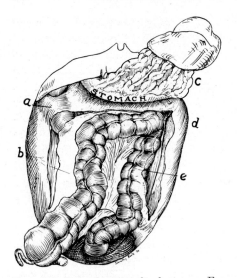

FIG. 117. Second stage of colectomy: Further mobilization of the colon; *a*, kidney; *b*, peritoneum; *c*, omentum; *d*, transverse colon; *e*, descending colon.

waiting three months during which time the polyps are destroyed, and then doing a subtotal colectomy and finally the anastomosis at a subsequent operation. Then, when one is assured of the adequate function of the anastomosis, the ileostomy may be closed under local anesthesia.

Recently it has been proposed to leave longer segments of the colon, the sigmoid, and descending colon above the site of the proposed anastomosis, with the ileum. It is difficult to see the advantages of this, and there are several apparent disadvantages to such a procedure. The added loop or segment proximal to the anastomosis is unnecessary as a reservoir, and, of greatest significance, it is beyond the reach of the investigating protoscope or sigmoidoscope which is the only means of maintaining strict observation over this field, which of course is subject to recurrent polyp formation.

The short rectal stump, as we advocate, supplies adequate storage space with the spacious ampulla of the rectum to serve as a reservoir to permit the patient the convenience of two or three stools a day under control. This short colonic stump is well within the range of investigation and can be frequently checked for the presence of any polyps, and treatment in the instance of recurrence can be rendered by fulguration.

Colectomy in three stages.—*First stage* (ileostomy).—This procedure is described elsewhere. Ileostomy should invariably, in our opinion, precede the other technical steps by a matter of at least three months because of the serious disturbances of fluid balance which is a necessary sequel to it. As time progresses and the ileostomy assumes some of the functions of the colon, hypertrophy takes place in its musculature, dilatation accompanies this change, and the stools become semisolid or even formed.

Second stage (subtotal colectomy).—Through a long left rectus incision, the colon is removed from right to left (Figs. 116 to 118). For the right half of the colon this is accomplished in the manner described elsewhere for resection of that portion of the bowel. Beginning to mobilize the right colon one cuts the outer leaf of the peritoneum in the bloodless area, rotates the bowel mesially and ligates the blood vessels as they appear. It is helpful to accomplish the peritonealization of raw surfaces as the different segments of the bowel are mobilized. The first mobilization goes up to the hepatic flexure where the retroperitoneal duodenum is identified to safeguard it against injury. When the blood supply to this area has been ligated and divided, the raw surfaces are easily covered over by a running suture, bringing the parietal and visceral layers of the peritoneum together. From the hepatic flexure to the splenic flexure little trouble is encountered if one leaves the omentum. There is no difficulty in separating the omentum from the colon and it is very advantageous to have subsequently as a protection against infection and occasionally as a covering for denuded areas.

The splenic flexure is somewhat more difficult to mobilize as it lies high and is often adherent, but by cutting the splenocolic ligament and the lateral parietal peritoneum down along the margin of the descending colon, one may rotate it mesially and get at the blood supply accurately. Again, the peritonealization of this segment is accomplished by a running suture adjoining the visceral and parietal layers of the peritoneum, and the dissection is carried on to the lower third of the sigmoid. Here the bowel is cut across and the lower end invaginated, the remaining raw surfaces covered, and the abdomen closed without drainage.

The turning in of the lower end of the bowel is a pro-

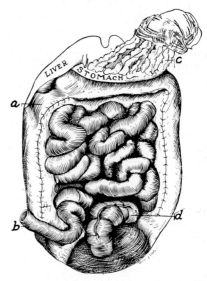

Fig. 118. Second stage completed: The ileostomy is shown in the right iliac fossa. The rectal stump including the lower part of the sigmoid just behind the rectosigmoid is shown, as well as coils of small intestine. The peritonealization is accurately completed. *a*, kidney; *b*, ileum; *c*, omentum; *d*, sigmoid.

cedure often fraught with considerable difficulty and danger in either the diffuse adenomatosis cases or in the chronic ulcerative colitis variety. In the former the polyps may be so dense and thick that a crushing clamp will cut through the attenuated wall of the bowel if it is applied vigorously. Certainly, in all chronic ulcerative colitis cases a heavy Payr clamp will cut through the friable wall if applied at all. It has been found more desirable to clamp the bowel between two soft gastro-enterostomy clamps covered with rubber, divide it with a cautery, and then suture the lower end over and over, closing it snugly as possible and turning it in as well as might be. This end of the bowel is then wrapped in a piece of iodoform gauze and the whole surrounded with rubber tissue which is brought out through the abdominal wound. Where there is any question of accurate closure, regardless of the pathology, it is well to drain as in the case of chronic ulcerative colitis. In the case in our series of 13 resections which succumbed, drainage in this manner was not established and the resulting pelvic abscess was the indirect cause of death.

Third stage (1, ileosigmoidostomy or 2, perineo-abdomoninal resection of the rectum).—(1) Ileosigmoidostomy: We do this step by one of two methods, one of which is an aseptic anastomosis over the Rankin clamp, and the other by the open technic. The former is quite easily and satisfactorily executed if there is sufficient rectal stump, or if the patient is the thin type and the bowel is mobile. The technic is identical with that described above for the end-to-side ileocolostomy. If difficulties are encountered owing to narrow pelvis or excess deposits of fat in the bowel wall, one may always resort to open anastomosis.

As a rule, the anastomosis is clean and there is no necessity for drains. The ileostomy is still present and serves as an added safeguard and sidetracks the fecal current from the recent anastomosis until sufficient time has elapsed for its safe and firm healing. Within two weeks, the ileostomy having served its purpose can easily be closed under local anaesthesia. The patient is now returned to a normal anal control and has on the average of two or three semisolid stools a day.

(2) Perineo-abdominal resection of the rectum: This is described elsewhere in relation to carcinoma of the rectum. The operation is commenced from the posterior aspect, the patient lying in a prone position with hips elevated. The rectum is mobilized up to the peritoneum just as in posterior excision of the rectum, but without entering the peritoneal cavity, and is encased in a rubber glove which is tied tightly about the cuff. This is pushed up into the hollow of the sacrum and the wound is then closed. Next the patient is turned on his back, an incision is made low in the medium line, the inferior mesenteric vessels are ligated, the pelvic peritoneum is incised and the rectosigmoid is freed by blunt dissection in the hollow of the sacrum; the rubber glove is grasped and the entire segment of sigmoid, rectum, and anus is lifted out of the abdomen. A new pelvic floor is established and the posterior wound drained.

Rehabilitation following these formidable procedures is slow, and adequate dietary measures, transfusions, and other steps for increasing the patient's resistance, which are considered fully elsewhere, are urgently indicated.

REFERENCES

1. COLE, WARREN H.: Quoted by Graham.[7]
2. DANIEL, W. H.: Quoted by Graham.[7]
3. DAVID, VERNON C.: Quoted by Graham.[7]
4. FRASER, JOHN, and DOTT, N. M.: Aseptic intestinal anastomosis; with special reference to colectomy. *Brit. Jour. Surg.*, **11**: 439–454 (Jan.), 1924.
5. FURNISS, H. D.: Instrument for anastomosis of intestines. *Am. Jour. Surg.*, **24**: 863–877 (July), 1934.
6. GRAHAM, A. STEPHENS: Quoted by Rankin.[13]
7. GRAHAM, A. STEPHENS: Current trends in surgery of the distal colon and rectum for cancer. *Ann. Surg.*, **127**: 1022–1034 (May), 1948.
8. JONES, T. E.: Quoted by Graham.[7]
9. KERR: Quoted by Rankin.[7]
10. LAHEY, and CATTELL: Quoted by Graham.[7]
11. MACFEE, W. F.: Quoted by Graham.[7]
12. PFEIFFER, DAMON B., and PATTERSON, F. M. SIMMONS: Congenital or hereditary polyposis of the colon. *Ann. Surg.*, **122**: 606–624, (Oct.), 1945.
13. RANKIN, F. W.: Resection and obstruction of the colon (obstructive resection). *Surg., Gynec., and Obstet.*, **50**: 594–598 (March), 1930.
14. RANKIN, F. W., and GRAHAM, A. STEPHENS: Aseptic end-to-side ileocolostomy: clamp method. *Ann. Surg.*, 1934 (April), 676–681.
15. RANKIN, F. W., and GRAHAM, A. STEPHENS: Closure of Colostomy. *Surg.. Gynec., and Obstet.*, **64**: 59, 1937.
16. RANKIN, F. W., and GRIMES, A. E.: Diffuse adenomatosis of the colon. *Jour. Am. Med. Assn.*, **108**: 711–715 (Feb. 27), 1937.
17. RAVDIN, I. S., ZINTEL, HAROLD A., and BENDER, DORIS H.: Adjuvants to surgical therapy in large bowel malignancy. *Ann. Surg.*, **126**: 439–447 (Oct.), 1947.
18. STONE, H. B., and MCLANAHAN, SAMUEL: Resection and immediate anastomosis for carcinoma of the colon. *Journ. A.M.A.*, **120** (Dec. 26) 1942.
19. WHIPPLE, A. O.: The use of the Miller-Abbott tube in surgery of the large bowel. *Surgery*, **8**: 289–293 (Aug.), 1940.

CHAPTER XIV

PROCEDURES FOR EXTIRPATION OF LESIONS OF THE RECTOSIGMOID, RECTUM, AND ANUS

The problem of selecting operations to suit individual cases has been discussed at some length under "Choice of Operation." The acceptance of the principle so strongly advocated by Miles that carcinomas that can be extirpated should be dealt with radically, not alone by their removal, but by removal of the contiguous gland-bearing tissue as well, predicates a formidable procedure in dealing with malignancy in this situation. In the first edition of this book we considered Miles's proposition to be highly laudable but, unfortunately, not always practical. At that time even his operability rate for the one-stage operation was only 35 per cent; many qualifying factors determined the feasibility of the one-stage operation such as, age, general condition of the patient, presence or absence of concurrent disease in other organs and the extent of metastatic involvement, local and hepatic. In recent years, however, owing to a better understanding and utilization of preoperative measures of rehabilitation, improved anesthetic methods and the advent of chemotherapy, the elderly, the depleted, and even the "inoperable," have been submitted to the radical resection with increasing frequency and with a steadily decreasing mortality rate.

The types of operation which we believe may fill most of the needs of the operating surgeon are, in the order of their desirability: first, abdominoperineal resection in one-stage (Miles's operation); second, a two-stage procedure consisting of preliminary cecostomy or colostomy (in cases of unrelieved obstruction, subabute perforation or fixation of the growth) followed by the Miles operation; third, perineo-abdominal resection in one-stage (Gabriel's operation); fourth, colostomy and posterior excision (Lockhart-Mummery's operation); fifth, anterior resection of the rectosigmoid (resection and primary anastomosis or by the procedures of David or Hartmann) and, sixth, local excision of the growth with or without preservation of the sphincter muscle, a procedure which we consider wholly palliative.

The following recent statement by T. E. Jones reflects the opinion of most surgeons of wide experience in this field: "As I first believed with firm conviction even though with temerity, I am now more convinced than ever that the procedure of choice for this le-

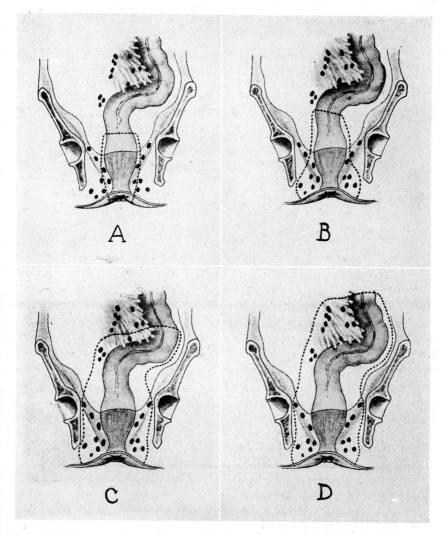

Fig. 119. Diagrams showing the evolution of the combined abdominoperineal excision of the rectum (after Miles). *A*, Shows the restricted nature of Kraske's operation; *B*, perineal excision of the rectum with wide removal of peri-anal skin and ischiorectal fat; *C*, abdomino-anal operation in which all of the levator ani muscles and the lower part of the pelvic mesocolon is excised, but the upper zone of spread is left behind; and *D*, the final stage in the evolution of the radical operation in which all the vulnerable tissues of the three zones of spread (Miles) is removed by a combined abdominoperineal maneuver.

sion [rectal cancer] and those in the rectosigmoid, as I interpret it, is the one-stage abdominoperineal resection, the Miles operation. It offers the best hope of cure, the lowest mortality and morbidity and the greatest palliation of all procedures."

COMBINED ABDOMINOPERINEAL OPERATION
IN ONE STAGE (MILES)

The details of technic in performing this operation have been very slightly modified from those originally employed by Miles in the first planned operation of the kind on January 7, 1907. The story of the evolution of this operation is a classic in surgical annals (Fig. 119).

Technic.—The incision is made low in the median line and if necessary, in order to secure ample exposure, is extended upward and to the left of the umbilicus. Beginning at the liver, the surgeon

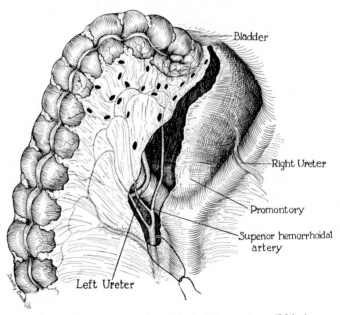

FIG. 120. Abdominoperineal excision of the rectum (Miles) employing Cope clamp. Division of peritoneum for mobilization of sigmoid and upper rectum; in order to insure a relatively bloodless field the inferior mesenteric artery is ligated as an initial step.

explores the surface of the two lobes for nodules as quickly as possible, and explores down the aorta, feeling the nodes around the pancreas and those on each side of the aorta, down into the bifurcation of the common iliac vessels and then down into the pelvis. Lastly, the growth is palpated gingerly and if it is deemed resectable the operating table is then adjusted to a moderate Trendelenburg position, a self-retaining retractor is placed, and the small bowel is retained in the upper part of the abdomen with the aid of large, moist packs (Figs. 120–128).

In order to assure a relatively bloodless operative field, the inferior mesenteric vessels are ligated as an initial step (Fig. 120).

The site of ligation should be between the left colic and hemorrhoidal branches in order to preserve adequate vascularization of the descending colon and upper portion of the sigmoid. With the sigmoid retracted toward the left side, the peritoneum over the inferior mesenteric vessel is incised after identification of the left ureter. This runs rather close to the vessels, but the right ureter is far distant and is never in danger of being ligated with them. On opening the peritoneum over the vessels, they are hooked up over a finger,

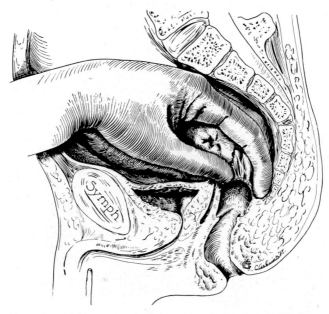

Fig. 121. Abdominoperineal excision of the rectum (Miles) employing Cope clamp. Cleaning out the hollow of the sacrum by blunt dissection, which is easily accomplished after ligation of the mesenteric vessels and mobilization of the peritoneal flaps, usually with only slight oozing. The hand introduced at the promontory of the sacrum is carried forward on each side of the bladder in the male and in the female to the utero-sacral attachments.

close to their origin and doubly ligated and divided. With the exception of the middle sacral artery, this is practically all of the blood supply to the rectum and sacral region, but the middle sacral artery, which is the terminal branch of the abdominal aorta, will frequently require a ligature of its own.

The peritoneum of the mesentery of the sigmoid is now incised forward, toward the base of the bladder on both sides, and the bladder is separated from the rectum. At this stage both ureters should be identified and carefully avoided. The bowel is then elevated, and with a hand behind it in the hollow of the sacrum, the node-bearing tissue, including the fat in this area, is freed by blunt dissection. There is seldom any bleeding of consequence following this dissection, but a hot pack placed in the pelvis will stop any venous oozing during the stage in which colostomy is established (Figs. 121–125).

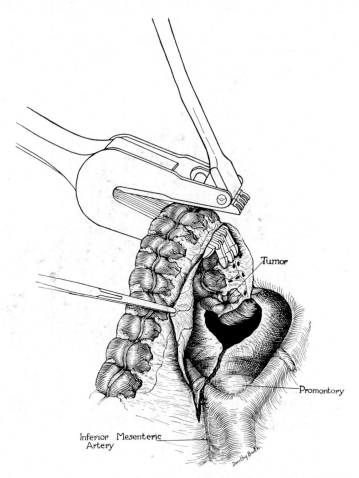

Fig. 122. Abdominoperineal excision of the rectum (Miles) employing Cope clamp. The crushing clamp containing three hinged segments is shown being applied to colon proximal to growth.

With the sigmoid elevated, a suitable place for colostomy is selected, at a point at which the blood supply is visible in the appendices epiploicae. The bowel here is divided between clamps, and a single-barreled colostomy stoma is established in the left groin in a manner identical to that described for the procedure in two stages. In this procedure a Payr clamp is thrust through a stab wound in the groin and applied to the sigmoid; through the abdominal

wound a second clamp is applied in the opposite direction and
the bowel between the two is divided with a cautery. The proximal
end is drawn out onto the abdomen and the clamp left on, completely obstructing the bowel for twenty-four to sixty hours. Miles

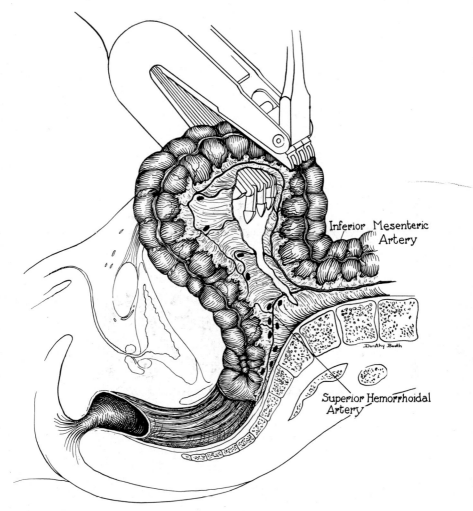

FIG. 123. Abdominoperineal excision of the rectum (Miles) employing Cope clamp.
Same stage as Figure 122, Sagittal view.

now removes a circle of skin instead of making a linear incision
when establishing the colostomy, in order to prevent the subsequent tendency to stenosis of the stoma. The rectal end of the
bowel is now turned in and dropped back into the pelvic cavity,
after which a new pelvic floor is formed by approximation of the
lateral peritoneal flaps. If the patient is a woman there is no diffi-

culty, because of the utilizable broad ligament and uterus; if a male there is almost as little trouble. The omentum is now brought down into the pelvis as the operating table is made level; this tends to keep the small bowel away from the site of operation. The abdomi-

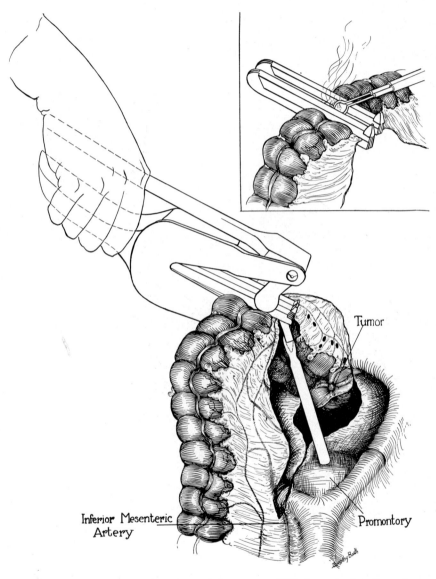

Tumor

Inferior Mesenteric
Artery

Promontory

Fig. 124. Abdominoperineal excision of the rectum (Miles) employing Cope clamp. Crushing force is applied to the distal end of the hinged segments until each is locked by a special catch. After removal of the crusher the middle segment of the clamp is unlocked and removed and the exposed thin lamella of crushed bowel divided by the cautery (insert).

nal wound is closed without drains inserted in the peritoneal cavity.
The two wounds should be carefully separated in order to prevent
subsequent infection of the median incision after the colostomy
commences to function. The patient is now turned on his side, or
on the abdomen with hips elevated and the lower segment of bowel
is extirpated by a relatively simple procedure that requires only a

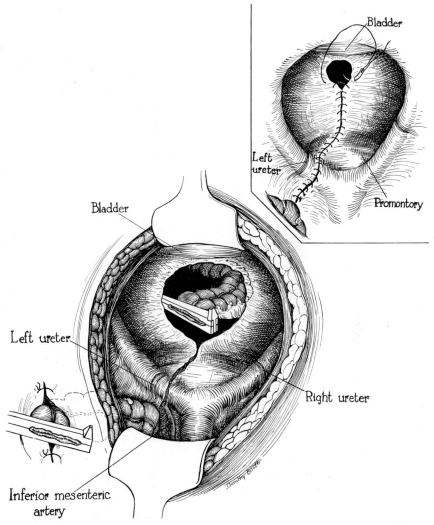

FIG. 125. Abdominoperineal excision of the rectum (Miles) employing Cope clamp.
The hinged segment of the proximal end of divided bowel is pushed lengthwise
through a small stab wound in the left iliac region to establish a single-barreled
colostomy; the distal end of bowel with its attached segment is pushed down below
the pelvic peritoneum and a new pelvic floor is established (insert). See also
Figures 126–130.

few minutes (Figs. 126–128). Because of extensive mobilization of the rectum in the abdominal stage of the operation, it comes out readily, once a line of cleavage has been established. Elliptical incisions are made about the anus which is closed by a purse-string

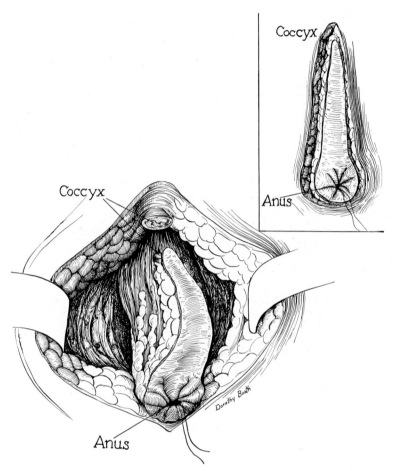

FIG. 126. Abdominoperineal excision of the rectum (Miles) employing Cope clamp. The incision starts over the middle of the sacrum and circles the anus which has been closed with a purse-string suture of heavy silk, (insert). The coccyx has been disarticulated from the sacrum, the fascia propria incised, and dissection of the hollow of the sacrum begun.

suture, and dissection about the rectum is carried out, all just as in posterior resection, except that in the combined operation it is seldom necessary to remove the coccyx. If oiled silk or rubber dam is placed in the hollow of the sacrum and gauze is packed tightly into it, several purposes are served. First, oozing is controlled; second, support is afforded the newly made pelvic floor; and third, by the use of the oiled silk or rubber, the removal of the gauze packing is simple and painless. The wound may be closed with several interrupted stay sutures or left open. The pack is removed at the end of forty-eight or seventy-two hours, after which there are instituted daily irrigations of normal saline as described under "Postoperative Treatment."

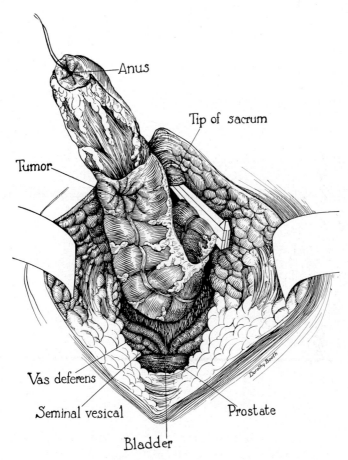

FIG. 127. Abdominoperineal excision of the rectum (Miles) employing Cope clamp. The anterior portion of the dissection has been carried down to the membranous urethra, and the prostate gland and seminal vesicles are shown dissected clear.

ALTERNATIVE PROCEDURE (ZACKARY COPE CLAMP TECHNIC)

Zackary Cope, in 1934, described a crushing clamp for the large intestine which we have employed routinely in performing the Miles operation during recent years (Figs. 120 to 128).

Cope describes his clamp and its application as follows:

"In the operation of abdominoperineal resection of the rectum for carcinoma the sigmoid colon has to be divided. The division of the bowel is usually made through a part which has been crushed so that little but peritoneum remains. When the bowel is hypertrophied or oedematous it may be difficult to crush the gut satisfactorily. With clamps of the usual scissor-type the distal part does not get so completely crushed as the part near the hinge and

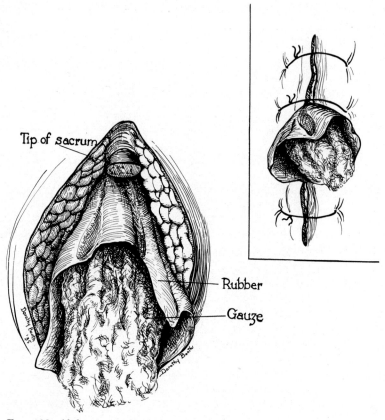

FIG. 128. Abdominoperineal excision of the rectum. A square of oiled silk has been thrust into the hollow of the pelvis and then packed with gauze.

the division is not made so clearly. Moreover, the wrapping of the cut ends may work off and soiling take place. With a view to the more easy division of the bowel and manipulation of the cut ends, I have devised a clamp made something on the pattern of Martel's and consisting of three narrow-hinged segments which fit closely into a powerful crushing lever. The crushing force being applied to the distal end of the hinged segments an equable effect on the whole circumference of the bowel is assured. Crushing continues till each segment is locked by a special catch. After removal of the crusher the middle segment of the clamp is unlocked and removed and the exposed thin lamella of crushed bowel divided by the cautery. The lateral segments of the clamp remain, one on the proximal and the other on the distal ends of the severed bowel. They do not slip off, for they are ridged longitudinally and grip the bowel tissue firmly. They can be covered with gauze, enabling manipulation of the bowel ends to be carried out with greater ease. The proximal clamp is easily pushed lengthwise through a small stab wound in the left iliac region, whilst the distal clamp is pushed down below the pelvic peritoneum and can readily be felt and seized during the perineal stage of the operation. Two lengths of clamp are made; one for the large and one a perfect crusher for the small gut. The Genito-Urinary Manufacturing Company, Devonshire Street, London, W., are the makers."

COMBINED PERINEO-ABDOMINAL OPERATION IN ONE STAGE

To Grey Turner should go credit for originating the perineal approach as the initial maneuver in carrying out the radical combined operation. He reported 7 such successful operations in 1920. Gabriel, in 1934, reported 25 perineo-abdominal operations done in one stage, and in England, he is its most enthusiastic advocate as the operation of election in cancer of the rectum. He contends that it is less technically difficult than the abdominoperineal procedures, that the dangers of sepsis and shock are largely eliminated, the former by avoiding intraperitoneal section of the colon, and shock by doing the perineal part of the operation first, so that no turning of the patient is required after completion of the abdominal operation; and that it fulfils all the requirements of a radical operation in regard to high section of the vascular and lymphatic pedicle, even permitting a slightly more radical procedure than that of Miles. The merits of these claims have been discussed under "Choice of Operation."

Technic.—The details of technic are adequately covered in the description of the Rankin two-stage perineo-abdominal operation. As performed by Gabriel the operation in one stage is carried out in the following distinct steps:

1. In all cases, regardless of grade of malignancy or location of the rectal growth, a preliminary abdominal exploration is done through a right paramedian subumbilical incision, in order to determine operability. If there is no evidence of metastasis the wound is closed temporarily by through-and-through silkworm-gut sutures with an anchored gauze dressing.

2. The patient is turned into the left lateral position, the anus is closed by purse-string sutures of stout silk or linen, and the perineal

excision is proceeded with in the usual manner, after disarticulation of the coccyx. Before opening the peritoneum the anus and rectum are covered with a rubber glove which is tied in place. The peritoneum is opened and the mobilized rectum is pushed up into the pelvis. The perineal wound is packed with gauze and covered with a towel. The patient is then turned on his back.

3. Trendelenburg position. The abominal wound is reopened and the small intestine packed out of the pelvis. The glove-covered rectum is grasped and delivered upward as the sigmoid is freed by lateral incision in the peritoneum at the base of the mesocolon. The inferior mesenteric pedicle is now ligated at the point of election, as described above for Miles operation.

4. A left iliac muscle-splitting incision four inches in length is made through which the rectum and sigmoid are pulled until a point near the junction of the sigmoid with the descending colon is reached.

5. The pelvic floor is re-established by approximation of the divided lateral flaps of peritoneum, the paramedian incision is closed without drainage and the oblique incision is closed in layers around the emerging colon, without placing sutures in the bowel.

6. The extruded colon is divided between clamps applied $1\frac{1}{2}$ inches external to the skin. It is our practice to leave the bowel obstructed for forty-eight or seventy-two hours in order to avoid wound infection, establishing a cecostomy if this is necessary. Gabriel, however, sutures a catheter into the opened end of bowel at once, into which he injects five ounces of warmed olive oil.

7. The median wound is sealed to prevent contamination from the colostomy and, finally, the legs are held up by an assistant on each side, hemostasis is verified, and a rubber bag or sheet is inserted and packed with gauze. The wound is partially closed with interrupted sutures and a dressing applied.

Alternative procedure (incision of the pelvic peritoneum from above).—Gabriel recently stated that "In a few cases it is advisable to incise the peritoneum at the bottom of the pelvis, in front of the rectosigmoid, *from above* as in abdomino-perineal excision. For instance, in women, if a hysterectomy has been done previously the level of the pouch of Douglas tends to be raised, and in addition there may be adhesions which make it extremely difficult to find the peritoneum from below. Again, in some male cases where an indurated edge of carcinoma can be felt infiltrating the peritoneum at the recto-vesical reflection, it is difficult by touch alone to be sure whether only the peritoneum is involved, or whether the base of the bladder has been invaded and the growth is in consequence inoperable. In such cases a transverse incision is made through the peritoneum about $\frac{1}{2}$ inch above the edge or lip of the malignant infiltration. Then with scissors and blunt dissection it is soon apparent if the growth can be stripped from the bladder. If so, the dissection is carried down a little farther, the abdominal incision is temporarily closed, and the perineal part of the operation is proceeded with in the usual way. The opening already made into the peritoneum is found quite readily from below and in a difficult case this is found to be a considerable help."

COMBINED OPERATION IN TWO STAGES

The procedure of choice in dealing with cancer of the rectum and rectosigmoid, viewed from the operative standpoint as well as from the standpoint of end-results, is, in our opinion, the one-stage abdominoperineal resection of the rectum following the technic of Miles. There are occasions, however, when obstruction, subacute perforation or fixation of the bowel may influence even the staunchest advocate of the one-stage procedure to resort to graded measures. When faced with infection or fixation, it was our practice formerly to employ a two-stage operation which was first described by one of us (Rankin) in 1929. In 1931 there were reported 23 consecutive operations of this type with but one death. Subsequently, however, as the number of cases in the series materially increased the mortality rate rose to a level higher than that which attended the abdominoperineal operation in one-stage. In 1948 one of us (Rankin) reported that during the seven year period from 1934 to 1941 the two-stage combined operation was performed only nine times, with a mortality of 22.2 per cent, whereas the Miles operation was undertaken on 167 occasions with a mortality of only 5.3 per cent. Now on the rare occasion when we feel a graded operation is indicated, our preference is cecostomy or transverse colostomy followed by an abdominoperineal resection in one stage when obstruction is completely relieved or fixation of the bowel has receded.

Rankin's operation.—The two stages are as follows:

1. Single-barreled colostomy.—Abdominal exploration having been carried out through a low paramedian incision, as described in the Miles operation, a small split-muscle incision is made in the left iliac region. Ordinarily it will not be necessary to adjust the table to the Trendelenburg position or to pack-off carefully the small intestine into upper abdomen, unless the mesocolon of the sigmoid is very short. With the sigmoid pulled well out of the paramedian incision, a convenient site in the mesentery is selected and the blood vessels close to the bowel divided, but only sufficiently to permit the proximal end of the subsequently divided sigmoid to be drawn out through the iliac incision (Fig. 129). In the presence of a considerable amount of fat in the mesentery, unusual care

should be exercised in order to preserve adequate blood supply to the two ends of bowel.

The bowel is divided between two Payr clamps, the upper one of which is thrust through the iliac incision to grasp the sigmoid at the point where the mesenteric vessels were divided (Fig. 130). The lower clamp is applied as close as possible to the other, but in the opposite direction, the bowel is cut across with a cautery, and the proximal end is drawn out onto the abdomen, whereas the distal end is inverted and dropped back into the abdomen. In making the colostomy incision the various layers of the abdominal wall are not dissected out. A small stab wound is made and is large enough only to permit the bowel to be pulled out easily; the peritoneum will hug the bowel closely and at most only one or two sutures in the skin will be necessary. Sutures are never used to attach the peritoneum or any other layer of the abdominal wall to the bowel. Retraction of the bowel end into the abdominal cavity is a theoretical danger that need cause no concern; in our experience with approximately five hundred such colostomies, performed in connection with the abdomino-perineal or perineo-abdominal operation in one or two stages, this has not occurred.

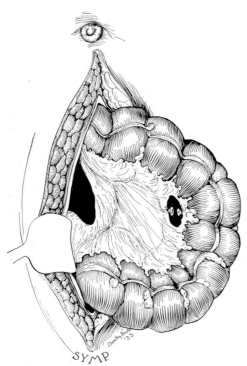

Fig. 129. Perineo-abdominal excision of rectum (Rankin), first stage: The ligation of the blood supply close to the lumen of the bowel is shown. The vascular arcs are preserved. Sufficient space is made to permit the division of the bowel and inversion of the distal end.

The clamp is held on the abdomen by tape, after the incision in the median line has been closed, and is left in place, to be opened at the end of sixty hours or more, as is necessary. If the preoperative cleansing measures have been adequate, the patient will tolerate obstruction well for sixty to seventy-two hours or longer; if it has not been adequate and evidences of obstruction exist, a cecostomy should invariably precede the establishment of the single-barreled colostomy. A period of rehabilitation of from three to

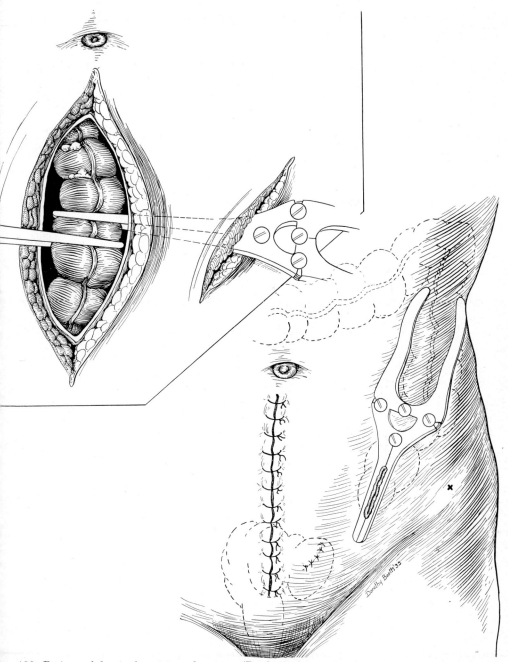

G. 130. Perineo-abdominal excision of rectum (Rankin), first stage: Insert shows the exploratory idline incision, and lateral to it is a stab wound made for bringing out the proximal loop for a lostomy. A Payr clamp is thrust through this wound and grasps the bowel at a selected point. A cond Payr clamp is put on parallel to it, the bowel is divided with a cautery, the proximal end is lled out through the stab wound, and the distal end inverted. On the right is shown the completed st stage of the operation with the Payr clamp left on.

five weeks is desirable before attempting the second stage. During
this time rectal irrigations are instituted from about the tenth day
until the day before the second stage. By using a two-way rectal
tube the bowel is cleansed without undue pressure on the blind end
and the warm solution used, together with the by-passing of the

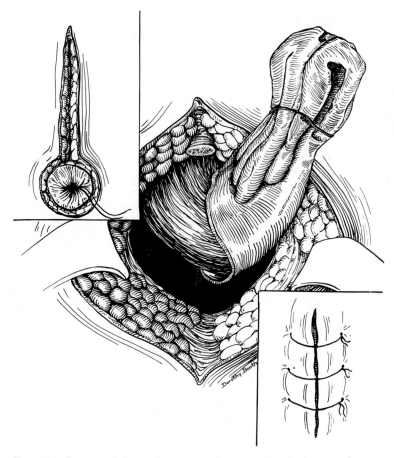

Fig. 131. Perineo-abdominal excision of rectum (Rankin), second stage,
upper insert: Posterior incision for removal of segment of bowel to be
sacrificed. This is identical with incision for posterior excision of rectum.
The rectum is shown completely mobilized and encased in rubber glove.
Lower insert: the wound is shown closed after mobilized rectum is pushed
up into hollow of sacrum.

fecal current, assists in reducing the inflammatory resection around
the growth. Criticism to the effect that the stump may open up as a
result of secretions and gas accumulating between the closed end
and an annular growth can be answered only by stating that this
has not occurred in our experience of well over 100 operations of
this type.

2. Perineo-abdominal resection.—The principal advantage this maneuver possesses over an abdominoperineal sequence is that shock is largely eliminated, because no turning of the patient is required after completion of the abdominal operation. The perineal dissection up to the peritoneum is carried out in a manner identical

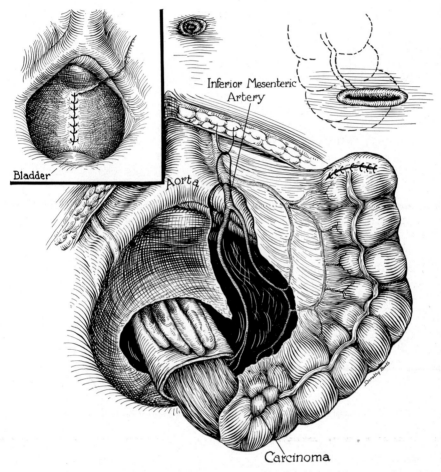

FIG. 132. Perineo-abdominal excision of rectum (Rankin), second stage: Anterior approach. Entire rectum being lifted out of hollow of sacrum. Insert shows pelvic floor re-established.

with that described in detail for posterior excision after colostomy. In brief, the technic is as follows: with the patient face downward on the table, with the hips elevated, and with the anus closed with a purse-string suture, two concave incisions are made which extend from a little above the sacrococcygeal joint, around to the center of the perineum. The dissection follows disarticulation of the coccyx from the sacrum and the division of the fascia pro-

pia opposite this joint. Dissection of the tissues in the hollow of
the sacrum is a blunt one, done with the gloved hand. The lateral
incisions are carried downward, taking away as much fat and node-
bearing tissue as is warranted and the levati ani muscle is removed
as high toward its bony attachment as possible. Anteriorly the rectum is separated from the prostate gland and seminal vesicles in the
male and the posterior vaginal wall and cervix in the female. When
the dissection has been completed up to the peritoneum but without opening it, the entire rectum is encased in a rubber glove, which
is tied tightly around the cuff (Fig. 131). The segment is dropped
back into the hollow of the sacrum and the posterior wound is
closed with stay-sutures after a temporary pack is inserted.

The patient is then turned on his back, and the latter part of the
second stage, or the abdominal portion, is consummated quickly
and easily through a low mid-line incision which is an enlargement
of the one used for exploration. There is no necessity for exploration
at this time and the operation is done entirely within the pelvis
which is isolated with the aid of wet gauze packs. The peritoneum
over the inferior mesenteric vessels is incised, and after identification of the left ureter, which is often in close proximity to the vessels, these vessels are doubly ligated close to their origin (see Miles's
operation for details of the abdominal procedure). Excepting only
the middle sacral artery, the terminal branch of the aorta, practically all the blood supply is thus tied. The peritoneum is now
incised forward toward the base of the bladder on both sides, and
the bladder is separated from the rectum. The node-bearing tissue
is wiped mesially from both sides with gauze, and the entire segment is lifted out through the abdomen (Fig. 132).

There is little or no difficulty in restoring the pelvic floor by approximation of the divided portions of the peritoneum. In the female, the broad ligaments and the uterus may be utilized if
necessary. The abdominal wound is now closed without drainage
and with the legs elevated by assistant, the posterior wound is reopened. A piece of oiled silk or rubber tissue is inserted into the
hollow of the sacrum and this is packed with gauze.

Lahey's operation.—Lahey, in 1930, described a modification of
the technic given above as the Rankin Operation. Instead of
inverting the divided distal end of colon he brings it out of the
lower end of the incision in the median line, or through a separate
stab wound, for purposes of irrigation of the rectum between stages.
At the second stage the fistula thus established is dissected out of
the abdominal wall and inverted, and an abdominoperineal resection carried out, as in the Miles's operation.

We have not utilized this procedure for several reasons: (1) If
an initial abdominal approach (other than to establish a cecostomy

seems desirable, the Jones' operation offers the advantage of avoiding the peritoneal cavity twice; (2) the Rankin perineo-abdominal procedure, which also provides a single-barreled colostomy, avoids the danger of contamination which the rectosigmoid fistula established in the abdominal wound potentiates, yet offers ample and satisfactory access to the rectum and lower sigmoid for cleansing irrigations between stages; and (3) because we now believe that the best maneuver on the rare occasion when a graded operation is indicated is cecostomy or transverse colostomy followed after a suitable interval by a one-stage abdominoperineal resection.

Jones' operation.—The principal objection to this procedure lies in the necessity of leaving a blind loop of bowel below the colonic stoma, and the technical handicap that may be encountered in attempting to invert the bowel in the event of a narrow pelvis.

Through a paramedian incision on the left, and after retraction of muscles, the abdomen is explored, the sigmoid and rectum are freed from their attachments by scissors and blunt dissection, and the superior hemorrhoidal artery is ligated at the level of the bifurcation of the aorta, below the left colic artery, great care being taken to preserve the sigmoidal arches. A permanent loop type of colostomy is performed, employing the upper end of the wound and the upper limits of the sigmoid, the latter in order to insure a maximum length of bowel below the colonic stoma. The peritoneal flaps are then sutured over the pelvis, and about the sigmoid, as high as possible. The blood supply to the bowel below the new peritoneal diaphragm is maintained through the marginal vascular arch and its communication with the left colic artery. This method permits irrigation and cleansing of the lower part of the bowel in the interval between operations.

At the second stage, the usual perineal excision is undertaken. After freeing the bowel, and bringing all that portion which has been placed in the pelvis down as far as possible, the bowel is clamped well above the growth, just beneath the peritoneal diaphragm, and sectioned. The end is either inverted by suture or simply tied, depending on the ease with which the sutures can be placed. The posterior wound is then closed in the usual manner.

ANTERIOR RESECTION OF THE RECTOSIGMOID

The difficulty in standardizing a nomenclature for the rectosigmoid juncture leads to confusion but any sphincter-saving operation for a cancer below the peritoneum certainly is excessively vulnerable. When the lesion is entirely intraperitoneal and at least 5 cm. above the peritoneal fold, an anastomosis, open or closed, or by David's obstructive method, can be employed in carefully selected cases with satisfaction. Nevertheless, we do not lose sight of the fact that even in instances of a low sigmoidal growth the ideal procedure, in the absence of contraindications, is the combined abdominoperineal operation.

Factors determining selection of procedure for lesions of the rectosigmoid have been considered under "Choice of Operation." The decision is often difficult to make. Too frequently the surgeon is influenced in border-line cases (lesion nearer than 5 cm. to the reflection of peritoneum on the bowel, short sigmoid, marked obesity) by the urgent plea of the patient to preserve bowel continuity. For this reason we believe that it is unwise to discuss with the patient the pros and cons of an abdominal anus versus perineal colostomy or the doubtful possibility of retaining the use of the anal sphincter in borderline cases. It is this uncertainty that a colostomy is essential which leads to hesitation, dissatisfaction and maladjustment among those who remain unconvinced that an abdominal colostomy is absolutely necessary. Under the best circumstance one may expect for anterior resection of the rectosigmoid with restoration of bowel continuity a higher morbidity and mortality.

The choice of operation lies between three procedures: (1) Obstructive resection with subsequent reestablishment of bowel continuity; (2) anterior resection and immediate anastomosis, with or without preliminary or simultaneous cecostomy or colostomy, and, (3) anterior resection without reestablishment of bowel continuity.

1. *Obstructive resection.*—In 1934, David described a technic of anterior resection for low sigmoidal growths based on the principle of obstructive resection. In 1936, we described a similar procedure which differed chiefly in that we employed the Rankin clamp on the exteriorized ends of bowel, whereas David used two Payr clamps which he removed the next day in order to apply a spur crushing clamp. Our indications for this operation were the same as those of David: (1) small growths of a low-grade of malignancy, as determined by biopsy through the sigmoidoscope; (2) polypoid growths of doubtful benignancy; and (3) refusal of permanent colostomy, an indication for which we have never been required to use this procedure. Owing to a better understanding of preoperative measures of rehabilitation, by which anemia and serum protein deficiency can be rapidly corrected, improved anesthetic methods and the advent of chemotherapeutic agents, we have in recent years substituted for this measure primary resection and immediate anastomosis.

Technic. The technic consists of three steps: (1) the rectosigmoid is thoroughly mobilized as in the Miles operation or in primary resection and anastomosis (Fig. 133); (2) obstructive resection, employing the three-bladed Rankin clamp, is carried out as described for mobile segments of colon on page 346; and, (3) a new

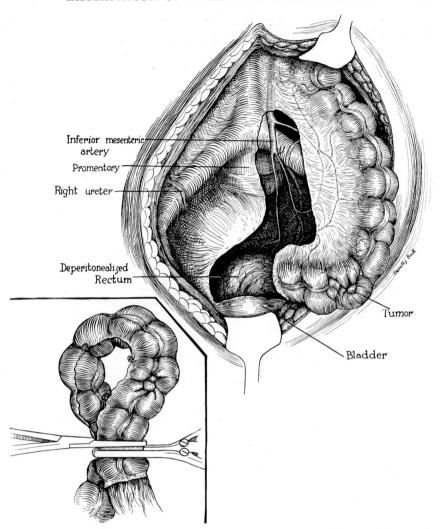

Inferior mesenteric
artery

Promentory

Right ureter

Deperitonealized
Rectum

Tumor

Bladder

FIG. 133. Anterior resection of rectosigmoid (obstructive resection method): Involved segment of sigmoid elevated several inches above its original position following division of peritoneal attachments of bowel and blunt dissection of rectum
from the hollow of sacrum. Point of ligation of sigmoid artery indicated. (Insert)
Rankin clamp applied to two limbs of sigmoid; the exteriorized portion to be removed with a cautery.

pelvic floor is reestablished at a higher level in order to cover the
denuded, deperitonealized rectum (Fig. 134).

2. *Anterior resection with immediate anastomosis.*—Our indications for this procedure are the same as those listed above for obstructive resection of rectosigmoidal growths. Although we believe
that this maneuver may be advantageously employed in certain
carefully selected cases, we do not lose sight of the fact that even

in instances of a low sigmoidal growth the ideal procedure, in the absence of contraindications, is the combined abdominoperineal operation.

Technic. The anastomosis may be accomplished by any of the various methods described in the chapter on "Procedures for Extirpation of Lesions of the Colon," or which have recently been described in detail by Dixon (Figs. 135–137), Wangensteen or by

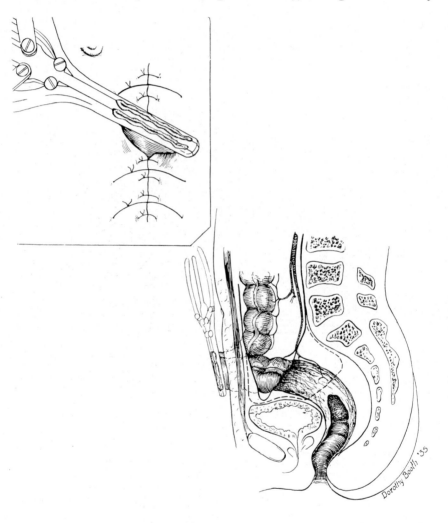

Fig. 134. Anterior resection of rectosigmoid (obstructive resection method): Sagittal section of the obstructive resection showing approximation of two limbs of bowel after removal of growth. The original pelvic floor, shown by the dotted line, has been re-established on a level with the promontory of sacrum in order to retroperitonealize the elevated deperitonealized rectum. (Insert) Anterior view showing the clamp *in situ*, the proximal blade of which is opened in forty-eight to seventy-two hours in order to establish the temporary colostomy

Waugh, who are the principal advocates of anterior resection of the rectosigmoid. Our own preference is a closed anastomosis which employs the Rankin narrow blade clamp (Figs. 111–114).

3. *Anterior resection without restoration of bowel continuity.*— This is a useful expedient for certain poor-risk patients. Series of cases have been reported by Hartmann, Gabriel, Muir and one of us (Rankin). Hartmann, by whose name the operation is commonly known, in 1923 demonstrated that by high ligation of the

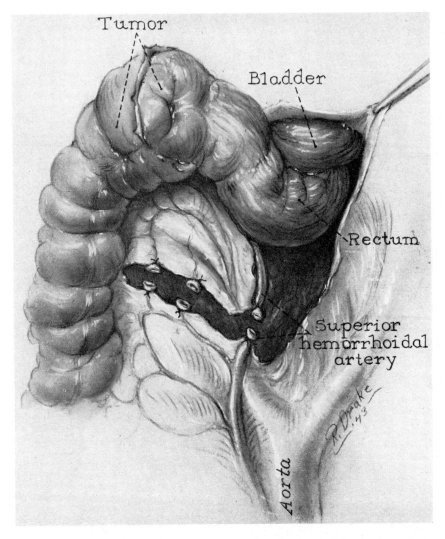

Fig. 135. After mobilization of rectum and sigmoid the site for the ligation of the superior hemorrhoidal or inferior mesenteric vessels is selected and a V-shaped section of mesentery is excised. (From Dixon: courtesy of *Annals of Surgery*.)

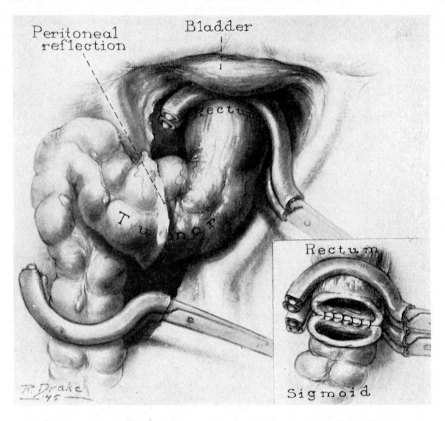

Fig. 136. Curved intestinal clamps are placed beyond the lines of resection of the intestine. After the segment is resected the clamps are placed side by side and the open colorectostomy is performed as indicated in the insert. (From Dixon: courtesy of *Annals of Surgery*.)

superior hemorrhoidal vessels the operation could be rendered thoroughly radical. From the standpoint of mortality, both immediate and remote from metastasis, the procedure is satisfactory. The morbidity, however, is higher than for the Miles operation owing to the occasional failure of the blood supply to the inverted upper end of the rectum, or to abscess formation. Moreover, Gabriel has mentioned as a late sequel the formation of hard, rounded masses of inspissated mucus in the rectum which are difficult to remove, as the anal canal becomes stenosed from disuse. He quoted Muir as having referred to another sequel, which is the development of a second carcinoma on the stump. Baker has also recently emphasized the malignant potential of the entire rectum when a single area of malignancy has been observed. He suggested that perhaps the high incidence of so-called local recurrence which accompanies anterior resection of the rectosigmoid might in part be due to the development of new cancers on the basis of satellite polyps which are frequently noted in specimens of rectum.

We now employ the Hartmann procedure only as an expedient on rare occasions when during the resection it is determined that completion of an abdominoperineal operation would be too hazardous. We have also used this maneuver as a palliative measure in the face of hepatic metastasis in elderly individuals who were considered particularly unsatisfactory risks.

This operation is carried out in a manner identical to that described for the combined abdominoperineal resection with the exceptions that mobilization of the rectum from the sacrum, prostate and bladder, or vagina, need not be so extensive and the bowel is divided *below* the growth which is removed anteriorly. Gabriel has

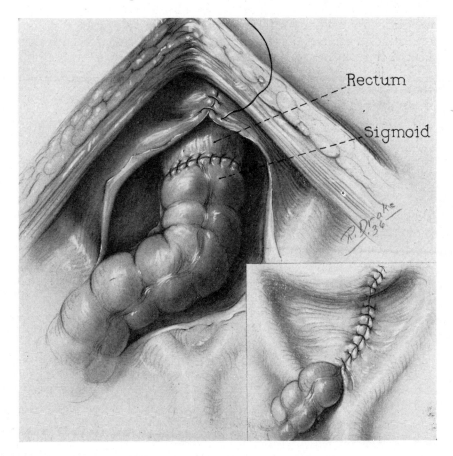

Fig. 137. The pelvic peritoneum is closed at a higher level, which makes the anastomosis retroperitoneal. The drain, which is brought-out suprapubically, has been omitted from the drawing. (From Dixon: courtesy of *Annals of Surgery*.)

suggested that the question of drainage be decided for the individual case in the course of the operation. If there is no gross soiling during the suturing, he believes it is not necessary. It was not used in his 11 cases, in all of which uneventful recoveries were made. In 1928, one of us (Rankin) reported 26 consecutive cases with but one death. Anterior drainage was instituted in all of these cases. In three instances failure of the blood supply to the inverted and retroperitonealized upper portion of the rectum necessitated removal of the rectal stump several days after the anterior resection.

COLOSTOMY AND PERINEAL EXCISION (LOCKHART-MUMMERY)

This procedure, in this country and England, was until recent years the most commonly performed operation for cancer of the rectum. Owing chiefly to the efforts of Lockhart-Mummery, the perineal excision was changed from a purely palliative procedure to one of distinct usefulness in the cure of low rectal growths. Lockhart-Mummery considers the operation suitable "in any case where the growth is at the anus or anywhere in the rectum proper, provided that it is not fixed to important structures. It cannot be performed if the growth is at or above the rectosigmoid junction, unless the growth is small and the sigmoid fairly lengthy."

The operation can be performed in one stage, but there is a distinct advantage in establishing the colostomy two or three weeks before actual excision; besides, the two-stage procedure is much safer.

Technic.—(1) *Colostomy*, the first stage has been described. We prefer left inguinal colostomy, which recommends itself because of the relative ease of its accomplishment, because of the convenience of an artificial anus so situated, and because of the simplicity of the involved mechanism. The second stage of the operation is consummated after an interval of two or three weeks, during which time the rectum is thoroughly cleansed by repeated irrigation instituted through the lower loop of the colostomy.

(2) *Posterior resection* may be accomplished in either of these positions: prone, with the hips raised by a kidney elevator or pillow (our preference), semi-prone, with buttocks over edge of table, and the knees well drawn up (Lockhart-Mummery), and an extreme lithotomy position. If the patient is a man, a catheter can be placed in the urethra to insure against injury, although it is not entirely essential and is seldom employed by us because of the possibility of a urethral chill.

The technic employed by us is almost identical with Lockhart-Mummery's description of the operation, which we will give here almost verbatim (Figs. 138 and 141).

The anus is accurately and securely closed with a stout suture of linen or silk, the ends of which are cut short in order to avoid the temptation of utilizing them for retraction purposes, an unsafe procedure. Discarding the instruments used in this step and changing gloves, an antiseptic solution is again applied to the operative field which is now draped. If the patient is a woman, the vagina should be rendered sterile by irrigating it with an antiseptic solution. If

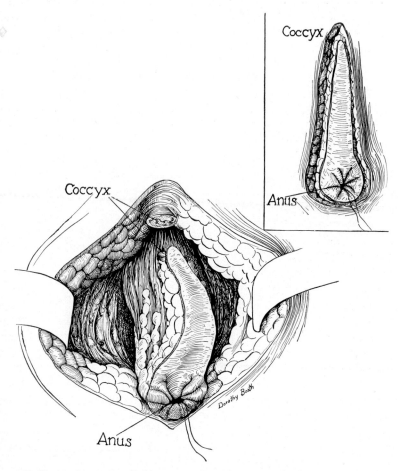

FIG. 138. Perineal excision of the rectum (Lockhart-Mummery). The incision starts over the middle of the sacrum and encircles the anus which has been closed with a purse-string suture of heavy silk. The coccyx has been disarticulated from the sacrum, the fascia propia incised, and dissection of the hollow of the sacrum begun.

reasonable caution is observed it is entirely possible to perform an absolutely aseptic operation from start to finish and thus avoid the chief cause of mortality; namely, sepsis in some form, such as cellulitis or peritonitis.

The slightly concave incisions are made on either side of the closed anus and extend from a little above the sacrococcygeal joint around the center of the perineum. The incisions are deepened and the base of the coccyx exposed. By pressing over the tip of the coccyx the sacrococcygeal joint can be found and the coccyx disarticulated with a knife. Although some difficulty may be experienced in dividing the meso-rectum and bowel due to a very narrow pelvis, we have always been able to surmount this difficulty without removing the lower end of the sacrum. However, if this expediency is resorted to it is most important that the peritoneum on the front of the sacrum be preserved and divided in the line of the spine, so

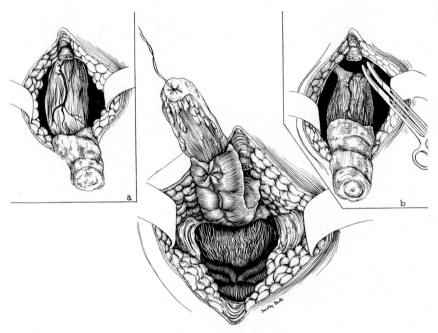

Fig. 139. Perineal excision of the rectum. The anterior portion of the dissection has been carried down to the membranous urethra, and the prostate gland and seminal vesicles are shown dissected clear. The peritoneum is opened to permit further mobilization of the bowel after divison of the superior hemorrhoidal vessels (insert *a*) and its lateral attachments (insert *b*).

that it can be sutured afterwards. This serves the dual purpose of minimizing the subsequent danger of osteomyelitis and the development of a hernia. Once the coccyx is removed, an incision is made through the connective tissue immediately below it, and the fascia propria of the rectum is cut across. By blunt dissection with the fingers, the hollow of the sacrum is cleaned out with little bleeding, except that the terminal branch of the aorta, the middle sacral vessel, is well developed and necessitates ligature.

After the posterior attachments of the rectum are separated, the surgeon now passes the first finger of his left hand beneath the fascia and pushes his finger forward under the left levator ani muscle and between it and the rectum. The structures between his finger and the skin are now divided with blunt-pointed scissors or a scalpel. These consist of muscle, fascia, and fat. The bleeding-points are clamped as divided by an assistant. This procedure is then repeated on the opposite side. The rectum is now mobilized posteriorly and laterally.

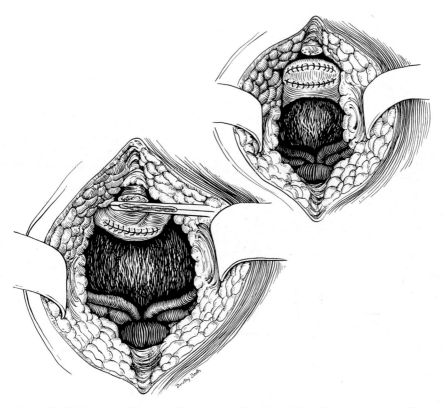

Fig. 140. Perineal excision of the rectum. The bowel has been removed with a cautery between clamps and the peritoneum has been attached higher on the sigmoid. Insert shows divided end of sigmoid inverted.

The anterior dissection is next commenced and is facilitated by traction exerted on forceps attached to the edge surrounding the inverted anus. With scissors or scalpel the perineal incision is deepened, and the dissection continued upward toward the pelvis until the membranous urethra and prostate capsule come into view. If the patient is a woman, one can obtain a line of cleavage by placing a finger in the vagina, dissecting close to the posterior vaginal wall, and thus one readily approaches the peritoneal fold. Great care must be taken at this stage to avoid injury to the rectum, which will result in contamination of the wound, or damage to the urethra or vagina. The rectum is separated from these structures in great measure by stripping with the finger covered with gauze assisted by an occasional use of the scalpel or snip of scissors. The lateral ligaments containing the middle hemorrhoidal vessels are next ligated and divided. At this stage the superior hemorrhoidal arteries, situated posteriorly, may be encountered and if so, must be

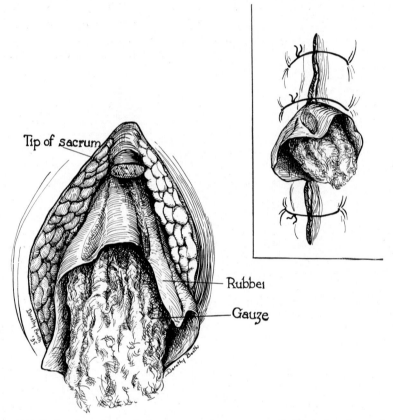

Fig. 141. Perineal excision of the rectum. A square of oiled silk has been thrust into the hollow of the pelvis and then packed with gauze.

divided and ligated. The last two maneuvers, the division of the blood vessels, completes the mobilization of the rectum.

The rectum is now retracted backward away from the bladder, and the peritoneal cavity sought for and opened as close to the rectum as possible, to avoid injury to the ureters which need not be looked for nor identified. The peritoneum is often quite high up and not easily isolated. As a rule, in women, it can be readily reached since the bottom of the pouch of Douglas usually is situated at about 3 to 4 cm. from the skin. The peritoneal cavity should be entered in practically every case, because thus more of the pelvic portion of the colon can be brought down and a wider removal of lymph nodes in the zone of upward extension is possible. The peritoneum on each side should be divided toward the back, along each side of the rectum, and a gauze pack is pushed into the cavity to prevent the entrance of any blood and to protect it. The rectum and the growth are now free except above and from the mesorectum behind. The latter, which becomes well defined as the rectum is drawn forward, is divided as high up and as far back as possible. Curved clamps, which are easier to tie off, are employed, care being taken not to injure the bowel, the edges of which should be closely defined with the finger.

At this stage Lockhart-Mummery divided the bowel as follows: A large pack soaked in an antiseptic is placed on either side of the bowel, above the point of division, so as to shut off the wound completely. The peritoneal and muscular coats of the colon are divided with a knife, leaving as far as possible only the mucous membrane undivided. The muscular coat is carefully stripped back for a quarter of an inch or so, and a large powerful clamp is placed on the bowel at the point of division. Another clamp is placed below this and between the two the bowel is divided with a cautery. The stump is ligated with stout catgut and the remaining clamp removed. A purse-string suture is now inserted and tied while an assistant pushes in the closed end of the colon, so as to make a firm closure of the blind end of bowel. The peritoneum is attached to the protruding segment of bowel. We prefer to reconstruct the pelvic floor before division of the colon. After removal of the pack, the peritoneum should be accurately sutured to the bowel at the highest point at which this can be conveniently accomplished. In inserting this suture care must be taken to leave the turned-in end of colon in the posterior wound and not in the peritoneal cavity, in case it should subsequently give way. The bowel is then divided between clamps with a cautery, and the tissues to be sacrificed are removed en masse. We have not found circular division of the coats of the colon down to the mucosa essential to accurate and permanent inversion of the divided end of sigmoid. Except for the most dexterous, such an undertaking is likely to be tedious, and entails considerable risk of entering the bowel. It is usually possible to invert the end of sigmoid, just as the duodenal stump is inverted following gastric resection, and in our experience mucous fistula has seldom developed following a closure of this type. Those few have closed spontaneously within a very short period of time. It remains now only to be certain the wound is dry and to insert a drain. If one thrusts a square of oiled silk or rubber dam into the hollow of the pelvis and then packs gauze tightly into it, several purposes are served. First, oozing is controlled (this is particularly important if spinal anesthesia has been used and the blood pressure is very low on completion of the operation); second, support is afforded the newly made pelvic floor; and, third, by use of the oiled silk or rubber tissue, the removal of the gauze packing is simple and painless. The upper end of the wound is approximated with several deeply placed stay sutures. It is our custom to remove all of the gauze at the end of about forty-eight hours and the oiled silk twenty-four or forty-eight hours later, at which time daily irrigations of warm normal saline solution are instituted (see "Postoperative Treatment").

REFERENCES

1. COPE, ZACKARY: *Lancet.*, **1**: 634 (March 24), 1934.
2. DIXON, C. F.: Anterior resection for malignant lesions of the upper part of the rectum and the lower part of the sigmoid. *Tr. Am. Surg. Assoc.*, **66**: 175–192, 1948.
3. GABRIEL, W. B.: Perineo-abdominal excision of the rectum in one stage. *Lancet*, **2**: 69–74 (July 14), 1934.
4. GABRIEL, W. B.: The principles and practice of rectal surgery. Springfield, Charles C Thomas, 3rd Ed., 1945, pp. 432.
5. JONES, D. F.: Malignant disease of the rectum. Thomas Nelson and Sons' Loose-Leaf Living Surgery, **5**: 219–241, 1929.
6. LAHEY, F. H.: Two-stage abdominoperineal removal of cancer of the rectum. *Surg., Gynec., and Obst.*, **51**: 692–699 (Nov.), 1930.
7. LOCKHART-MUMMERY, J. P.: Excision of the rectum for cancer. *Am. Jour. Cancer*, **18**: 1–14 (May), 1933.
8. MILES, W. E.: Cancer of the rectum. London, Harrison and Sons, 1926, 72 pp.
9. RANKIN, F. W.: Surgery of the colon. New York, D. Appleton and Company, 1926, 366 pp.
10. RANKIN, F. W.: An aseptic method of intestinal anastomosis. *Surg., Gynec., and Obst.*, **47**: 78–88 (July), 1928.
11. RANKIN, F. W.: Two stage resection for carcinoma of the rectosigmoid and rectum. *Surg., Gynec., and Obst.*, **53**: 670–675 (Nov.), 1931.
12. RANKIN, F. W.: Graded perineo-abdominal resection of the rectum and rectosigmoid. *Am. Jour. Surg.*, **27**: 214–222 (Feb.), 1935.
13. TURNER: Quoted by Gabriel.

CHAPTER XV

PALLIATIVE AND MISCELLANEOUS PROCEDURES

PROCEDURES FOR PARTIAL OR COMPLETE EXCLUSION OF THE RECTUM

These procedures are more generally employed as measures of palliation when, because of the obstructing lesion and evidences of metastasis, it is considered advisable to sidetrack the fecal current rather than to excise the bowel. The procedures more commonly employed are: colocolostomy, ileocolostomy (transverse colon), and ileosigmoidostomy, which may be made with or without division of the terminal ileum, and with or without bilateral mucous fistulas (Fig. 142).

Colocolostomy.—Lateral anastomosis in the large bowel is probably more often indicated between the transverse colon and the sigmoid, in instances of obstructing, inoperable lesions of the splenic flexure. Although employed as a stage preliminary to resection of the splenic flexure or descending colon for malignant lesions it is not, in our opinion, a safe maneuver, since chronic obstruction usually accompanies lesions situated in the left side of the colon. Cecostomy followed in ten days or two weeks by colocolostomy is a relatively safe procedure and offers greater palliation than a colostomy established in the proximal portion of the transverse colon.

Lateral anastomosis may be accomplished over the Rankin three-bladed clamp, by other closed, aseptic methods or by open anastomosis. The technical details of our closed method, which employs the Rankin clamp, is sufficiently covered in a description of ileocolostomy over the clamp. First a raised area in one of the segments of colon to be anastomosed is fixed by a blade of the clamp, then a similar area in the other segment is fixed by the second blade; the elliptical pieces of bowel above the clamp are removed with a cautery to establish openings in the lumen. Anastomosis is accomplished by continuous sutures applied separately, anteriorly and posteriorly.

Ileocolostomy.—This procedure has been described in connection with resection of the right half of the colon.

Ileosigmoidostomy.—This anastomosis may be accomplished in the following ways: (1) lateral anastomosis of the terminal ileum to the sigmoid without division; (2) lateral anastomosis after in-

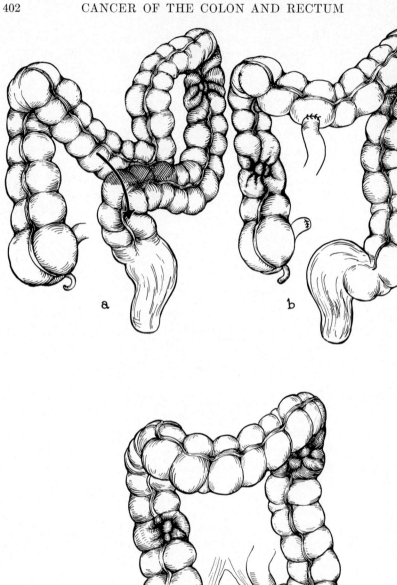

FIG. 142. Short-circuiting procedures. *a*, Colocolostomy; *b*, ileocolostomy; and *c*, ileosigmoidostomy.

version of the divided end of ileum; (3) end of ileum to side of sigmoid; and (4) in addition to the anastomosis, provisions may be made for external drainage at both ends of the colon—mucous fistulas of the cecum, or cecal end of divided ileum on the right and of the descending colon in the form of a colostomy on the left. The first type of operation has little to recommend it since the colon is not completely excluded unless the ileum is divided. More satisfactory, but still inadequate, is ileosigmoidostomy by the second method, in which the distal end of divided ileum is either brought out of a stab wound as a mucous fistula or inverted and dropped into the abdomen. Anastomosis of the end of the ileum to the side of the sigmoid appeals to us more than any other technic and this can be readily accomplished by the Rankin clamp method in the same way as has been described for ileocolostomy in which the transverse colon is involved. The disadvantages of ileosigmoidostomy, when mucous fistulas are not provided, is that occasionally the excluded ascending colon accumulates large quantities of fecal material. Permanent mucous fistulas are established by dividing the colon proximal to the anastomosis, and bringing the upper end out of a small stab wound in the left iliac region as a single-barreled colostomy, the technic of which is described elsewhere. The cecal end of divided ileum is brought out of a McBurney incision in much the same manner described for permanent ileostomy.

LOCAL EXCISION OF THE RECTUM

Local resection of the anus or the rectal ampulla without colostomy, in the form of such procedures as devised by Harrison Cripps, Quenu, Tuttle and others, is useful in a very limited group of cases. The operations, however, have a definite place in the surgeon's armamentarium, small though it may be. They have been much more commonly performed in European than in English speaking countries, where the more favorable outlook of a radical operation with abdominal colostomy has been considered preferable to limited excisions designed to conserve sphincteric mechanism.

Gabriel in an equitable evaluation of conservative, local resections in which he reviewed series of cases reported by Harrison Cripps, Swinford Edwards, and Grey Turner, concluded that these methods "would appear to be worthy of consideration only in *small and very early* cancers of the middle third of the rectum, which are judged to be undoubtedly of group A [Duke's classification], and in which there is therefore good reason for believing that a localized resection will suffice to eradicate the disease. Biopsy should prove the tumour to be of a low grade of malignancy, preferably grade 1."

Ordinarily, in our opinion, such procedures should be reserved for the extremely aged or for polypoid growths or strictures of a benign nature. In the latter instances both the morbidity and mortality will be improved by a preliminary colostomy.

Simple amputation of the anus.—In cases in which the anal canal is involved, the growth, with a wide margin of skin, the sphincter, perianal fat, the anal canal, and a sufficient amount of the ampulla are incised (Fig. 143). The rectum above is not loosened from its bed and no attempt is made to unite skin to the stump of the rectum. With care in the use of bougies in the third and fourth weeks, to prevent contracture, the functional results not infrequently are moderately satisfactory.

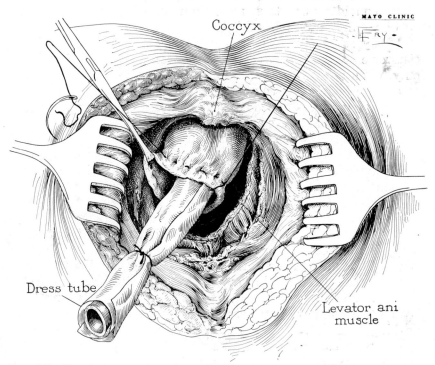

FIG. 143. Simple amputation of the rectum (palliative). (From Saunders: *The Colon, Rectum and Anus.*)

Segmental resection of the rectum.—When the ampullary portion is involved, the rectum is reached through a posterior straight incision extending from the tip of the coccyx to the posterior margin of the anus. The operation consists, with or without removal of the coccyx, of dissection of the entire rectum from the hollow of the sacrum (Fig. 144a), extention of the dissection anteriorly until the peritoneal cavity is open, freeing the rectum from its lateral attachments, and ligation of the posteriorly situated superior hemorrhoidal vessels. The mobilized segment containing the growth is delivered

into the wound and with a liberal portion of the invaded bowel is
excised between clamps (Fig. 144b). If the anal canal is to be preserved, one of several maneuvers can be executed; the well mobilized
sigmoid may be drawn through the anal canal and sutured, after

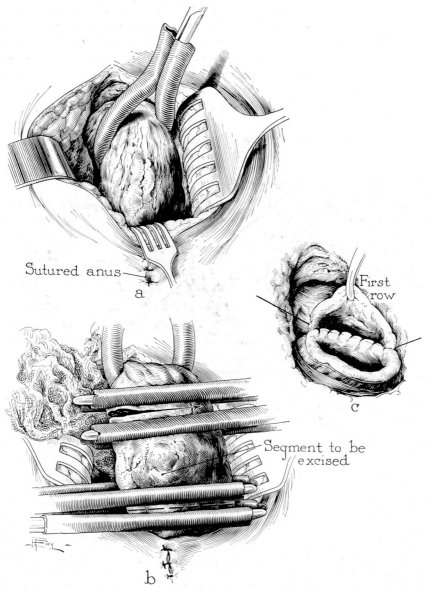

Fig. 144. Segmental resection of the rectum (palliative); a, the rectum mobilized;
b, the growth delivered into the wound and excised between clamps; c, approximation of divided ends of bowel by circular suture (see also Fig. 145). (From Saunders:
The Colon, Rectum and Anus.)

first denuding the latter of mucous membrane, or the divided ends of the bowel can be approximated by circular suture (Figs. 144c and 145). However, it may be found impossible to accomplish either of these procedures, necessitating the establishment of a perineal or even a sacral anus.

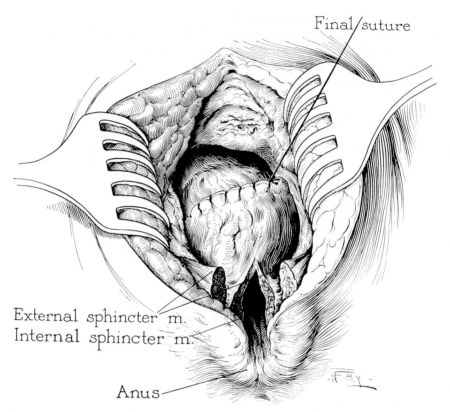

FIG. 145. Segmental resection of the rectum (palliative). Completion of the operation. (From Saunders: *The Colon, Rectum and Anus.*)

PRESACRAL NEURECTOMY FOR PELVIC PAIN AND VESICAL ATONY

For several years one of us (Rankin) has followed the suggestion of Abel, of London, in routinely performing presacral neurectomy after the combined abdominoperineal resection has been completed. There are two reasons for this: first, the influence on the atony of the bladder; and second, for relief of pain in the event of pelvic recurrence. The abdominal part of the abdominoperineal resection involves extensive dissection and there is small wonder that, in cleaning out the fat and soft tissues both from the lateral pelvic walls and the hollow of the sacrum, even greater injury is not done to the nerve supply of the bladder. It is a common experience that complications in the urinary tract following the bladder atony and necessary catheterization are of quite serious import. After this procedure the bladder seems to empty more readily and one can get away from prolonged catheterization in many cases.

The most reasonable explanation of the success of neurectomy seems to be that the hypogastric nerves in man carry inhibitory impulses to the bladder which may be sufficient to prevent its complete emptying when these nerves are intact and the pelvic nerves are injured. The reported results of sympathectomy carried out for the relief of pelvic pain seem to indicate that the same procedure would be useful for pain of recurrent malignancy. There is some controversy among neurologists as to the mechanism by which this is accomplished, the only proved contribution of the autonomic nerves in pain being in relation to referred pain in production of which only efferent fibers are utilized. The fact appears well established that pain impulses are mediated along the hypogastric plexuses, and whether they are transmitted over the autonomic nerves or pathways belonging to the spinal nerves is immaterial if by sectioning the hypogastric plexuses, pain impulses can be interrupted and intense pain of recurrent malignancy prevented.

The beneficial effects of lumbar sympathetic ganglionectomy and ramisection in the treatment of megacolon, as noted by Wade and Royle, Adson and Robertson, prompted a report by Rankin and Learmonth, in 1930, of a modification of the technic of operation, in which a transperitoneal division of the presacral and inferior mesenteric nerves is accomplished. This latter procedure, with which we have experienced success in the treatment of megacolon, is identical with the one that we describe here.

Technic.—Since the inferior mesenteric artery arises opposite the third lumbar vertebra, and the presacral nerve is to be found in front of the fifth lumbar vertebra, full exposure of these structures may be obtained through a left paramedian incision 15 cm. long, and centered on the umbilicus. A self-retaining retractor is adjusted, and the table is tilted to the Trendelenburg position. The small bowel is packed off upward and to the right, so as to expose and pull upward the root of its mesentery; the attachment of the mesentery to the posterior abdominal wall is above the field of the operation, save when the bifurcation of the abdominal aorta is unusually high. An assistant draws the sigmoid colon to the left and slightly downward, to expose the bifurcation of the aorta. In rare cases, the root of the mesosigmoid may be displaced medially, in front of the fifth lumbar vertebra, when it must be mobilized by division of the right leaf of its peritoneum. The promontory of the sacrum is now identified, and in most cases it is possible to see the strands of the presacral nerve as they descend in the middle line, immediately under the peritoneum. The peritoneum is picked up in the middle line, and is incised vertically from the level of the promontory to the origin of the inferior mesenteric artery (Fig. 133). The two edges of this incision are displaced by forceps to each side. The strands of the presacral nerve are not adherent to the membrane, and posteriorly they are separated from the great vessels by a layer of fine connective tissue. The nerve is first divided below, at the right border of the left common iliac vein; it is well to place a ligature on its distal end, as this is usually accompanied by a small artery. It is then raised upward by gentle dissection with moist gauze, and the branches which reach it from the fourth

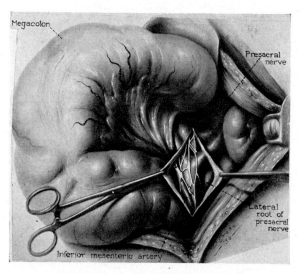

Fig. 146. Sympathectomy for pelvic pain and vesical atony (Rankin and Learmonth technic). After division of presacral nerve the inferior mesenteric nerves are removed by dividing them at the point indicated.

lumbar ganglia are divided on each side. Immediately below the bifurcation of the aorta, the connecting branches from the third lumbar ganglia are divided as they pass to join the nerve from beneath the common iliac arteries. When the nerve has been raised a little higher, its lateral roots, formed by the union of the branches from the first and second lumbar ganglia, may be severed; the middle root is preserved if possible to be used as a guide to the intermesenteric plexus. The trunk of the inferior mesenteric artery is now identified; by tracing upward the middle root of the presacral nerve the operator reaches the two large principal roots of the inferior mesenteric plexus, one on each side of the vessel, and joining it 1.5 cm. below its origin. If the middle root of the presacral nerve cannot be used as a guide, the main trunks of the inferior mesenteric plexus will be found at the positions of five o'clock and seven o'clock with reference to the origin of the artery. They are large and easily isolated. About 2.5 cm. of each are then resected if any ganglionic mass is present on either, it must be included in the resected portion. Any subsidiary periarterial strands are then sought for and, if any are found, they are divided. Bleeding is not to be expected during this part of the operation; the inferior mesenteric vein is too far to the left to appear in the field. The incision in the posterior peritoneum is now brought together with a continuous suture of catgut, and the abdominal wound is closed in the usual manner.

INTERPOSITION OF ILEUM FOR COLONIC DEFECT

Following anterior resection of the lower sigmoid or rectosigmoid for malignancy or diverticulitis, Stone advocates interposition of a loop of ileum between the descending colon and the rectum. His technic is as follows: the ileum is divided about 35 cm. from the ileocecal valve, because at this point the mesentery is long and freely movable. Ileum sufficient to bridge the gap is measured upwards, and again divided. The two free ends above and below are removed, loops are turned in, and lateral anastomosis is made between them in order to restore the continuity of the ileum. The rectum is then opened at its blind end, and a tube which is passed into the rectum, by way of the anus, is drawn up through the opening. The lower end of the free loop of ileum is passed down over the rectal tube and is attached to it by sutures of catgut. The tube is then pulled downward by an assistant, until the stump of ileum is invaginated into the upper end of the rectum, where it is fixed in position by a number of interrupted sutures, and the tube is left in place. The upper end of the transposed loop is now closed with a purse-string suture and joined to the descending colon by lateral anastomosis above the previously made terminal colonic stoma, which is not disturbed at this operation. Openings in the mesentery are accurately closed by suture.

EXCISION OF BENIGN POLYPS OF THE COLON
AND RECTUM

Single adenomas of the colon are being diagnosed and accurately localized more often in recent years as a result of the more frequent utilization of the double contrast method of visualizing the colon after expulsion of a barium enema. Exploration of patients in whom a polypoid tumor of the colon is suspected (on the basis of persistent bleeding) is seldom justified since these lesions are extremely difficult to palpate. Even when a polypoid growth is demonstrated roentgenologically, it may, as David has pointed out, be found on exploration to be six to eight inches from the site observed on the roentgenogram, owing to the long pedicle of normal mucosa which many of these growths develop.

Rectal polyps are readily demonstrated through the proctoscope. Pedunculated polyps of the lower sigmoid and rectosigmoid may even protrude from the anus. Malignant changes may be suspected if induration is noted either at the base, within the body of the adenoma, or at the periphery. The suspicion becomes greater if ulceration accompanies the induration. Gabriel states that he has never known a diagnosis of malignancy on these grounds to prove incorrect. A suspicion of malignancy may sometimes be confirmed by biopsy. A negative report, however, is by no means conclusive. Helwig (see page 137), Gabriel, and others have shown that malignant changes may occur in any portion of the adenoma. After removal of a polyp fixed sections should be carefully studied.

Colon.—The patient should be carefully prepared as if for a radical resection of the colon or rectum (See "Preoperative and Postoperative Preparation"). If the lesions is a readily movable, pedunculated polyp with no areas of induration or dimpling of the bowel at the site of attachment, which would suggest possible malignant changes, it may properly be excised at its base. If, however, malignancy is suspected or if the lesions is a large, sessile attached adenoma or papilloma, segmental resection is indicated.

In performing colotomy the utmost care should be exercised to prevent contamination. The small intestines are carefully excluded from the operative field with large moist gauze packs, and the involved segment, which is brought out of the abdominal wound, is incised in the area between the longitudinal bands, at a point opposite the tumor. The growth is delivered through the incision, a clamp is applied well beneath its base, and above this clamp the tumor is removed with a cautery. The wound in the mucous membrane is closed by a continuous suture of chromic catgut; the incision in the anterior wall of the bowel is closed in the usual manner, employing two rows of sutures.

Rectum.—Pedunculated adenomas may be removed by ligation of the pedicle if they can be prolapsed through the anus. Those that can be visualized through the proctoscope are usually removed by fulguration of the pedicle through the proctoscope. Large sessile papillomas are difficult to approach from above or below unless one decides to remove the rectum. David has treated 15 cases in the following manner: "The rectum is split open up to the coccyx (Fig. 147). The tumor is grasped by Allis forceps and gently pulled down-

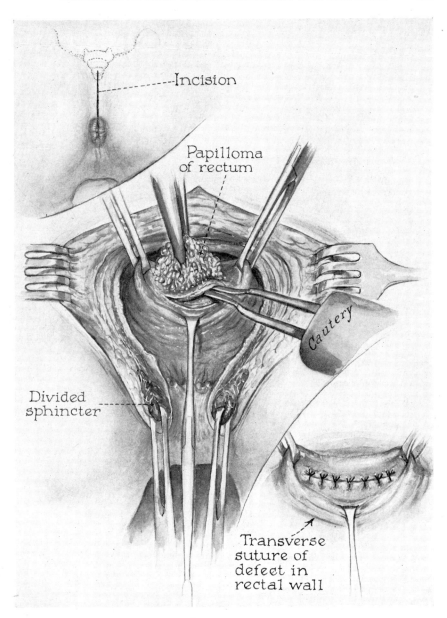

Fig. 147. Operation for removal of sizable benign lesions in the ampulla of the rectum showing the incision, removal of the growth, and suture of the mucosa. (Vernon C. David: courtesy of *Surgery.*)

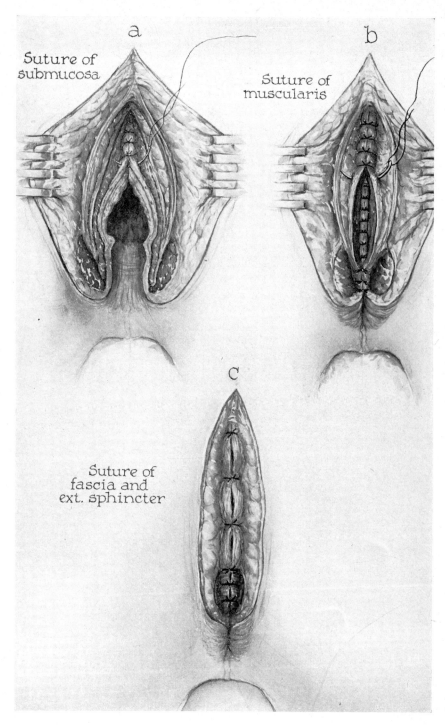

FIG. 148. (*a*) Suture of the bowel by interrupted catgut stitch going through the submucosa; (*b*) suture of the muscularis of the bowel; (*c*) suture of the sphincter and interrupted sutures through the extension of the sphincter muscle to the coccyx. (Vernon C. David: courtesy of *Surgery*.)

ward, intussuscepting the bowel mucosa. The normal, healthy mucosa surrounding the tumor is picked up by Allis forceps, to prevent retraction of the mucosa, and the tumor is completely removed by the cutting cautery going through the submucosa. Bleeding points are ligated and a running stitch of catgut approximates the mucosa on both sides of the defect. The completely incised bowel wall is then closed with fine catgut, taking care not to place sutures through the mucosa which would serve as avenues of infection from the lumen of the bowel (Fig. 142). The stitches are placed in the submucosa, which tends to invert the mucosa into the lumen of the bowel. The muscularis is then sutured with interrupted catgut and a third row of stitches is placed through the areola tissue over the bowel, which includes the extensions of the external sphincter muscle to the coccyx. The external sphincter muscle is united separately by two interrupted mattress stitches of catgut." Although there is some leakage along the suture line about the sixth day, in all David's cases healing took place without a fistula and with continence of the sphincter muscles.

REFERENCES

1. DAVID, VERNON C.: The management of polyps occurring in the rectum and colon. *Surgery*, **14**: 387–394 (Sept.), 1943.
2. GABRIEL, W. B.: The principles and practice of rectal surgery. Springfield, Charles C Thomas, 3rd Ed., pp. 432, 1945.
3. RANKIN, F. W.: Resection of the rectum and rectosigmoid by single or graded procedures. *Ann. Surg.*, **104**: 628–634 (Oct.), 1936.
4. RANKIN, F. W., and LEARMONTH, J. R.: Section of the sympathetic nerves of the distal part of the colon and the rectum in the treatment of Hirschsprung's disease and certain types of constipation. *Ann. Surg.*, **92**: 710–720 (Oct.), 1930.
5. LEARMONTH, J. R., and BRAASCH, W. F.: Resection of the presacral nerve in the treatment of cord bladder. *Surg., Gynec., and Obst.*, **51**: 494–499 (Oct.), 1930.
6. STONE, H. B.: Interposition of the loop of ileum to repair defects in the colon. *Ann. Surg.*, **88**: 593–596 (Sept.), 1928.

AUTHOR INDEX

(Bold face numerals refer to the pages upon which author's name appears in the references.)

SUBJECT INDEX

THIS BOOK

CANCER OF THE COLON
AND RECTUM

SECOND EDITION

By

FRED W. RANKIN, M.D. AND A. STEPHENS GRAHAM, M.D.

*was set, printed and bound by The Collegiate Press of Menasha,
Wisconsin. The type is 11 on 12 point Monotype 8A. The type
page is 27 x 46 picas. The text paper is 70-lb. White Deep
Falls Enamel. The binding is DuPont Fabrikoid;
Quality 700; Color 5027; Grain, C-5 (Roller);
Plia. Med.; Finish, S.B.*

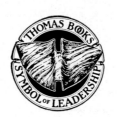

*With THOMAS BOOKS careful attention is given to all details of
manufacturing and design. It is the publisher's desire to present
books that are satisfactory as to their physical qualities
and artistic possibilities and appropriate for their
particular use. THOMAS BOOKS will be
true to those laws of quality that assure
a good name and good will.*